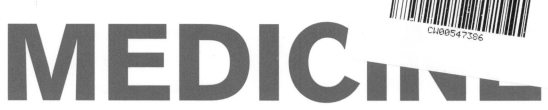

MEDICINE
A GRAPHIC HISTORY

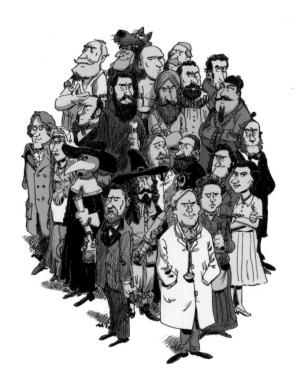

Artist: Philippe Bercovici
Writer: Jean-Noël Fabiani
Colourist: Isabelle Lebeau
Translator: Edward Gauvin

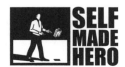

SELF MADE HERO

To Jane
For her love, her expertise,
and her patience during the writing of this book.

To the students and teachers
in the History of Medicine programme
at Paris Descartes University.

First published in English in 2020
by SelfMadeHero
139–141 Pancras Road
London NW1 1UN
www.selfmadehero.com

English translation © 2020 SelfMadeHero

Words by Jean-Noël Fabiani
Art by Philippe Bercovici
Translated from the French by Edward Gauvin

Publishing Director: Emma Hayley
Editorial & Production Director: Guillaume Rater
Sales & Marketing Manager: Steve Turner
Designer: Txabi Jones
UK Publicist: Paul Smith
With thanks to: Nick de Somogyi and Dan Lockwood

First published in French by Les Arènes
© Les Arènes, Paris, 2018

INSTITUT
FRANÇAIS
ROYAUME-UNI

This book is supported by the Institut français (Royaume-Uni)
as part of the Burgess programme

A CIP record for this book is available from the British Library

ISBN: 978-1-910593-79-0

10 9 8 7 6 5 4 3 2 1

Printed and bound in Slovenia

CONTENTS

FOREWORD

The history of medicine is an aspect of History with a capital H—inextricable from the vast progress of human thought, deeply entwined with the wars and politics of subsequent ages, and constantly subject to the myths that society imposes upon it. The physicians of ancient Greece or the Renaissance were all men (occasionally women) of their time, and necessarily shared the beliefs, struggles, and questions presented by those times, serving—and sometimes bravely disobeying—the powers that be.

To study this history, however, and to trace the many paths that medicine has taken, is to understand the ultimate goal it has always set for itself: to be recognized as a true science. And yet, born as a primitive instinct among prehistoric humans, it was first considered a mysterious magic—one of many in the dimly understood universe of those unfathomable times. Nor was this aura of magical therapy entirely abandoned through subsequent centuries, when, in the wake of Hippocrates' teachings, the "medical arts"—jeered at for so long—at last established themselves. But even as the years wore on, the attempts at a more rational science of medicine fell foul of a stubbornly persistent succession of myths, whether from alchemy, Christian doctrine, or symbolic representations of the unconscious. Although medicine has slowly, and with difficulty, accommodated the contributions of the so-called "hard" sciences, it still seems to falter as a genuine science unto itself. It is true that many a Nobel Prize in Medicine has been awarded to scientists more familiar with their laboratory bench than a stethoscope; true, too, that modern medicine increasingly demands a fundamental knowledge of biology...

And yet it is still the suffering human being—with their unpredictable demands, their doubts and their fears, their individual personalities and unique presentation of symptoms—who will always remain the central subject of medicine, and a far cry from any possible mathematical equation of ill health made from them. So medical practitioners must not only reason with the algorithms of evidential medicine, but also be expert in assessing the ineffably human idiosyncrasies that any single patient may present.

This history of doctors and medicine is, then, finally, a very serious one indeed, for today's society is, more than ever before in its history, confronted by major issues that place the very future of humankind at stake.

Happily, though, not all is doom and gloom. The long story of medicine is embroidered with a rich seam of anecdote—a succession of scenes, both poignant and laughable, from the familiar human comedy, where scholars and social climbers, charlatans and saints, amateurs and professionals merrily rub shoulders. With such an embarrassment of riches to choose from, this author's only regrets are those many stories and individuals he could not include.

The incredible story of medicine demands to be told not only in words but in pictures, because it is at once both deadly serious and essentially comic.

Jean-Noël Fabiani

CHAPTER 1

FROM PREHISTORIC TIMES TO ANTIQUITY

Ever since humans began walking the earth, they have sought to soothe ills. How could it have been otherwise?

How did they go about doing so? With whatever means were at hand, naturally. And these means came from nature, which was finite, and observation, which was vast.

As early as the Palaeolithic Era, nomadic hunter-gatherers knew how to use plants to reduce a fracture. Medicine men were wizards who healed through magic and a few recipes passed down by word-of-mouth.

In Neolithic times, the advent of agriculture and the raising of livestock led to settled and concentrated populations. Thus were society and religion established. And priests naturally became intermediaries of the gods when it came to the knowledge and the power to heal.

But with the rise in settled populations, humans exposed themselves to another scourge, one that up till then had been marginal: the risk of an epidemic, which would at that time have been blamed on divine wrath.

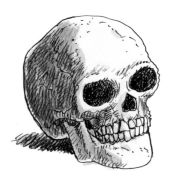

MEDICINE IN PREHISTORIC TIMES

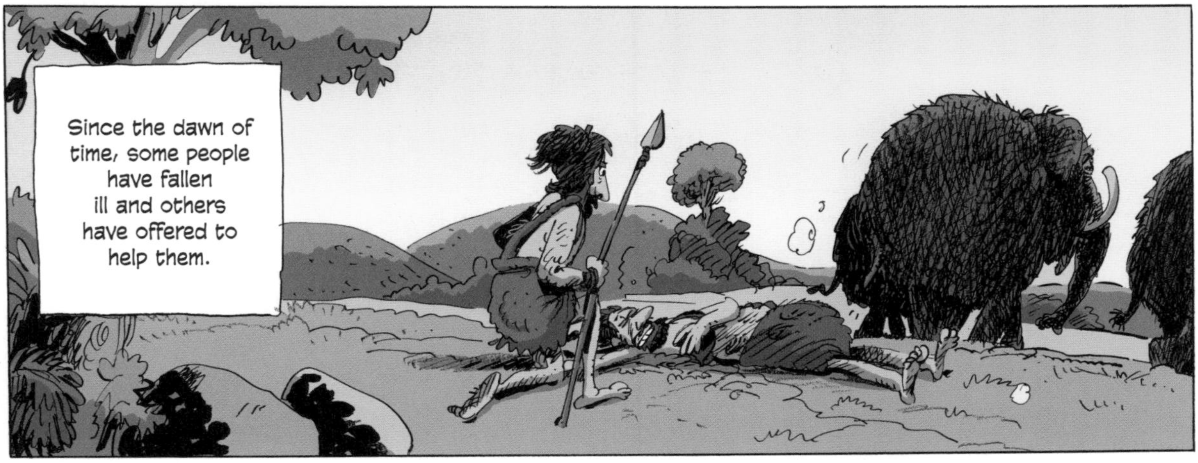
Since the dawn of time, some people have fallen ill and others have offered to help them.

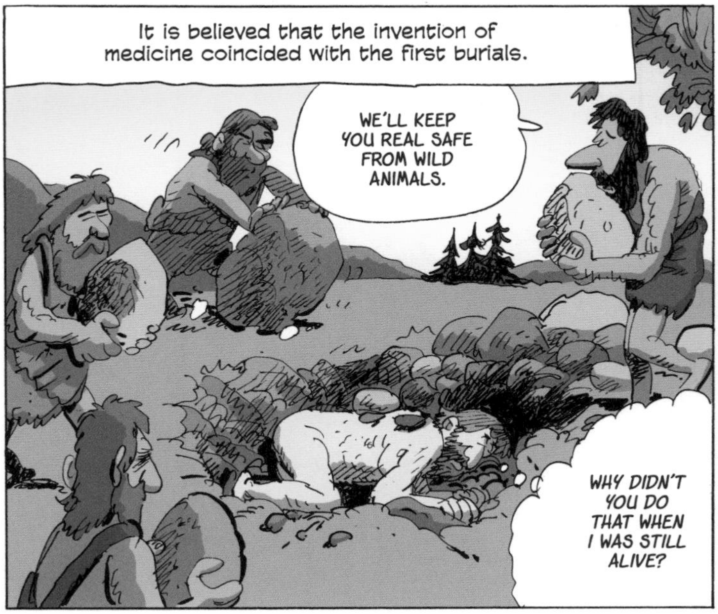
It is believed that the invention of medicine coincided with the first burials.
WE'LL KEEP YOU REAL SAFE FROM WILD ANIMALS.
WHY DIDN'T YOU DO THAT WHEN I WAS STILL ALIVE?

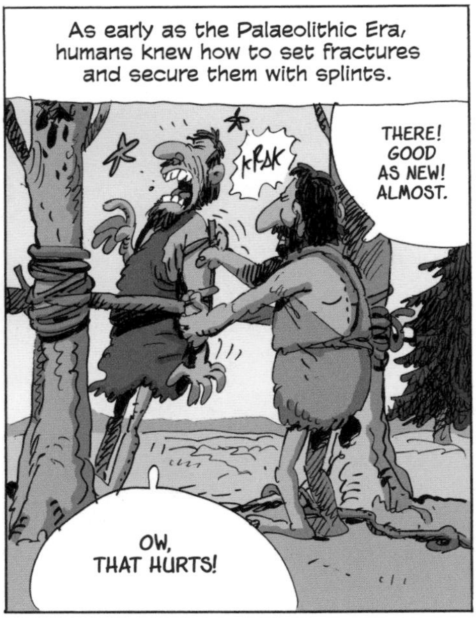
As early as the Palaeolithic Era, humans knew how to set fractures and secure them with splints.
KRAK
THERE! GOOD AS NEW! ALMOST.
OW, THAT HURTS!

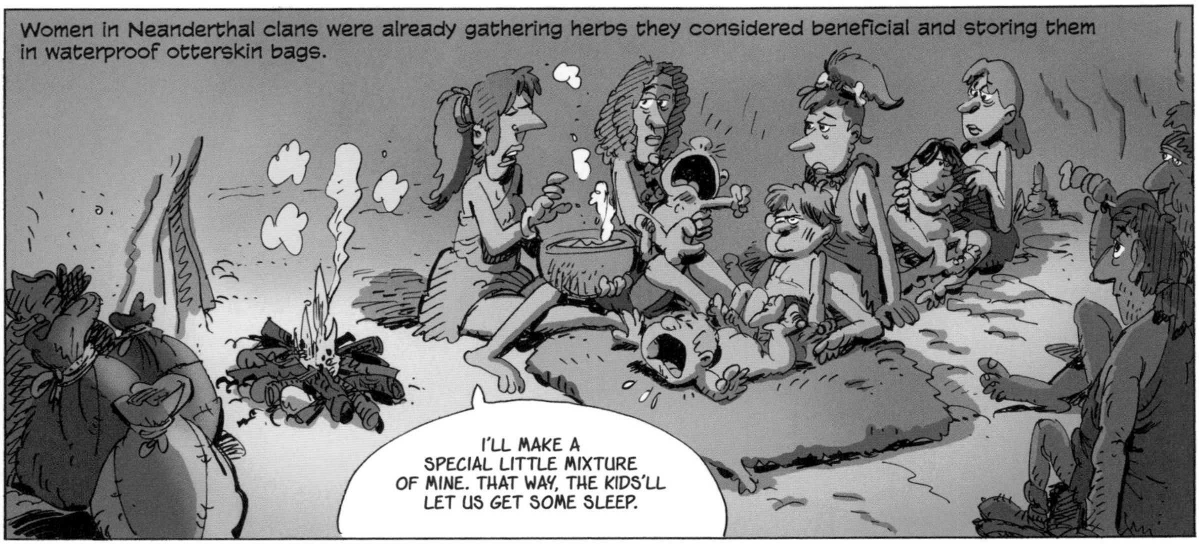
Women in Neanderthal clans were already gathering herbs they considered beneficial and storing them in waterproof otterskin bags.
I'LL MAKE A SPECIAL LITTLE MIXTURE OF MINE. THAT WAY, THE KIDS'LL LET US GET SOME SLEEP.

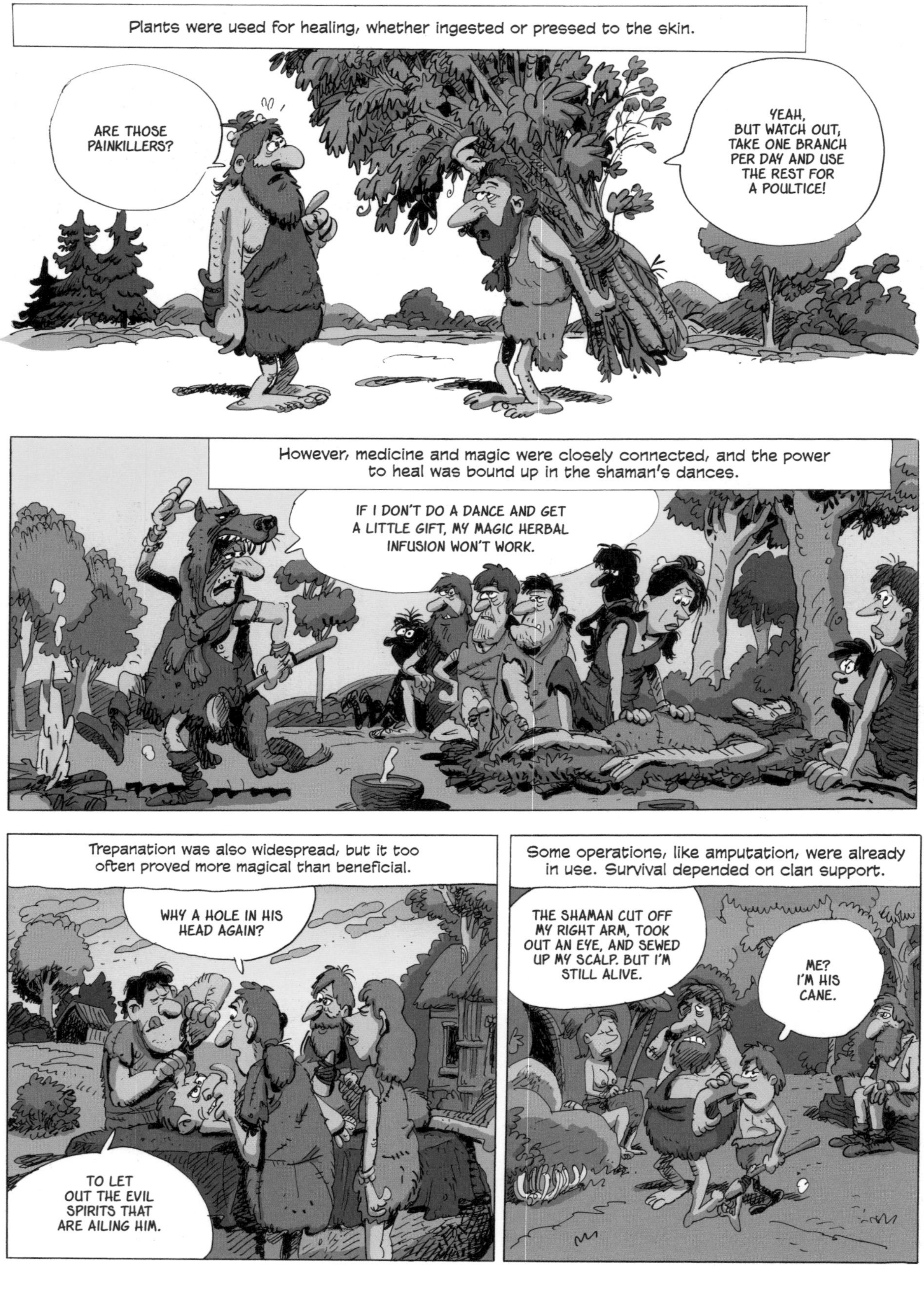
Plants were used for healing, whether ingested or pressed to the skin.
ARE THOSE PAINKILLERS?
YEAH, BUT WATCH OUT, TAKE ONE BRANCH PER DAY AND USE THE REST FOR A POULTICE!
However, medicine and magic were closely connected, and the power to heal was bound up in the shaman's dances.
IF I DON'T DO A DANCE AND GET A LITTLE GIFT, MY MAGIC HERBAL INFUSION WON'T WORK.
Trepanation was also widespread, but it too often proved more magical than beneficial.
WHY A HOLE IN HIS HEAD AGAIN?
TO LET OUT THE EVIL SPIRITS THAT ARE AILING HIM.
Some operations, like amputation, were already in use. Survival depended on clan support.
THE SHAMAN CUT OFF MY RIGHT ARM, TOOK OUT AN EYE, AND SEWED UP MY SCALP. BUT I'M STILL ALIVE.
ME? I'M HIS CANE.

MEDICINE IN ANTIQUITY

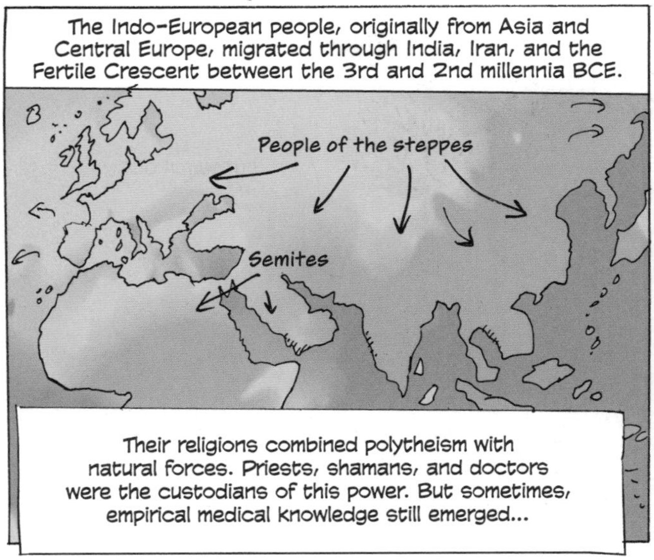
The Indo-European people, originally from Asia and Central Europe, migrated through India, Iran, and the Fertile Crescent between the 3rd and 2nd millennia BCE.
People of the steppes
Semites
Their religions combined polytheism with natural forces. Priests, shamans, and doctors were the custodians of this power. But sometimes, empirical medical knowledge still emerged...

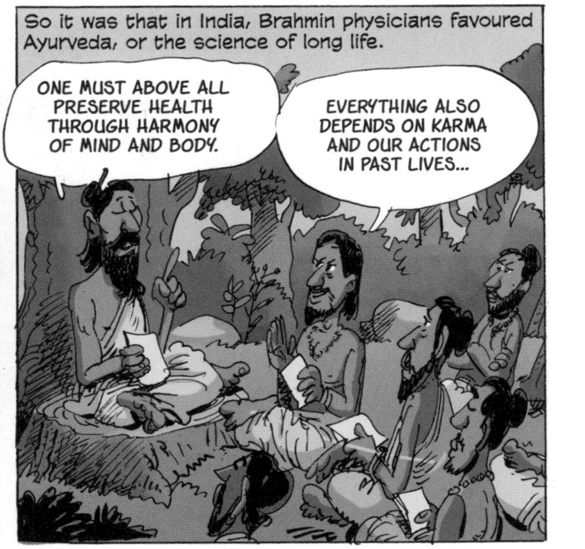
So it was that in India, Brahmin physicians favoured Ayurveda, or the science of long life.
ONE MUST ABOVE ALL PRESERVE HEALTH THROUGH HARMONY OF MIND AND BODY.
EVERYTHING ALSO DEPENDS ON KARMA AND OUR ACTIONS IN PAST LIVES...

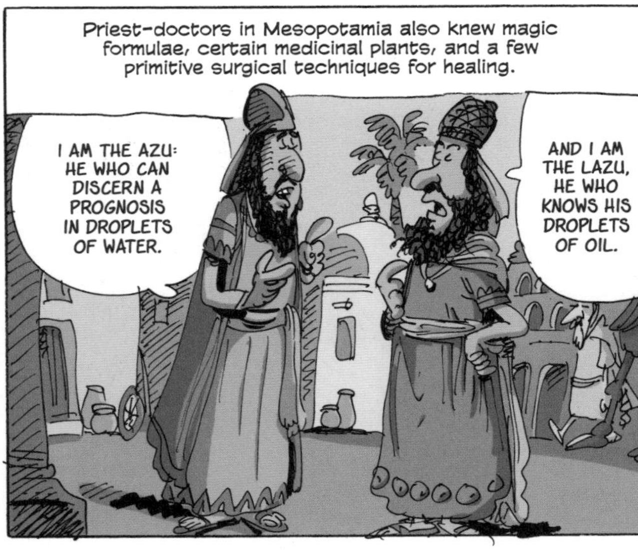
Priest-doctors in Mesopotamia also knew magic formulae, certain medicinal plants, and a few primitive surgical techniques for healing.
I AM THE AZU: HE WHO CAN DISCERN A PROGNOSIS IN DROPLETS OF WATER.
AND I AM THE LAZU, HE WHO KNOWS HIS DROPLETS OF OIL.

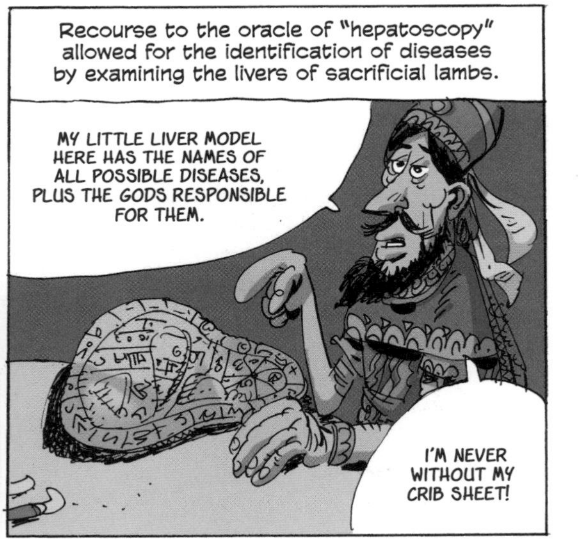
Recourse to the oracle of "hepatoscopy" allowed for the identification of diseases by examining the livers of sacrificial lambs.
MY LITTLE LIVER MODEL HERE HAS THE NAMES OF ALL POSSIBLE DISEASES, PLUS THE GODS RESPONSIBLE FOR THEM.
I'M NEVER WITHOUT MY CRIB SHEET!

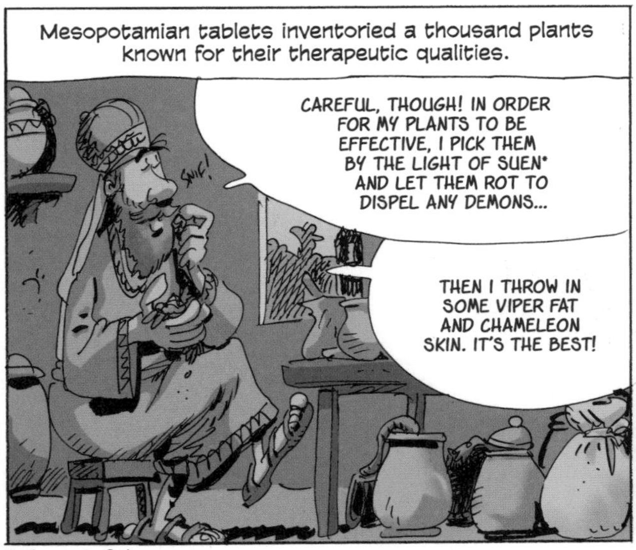
Mesopotamian tablets inventoried a thousand plants known for their therapeutic qualities.
CAREFUL, THOUGH! IN ORDER FOR MY PLANTS TO BE EFFECTIVE, I PICK THEM BY THE LIGHT OF SUEN* AND LET THEM ROT TO DISPEL ANY DEMONS...
SNIF!
THEN I THROW IN SOME VIPER FAT AND CHAMELEON SKIN. IT'S THE BEST!

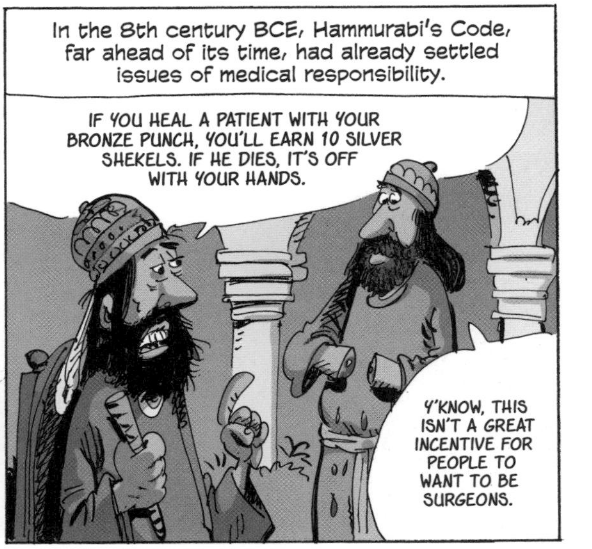
In the 8th century BCE, Hammurabi's Code, far ahead of its time, had already settled issues of medical responsibility.
IF YOU HEAL A PATIENT WITH YOUR BRONZE PUNCH, YOU'LL EARN 10 SILVER SHEKELS. IF HE DIES, IT'S OFF WITH YOUR HANDS.
Y'KNOW, THIS ISN'T A GREAT INCENTIVE FOR PEOPLE TO WANT TO BE SURGEONS.

* The god of the moon.

EGYPTIAN MEDICINE

Egyptian medicine was essentially religious, based on a creation myth: Osiris, the god of life, death, and resurrection.

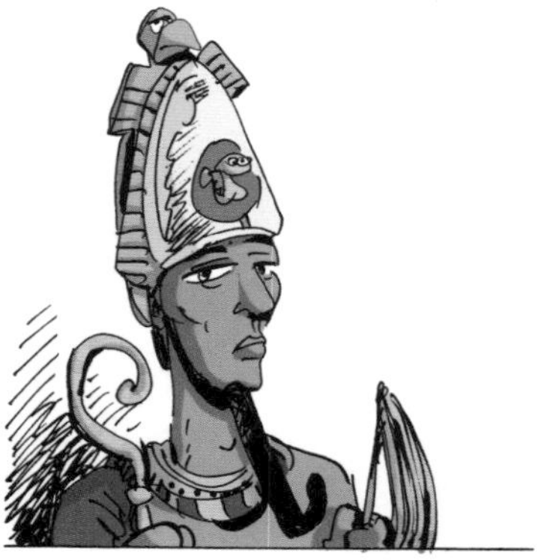

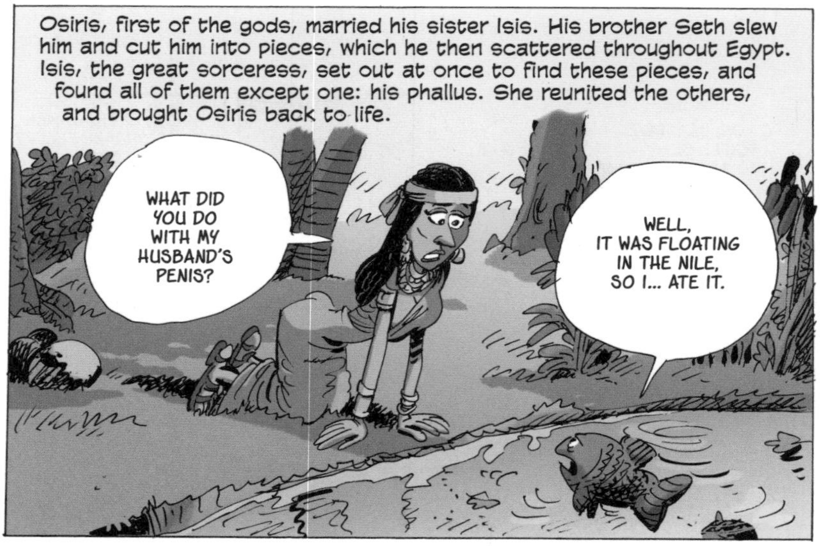
Osiris, first of the gods, married his sister Isis. His brother Seth slew him and cut him into pieces, which he then scattered throughout Egypt. Isis, the great sorceress, set out at once to find these pieces, and found all of them except one: his phallus. She reunited the others, and brought Osiris back to life.
WHAT DID YOU DO WITH MY HUSBAND'S PENIS?
WELL, IT WAS FLOATING IN THE NILE, SO I... ATE IT.

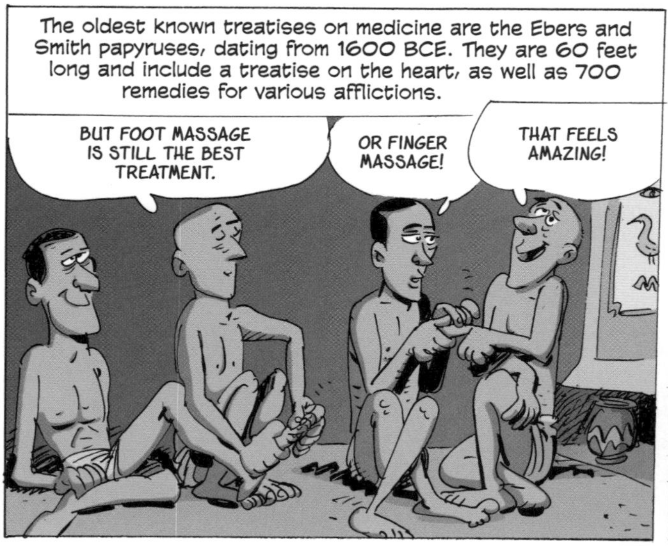
The oldest known treatises on medicine are the Ebers and Smith papyruses, dating from 1600 BCE. They are 60 feet long and include a treatise on the heart, as well as 700 remedies for various afflictions.
BUT FOOT MASSAGE IS STILL THE BEST TREATMENT.
OR FINGER MASSAGE!
THAT FEELS AMAZING!

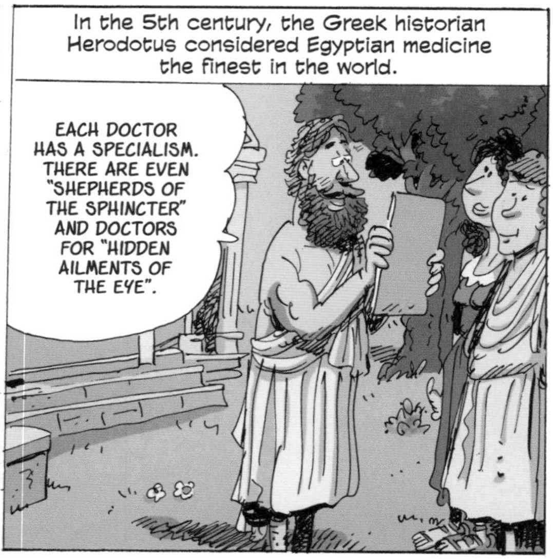
In the 5th century, the Greek historian Herodotus considered Egyptian medicine the finest in the world.
EACH DOCTOR HAS A SPECIALISM. THERE ARE EVEN "SHEPHERDS OF THE SPHINCTER" AND DOCTORS FOR "HIDDEN AILMENTS OF THE EYE".

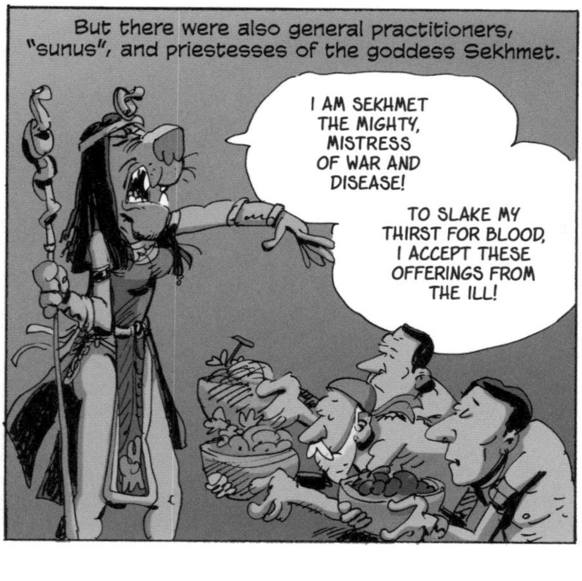
But there were also general practitioners, "sunus", and priestesses of the goddess Sekhmet.
I AM SEKHMET THE MIGHTY, MISTRESS OF WAR AND DISEASE!
TO SLAKE MY THIRST FOR BLOOD, I ACCEPT THESE OFFERINGS FROM THE ILL!

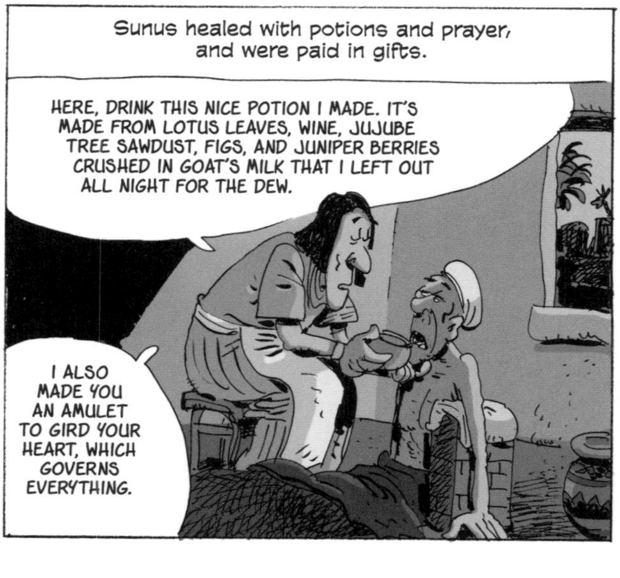
Sunus healed with potions and prayer, and were paid in gifts.
HERE, DRINK THIS NICE POTION I MADE. IT'S MADE FROM LOTUS LEAVES, WINE, JUJUBE TREE SAWDUST, FIGS, AND JUNIPER BERRIES CRUSHED IN GOAT'S MILK THAT I LEFT OUT ALL NIGHT FOR THE DEW.
I ALSO MADE YOU AN AMULET TO GIRD YOUR HEART, WHICH GOVERNS EVERYTHING.

Also widely practised was circumcision at puberty, for societal and religious reasons.

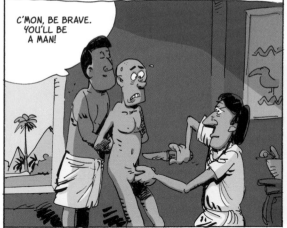

C'MON, BE BRAVE. YOU'LL BE A MAN!

Egyptians were good observers, and knew anatomy well, for their embalmers had seen to dead bodies for three millennia...

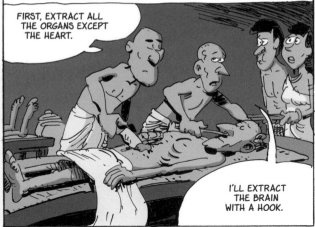

FIRST, EXTRACT ALL THE ORGANS EXCEPT THE HEART.

I'LL EXTRACT THE BRAIN WITH A HOOK.

The greatest physician of "the gods and men of Egypt" was Imhotep, Pharaoh Djoser's chancellor (2800 BCE).

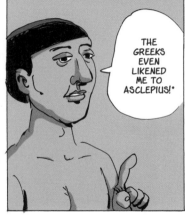

THE GREEKS EVEN LIKENED ME TO ASCLEPIUS!*

The priests of Sekhmet were remarkable observers of symptoms, especially cardiac, such as heart disease.

Egyptian doctors largely practised magical and religious healing, but with empirical and often very effective formulae.

HEBREW MEDICINE

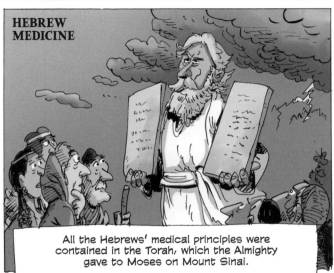

All the Hebrews' medical principles were contained in the Torah, which the Almighty gave to Moses on Mount Sinai.

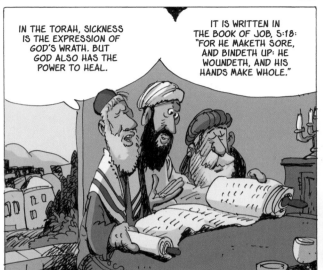

IN THE TORAH, SICKNESS IS THE EXPRESSION OF GOD'S WRATH. BUT GOD ALSO HAS THE POWER TO HEAL.

IT IS WRITTEN IN THE BOOK OF JOB, 5:18: "FOR HE MAKETH SORE, AND BINDETH UP: HE WOUNDETH, AND HIS HANDS MAKE WHOLE."

Hebrew medicine consisted of rules for prevention and hygiene.

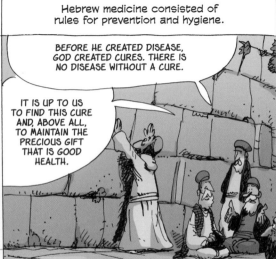

BEFORE HE CREATED DISEASE, GOD CREATED CURES. THERE IS NO DISEASE WITHOUT A CURE.

IT IS UP TO US TO FIND THIS CURE AND, ABOVE ALL, TO MAINTAIN THE PRECIOUS GIFT THAT IS GOOD HEALTH.

* The Greek god of medicine, struck down by lightning for resurrecting the dead.

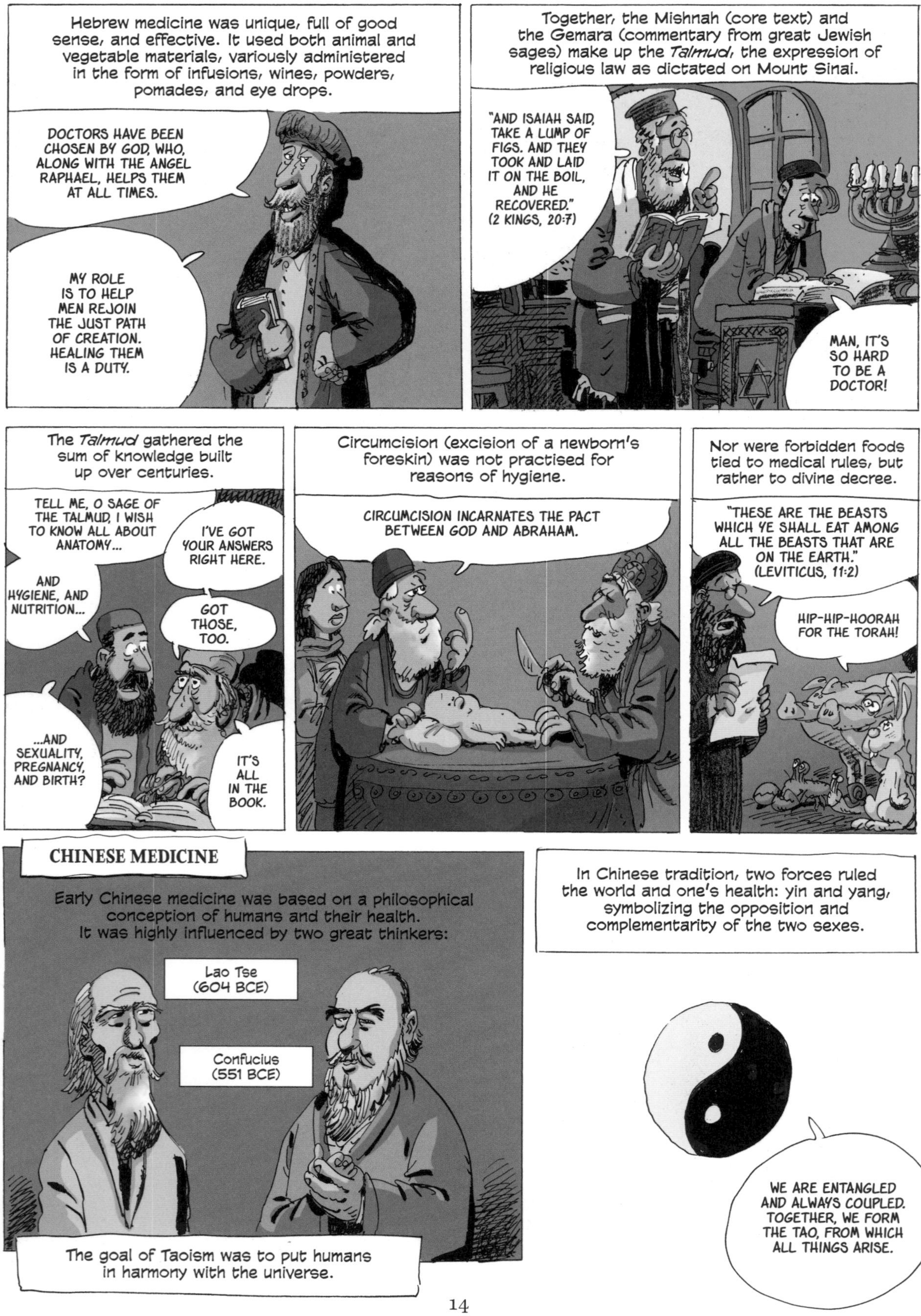
Hebrew medicine was unique, full of good sense, and effective. It used both animal and vegetable materials, variously administered in the form of infusions, wines, powders, pomades, and eye drops.
DOCTORS HAVE BEEN CHOSEN BY GOD, WHO, ALONG WITH THE ANGEL RAPHAEL, HELPS THEM AT ALL TIMES.
MY ROLE IS TO HELP MEN REJOIN THE JUST PATH OF CREATION. HEALING THEM IS A DUTY.
Together, the Mishnah (core text) and the Gemara (commentary from great Jewish sages) make up the *Talmud*, the expression of religious law as dictated on Mount Sinai.
"AND ISAIAH SAID, TAKE A LUMP OF FIGS. AND THEY TOOK AND LAID IT ON THE BOIL, AND HE RECOVERED." (2 KINGS, 20:7)
MAN, IT'S SO HARD TO BE A DOCTOR!
The *Talmud* gathered the sum of knowledge built up over centuries.
TELL ME, O SAGE OF THE TALMUD, I WISH TO KNOW ALL ABOUT ANATOMY...
I'VE GOT YOUR ANSWERS RIGHT HERE.
AND HYGIENE, AND NUTRITION...
GOT THOSE, TOO.
...AND SEXUALITY, PREGNANCY, AND BIRTH?
IT'S ALL IN THE BOOK.
Circumcision (excision of a newborn's foreskin) was not practised for reasons of hygiene.
CIRCUMCISION INCARNATES THE PACT BETWEEN GOD AND ABRAHAM.
Nor were forbidden foods tied to medical rules, but rather to divine decree.
"THESE ARE THE BEASTS WHICH YE SHALL EAT AMONG ALL THE BEASTS THAT ARE ON THE EARTH." (LEVITICUS, 11:2)
HIP-HIP-HOORAH FOR THE TORAH!
CHINESE MEDICINE
Early Chinese medicine was based on a philosophical conception of humans and their health. It was highly influenced by two great thinkers:
Lao Tse (604 BCE)
Confucius (551 BCE)
The goal of Taoism was to put humans in harmony with the universe.
In Chinese tradition, two forces ruled the world and one's health: yin and yang, symbolizing the opposition and complementarity of the two sexes.
WE ARE ENTANGLED AND ALWAYS COUPLED. TOGETHER, WE FORM THE TAO, FROM WHICH ALL THINGS ARISE.

The goal of Chinese medicine was thus to ensure balance between yin and yang.

Taking one's pulse was an art that allowed for the probing of one's qi, or the organs' vital energy.

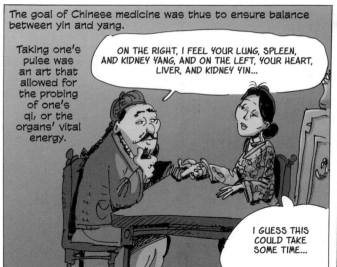

ON THE RIGHT, I FEEL YOUR LUNG, SPLEEN, AND KIDNEY YANG, AND ON THE LEFT, YOUR HEART, LIVER, AND KIDNEY YIN...

I GUESS THIS COULD TAKE SOME TIME...

Illness was considered a breach of harmony, and doctors had to prevent this descent into chaos.

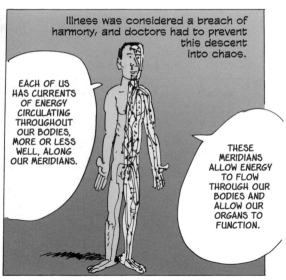

EACH OF US HAS CURRENTS OF ENERGY CIRCULATING THROUGHOUT OUR BODIES, MORE OR LESS WELL, ALONG OUR MERIDIANS.

THESE MERIDIANS ALLOW ENERGY TO FLOW THROUGH OUR BODIES AND ALLOW OUR ORGANS TO FUNCTION.

All along these meridians are points that can be stimulated with needles (acupuncture) or heat (moxibustion).

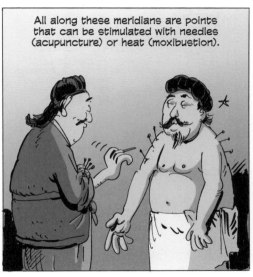

Some Chinese doctors have left their mark on history.

HUA TUO (110–207) was a surgeon who used acupuncture, moxibustion, and pharmacopoeia. He also developed products to relieve pain.

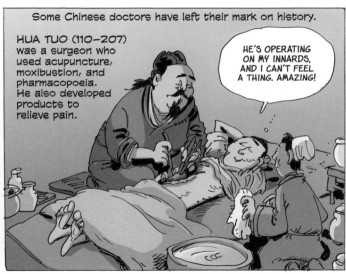

HE'S OPERATING ON MY INNARDS, AND I CAN'T FEEL A THING. AMAZING!

SUN SIMIAO (590–682) was a great physician who also described the benefits of acupuncture, moxibustion, and plants.

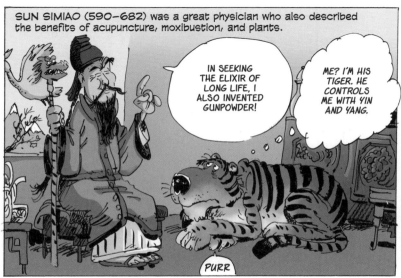

IN SEEKING THE ELIXIR OF LONG LIFE, I ALSO INVENTED GUNPOWDER!

ME? I'M HIS TIGER. HE CONTROLS ME WITH YIN AND YANG.

PURR

Unlike other ancient medicines, Chinese medicine was based on philosophy rather than religion. Doctors were thinkers, not priests.

And unlike other traditional medicines, Chinese medicine is still practised today, both in China and the West.

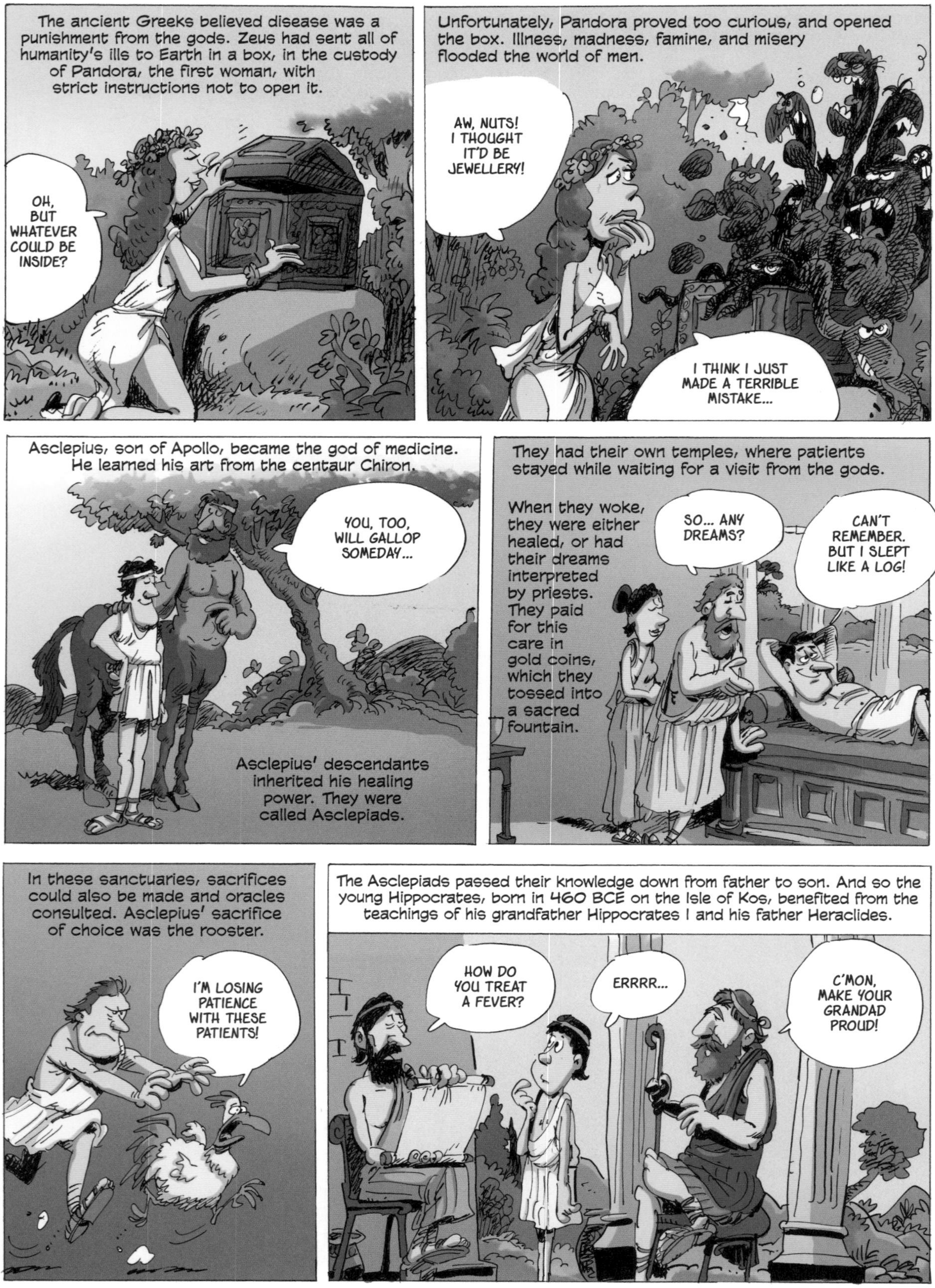
The ancient Greeks believed disease was a punishment from the gods. Zeus had sent all of humanity's ills to Earth in a box, in the custody of Pandora, the first woman, with strict instructions not to open it.
OH, BUT WHATEVER COULD BE INSIDE?
Unfortunately, Pandora proved too curious, and opened the box. Illness, madness, famine, and misery flooded the world of men.
AW, NUTS! I THOUGHT IT'D BE JEWELLERY!
I THINK I JUST MADE A TERRIBLE MISTAKE...
Asclepius, son of Apollo, became the god of medicine. He learned his art from the centaur Chiron.
YOU, TOO, WILL GALLOP SOMEDAY...
Asclepius' descendants inherited his healing power. They were called Asclepiads.
They had their own temples, where patients stayed while waiting for a visit from the gods.
When they woke, they were either healed, or had their dreams interpreted by priests. They paid for this care in gold coins, which they tossed into a sacred fountain.
SO... ANY DREAMS?
CAN'T REMEMBER. BUT I SLEPT LIKE A LOG!
In these sanctuaries, sacrifices could also be made and oracles consulted. Asclepius' sacrifice of choice was the rooster.
I'M LOSING PATIENCE WITH THESE PATIENTS!
The Asclepiads passed their knowledge down from father to son. And so the young Hippocrates, born in 460 BCE on the Isle of Kos, benefited from the teachings of his grandfather Hippocrates I and his father Heraclides.
HOW DO YOU TREAT A FEVER?
ERRRR...
C'MON, MAKE YOUR GRANDAD PROUD!

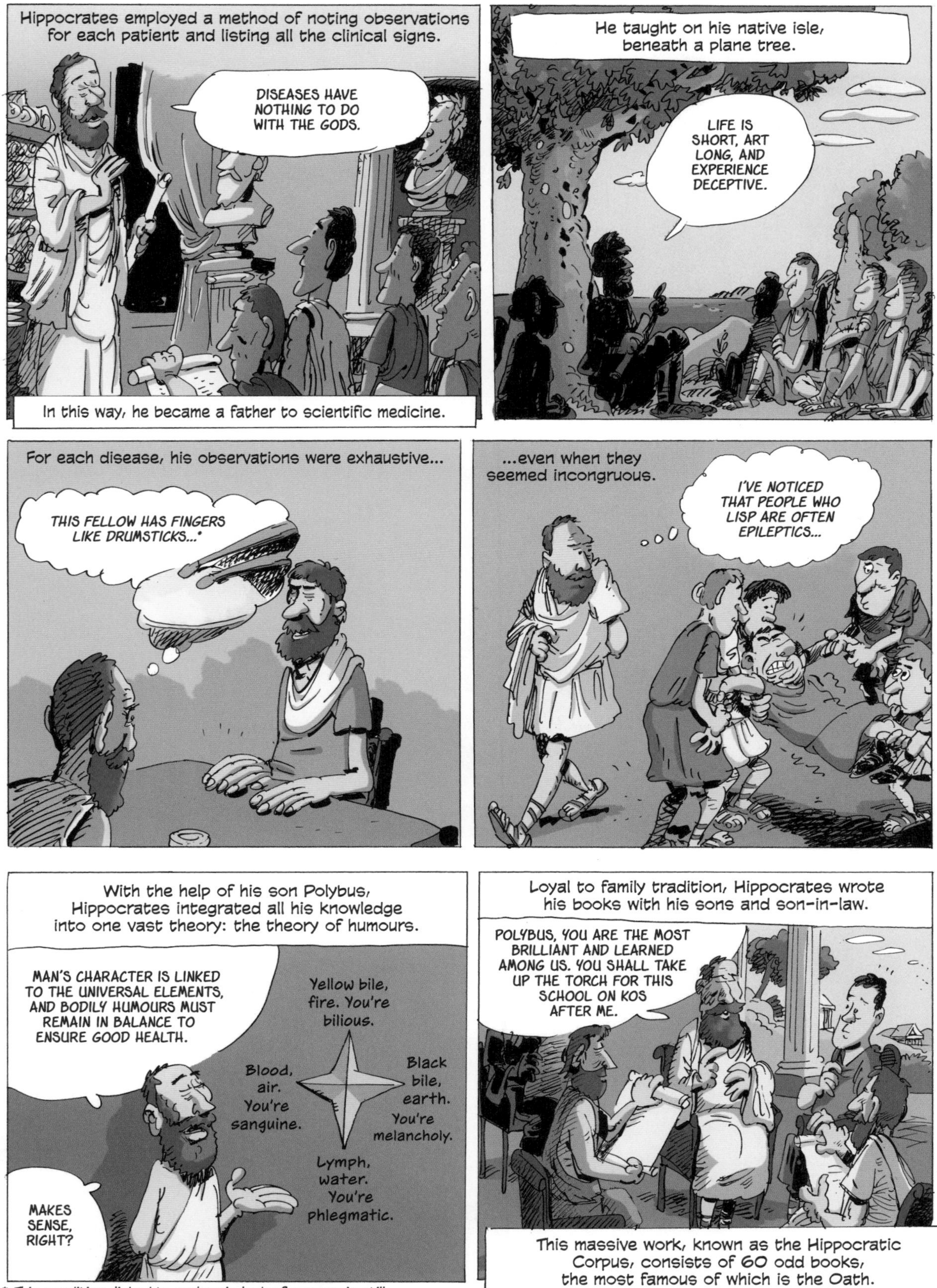
Hippocrates employed a method of noting observations for each patient and listing all the clinical signs.
DISEASES HAVE NOTHING TO DO WITH THE GODS.
In this way, he became a father to scientific medicine.
He taught on his native isle, beneath a plane tree.
LIFE IS SHORT, ART LONG, AND EXPERIENCE DECEPTIVE.
For each disease, his observations were exhaustive...
THIS FELLOW HAS FINGERS LIKE DRUMSTICKS...*
...even when they seemed incongruous.
I'VE NOTICED THAT PEOPLE WHO LISP ARE OFTEN EPILEPTICS...
With the help of his son Polybus, Hippocrates integrated all his knowledge into one vast theory: the theory of humours.
MAN'S CHARACTER IS LINKED TO THE UNIVERSAL ELEMENTS, AND BODILY HUMOURS MUST REMAIN IN BALANCE TO ENSURE GOOD HEALTH.
Yellow bile, fire. You're bilious.
Blood, air. You're sanguine.
Black bile, earth. You're melancholy.
Lymph, water. You're phlegmatic.
MAKES SENSE, RIGHT?
Loyal to family tradition, Hippocrates wrote his books with his sons and son-in-law.
POLYBUS, YOU ARE THE MOST BRILLIANT AND LEARNED AMONG US. YOU SHALL TAKE UP THE TORCH FOR THIS SCHOOL ON KOS AFTER ME.
This massive work, known as the Hippocratic Corpus, consists of 60 odd books, the most famous of which is the Oath.

* This condition, linked to a chronic lack of oxygen, is still known as "digital hippocratism", or "nail clubbing".

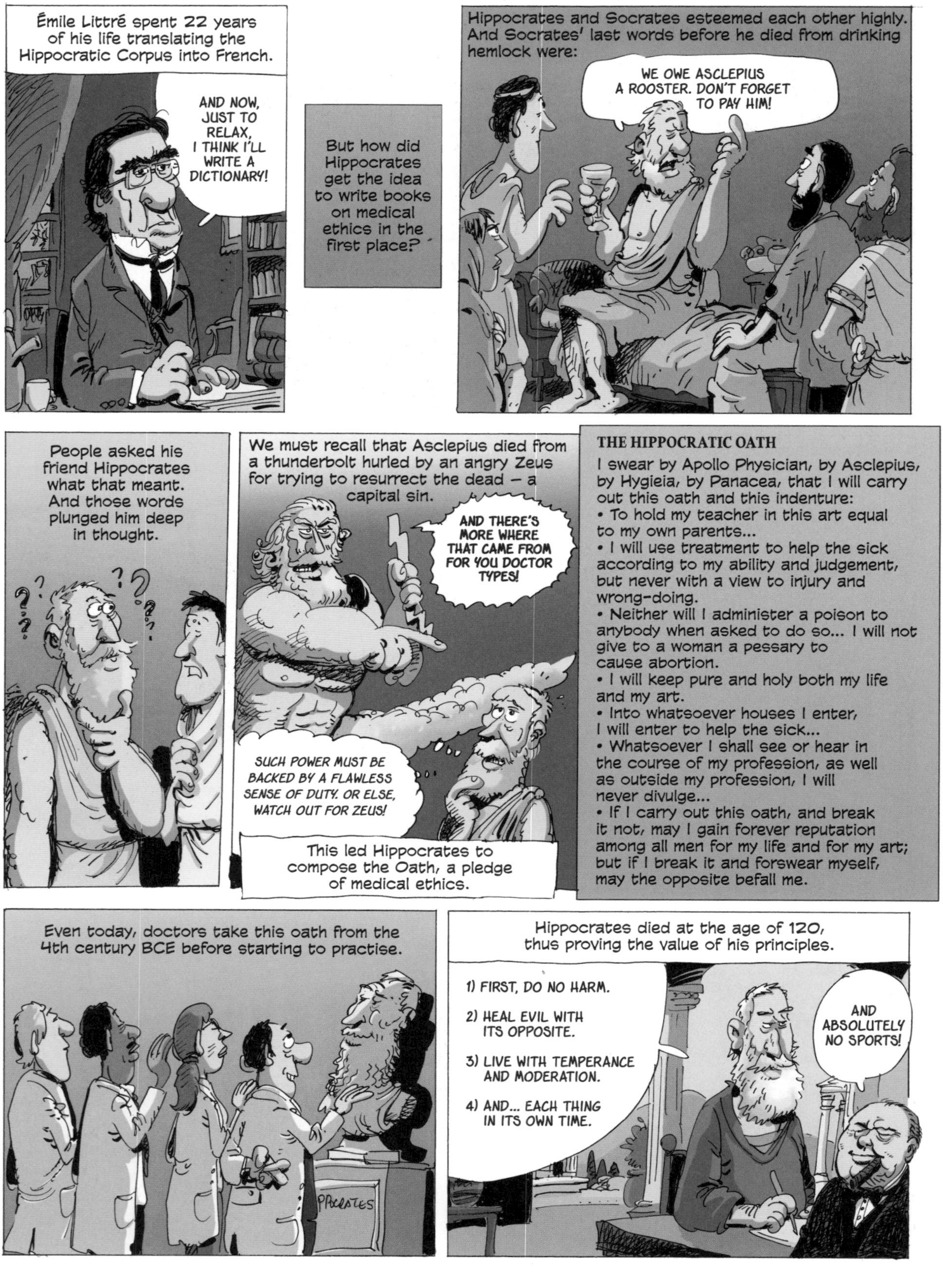
Émile Littré spent 22 years of his life translating the Hippocratic Corpus into French.
AND NOW, JUST TO RELAX, I THINK I'LL WRITE A DICTIONARY!
But how did Hippocrates get the idea to write books on medical ethics in the first place?
Hippocrates and Socrates esteemed each other highly. And Socrates' last words before he died from drinking hemlock were:
WE OWE ASCLEPIUS A ROOSTER. DON'T FORGET TO PAY HIM!
People asked his friend Hippocrates what that meant. And those words plunged him deep in thought.
We must recall that Asclepius died from a thunderbolt hurled by an angry Zeus for trying to resurrect the dead – a capital sin.
AND THERE'S MORE WHERE THAT CAME FROM FOR YOU DOCTOR TYPES!
SUCH POWER MUST BE BACKED BY A FLAWLESS SENSE OF DUTY. OR ELSE, WATCH OUT FOR ZEUS!
This led Hippocrates to compose the Oath, a pledge of medical ethics.
THE HIPPOCRATIC OATH
I swear by Apollo Physician, by Asclepius, by Hygieia, by Panacea, that I will carry out this oath and this indenture:
• To hold my teacher in this art equal to my own parents...
• I will use treatment to help the sick according to my ability and judgement, but never with a view to injury and wrong-doing.
• Neither will I administer a poison to anybody when asked to do so... I will not give to a woman a pessary to cause abortion.
• I will keep pure and holy both my life and my art.
• Into whatsoever houses I enter, I will enter to help the sick...
• Whatsoever I shall see or hear in the course of my profession, as well as outside my profession, I will never divulge...
• If I carry out this oath, and break it not, may I gain forever reputation among all men for my life and for my art; but if I break it and forswear myself, may the opposite befall me.
Even today, doctors take this oath from the 4th century BCE before starting to practise.
HIPPOCRATES
Hippocrates died at the age of 120, thus proving the value of his principles.
1) FIRST, DO NO HARM.
2) HEAL EVIL WITH ITS OPPOSITE.
3) LIVE WITH TEMPERANCE AND MODERATION.
4) AND... EACH THING IN ITS OWN TIME.
AND ABSOLUTELY NO SPORTS!

Aristotle was the student of Plato (himself a student of Socrates) and the private tutor of Alexander the Great.

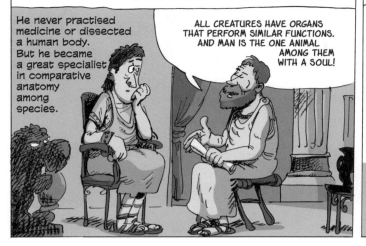

He never practised medicine or dissected a human body. But he became a great specialist in comparative anatomy among species.

ALL CREATURES HAVE ORGANS THAT PERFORM SIMILAR FUNCTIONS. AND MAN IS THE ONE ANIMAL AMONG THEM WITH A SOUL!

He would have a great influence on doctors in the centuries to come...

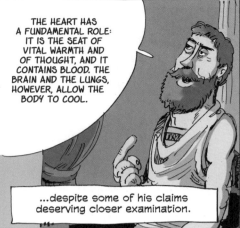

THE HEART HAS A FUNDAMENTAL ROLE: IT IS THE SEAT OF VITAL WARMTH AND OF THOUGHT, AND IT CONTAINS BLOOD. THE BRAIN AND THE LUNGS, HOWEVER, ALLOW THE BODY TO COOL.

...despite some of his claims deserving closer examination.

Alexander, a worthy pupil, conquered the world and founded the city and Library of Alexandria.

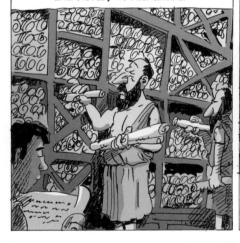

Such were the origins of a brilliant medical school.

WE ONLY CARRY THE SCROLLS AROUND. WE CAN'T READ THEM.

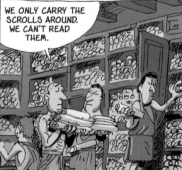

King Ptolemy, who encouraged the sciences, added to the Library, which came to hold over 700,000 works.

In Alexandria, Herophilus and Erasistratus greatly advanced the study of anatomy c. 300 BCE. For 50 years, human dissection was permitted... as well as the vivisections of criminals!

YOU GET A BETTER VIEW WHEN THEY'RE STILL ALIVE.

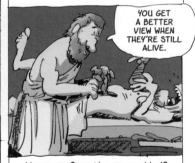

However, from the second half of the 3rd century, use of the human body was prohibited.

The pair of them were also great doctors. Erasistratus even discovered why Antiochus was ill: he was secretly in love with his stepmother.

THEREIN LIES WHAT AILS THEE!

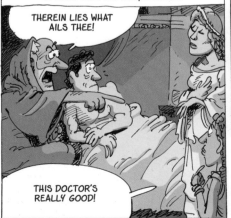

THIS DOCTOR'S REALLY GOOD!

Herophilus wrote nine anatomical treatises, but they were destroyed when the Library caught fire in 48 BCE.

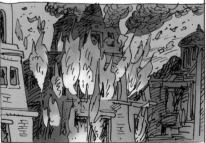

The loss of that Library, in which the sum of the learning of Antiquity lay gathered, without doubt led to the scientific obscurantism of the Christian Middle Ages.

The Romans proved uninterested in medicine, which they found too compassionate.

ROMANS DON'T NEED DOCTORS, ESPECIALLY NOT GREEK ONES WHO THINK WE'RE BARBARIANS.

AND CARTHAGE MUST BE DESTROYED!

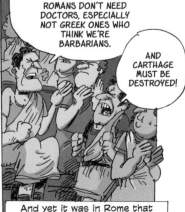

And yet it was in Rome that the Greek Claudius Galen made his name.

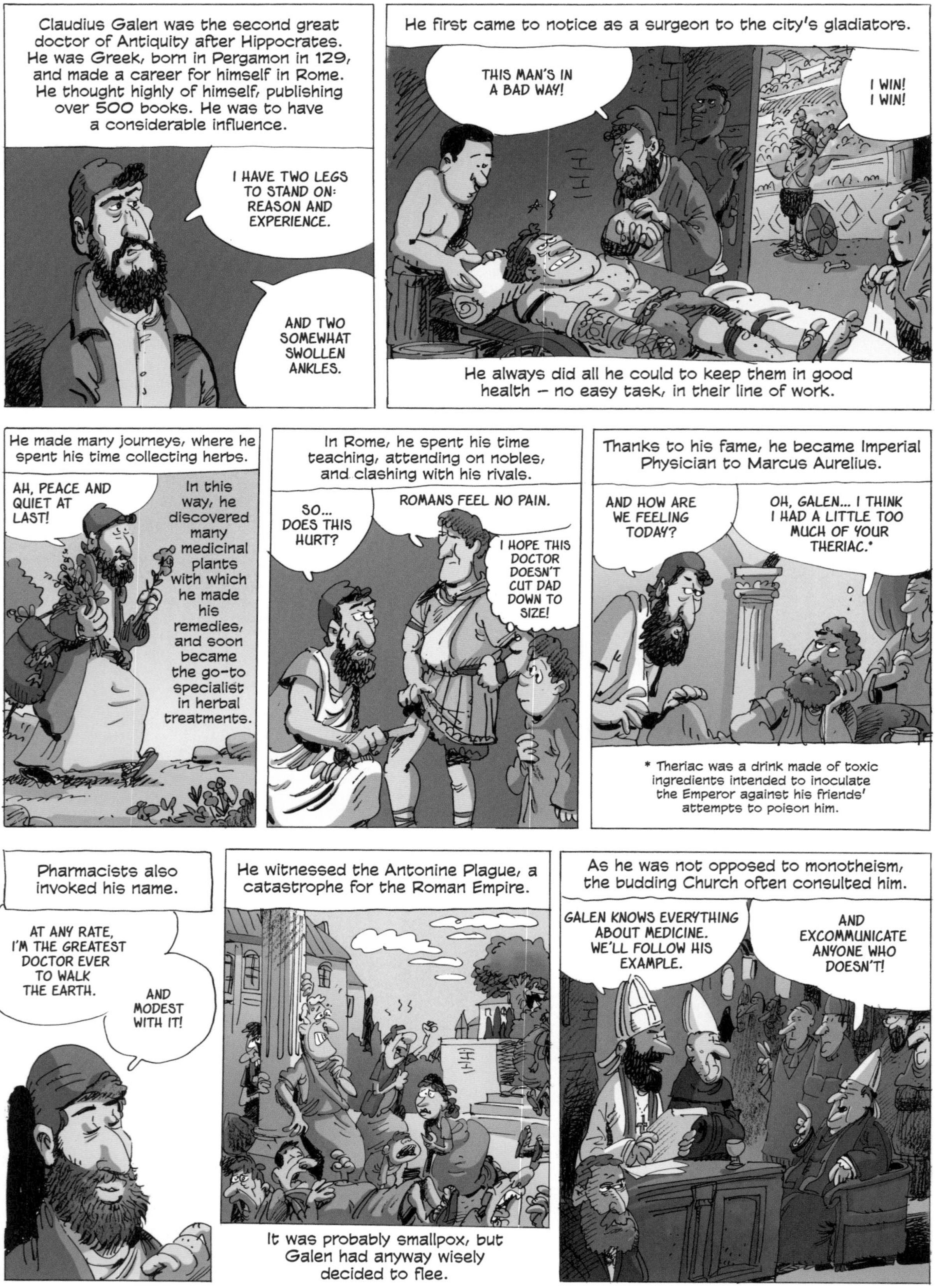
Claudius Galen was the second great doctor of Antiquity after Hippocrates. He was Greek, born in Pergamon in 129, and made a career for himself in Rome. He thought highly of himself, publishing over 500 books. He was to have a considerable influence.
I HAVE TWO LEGS TO STAND ON: REASON AND EXPERIENCE.
AND TWO SOMEWHAT SWOLLEN ANKLES.
He first came to notice as a surgeon to the city's gladiators.
THIS MAN'S IN A BAD WAY!
I WIN! I WIN!
He always did all he could to keep them in good health – no easy task, in their line of work.
He made many journeys, where he spent his time collecting herbs.
AH, PEACE AND QUIET AT LAST!
In this way, he discovered many medicinal plants with which he made his remedies, and soon became the go-to specialist in herbal treatments.
In Rome, he spent his time teaching, attending on nobles, and clashing with his rivals.
SO... DOES THIS HURT?
ROMANS FEEL NO PAIN.
I HOPE THIS DOCTOR DOESN'T CUT DAD DOWN TO SIZE!
Thanks to his fame, he became Imperial Physician to Marcus Aurelius.
AND HOW ARE WE FEELING TODAY?
OH, GALEN... I THINK I HAD A LITTLE TOO MUCH OF YOUR THERIAC.*
* Theriac was a drink made of toxic ingredients intended to inoculate the Emperor against his friends' attempts to poison him.
Pharmacists also invoked his name.
AT ANY RATE, I'M THE GREATEST DOCTOR EVER TO WALK THE EARTH.
AND MODEST WITH IT!
He witnessed the Antonine Plague, a catastrophe for the Roman Empire.
It was probably smallpox, but Galen had anyway wisely decided to flee.
As he was not opposed to monotheism, the budding Church often consulted him.
GALEN KNOWS EVERYTHING ABOUT MEDICINE. WE'LL FOLLOW HIS EXAMPLE.
AND EXCOMMUNICATE ANYONE WHO DOESN'T!

CHAPTER 2

THE MIDDLE AGES

The burning of the Library of Alexandria (which at the height of its glory held 700,000 scrolls) is often blamed for the loss of the knowledge accumulated in Antiquity. The social and military unrest that accompanied the fall of the Roman Empire, and the massive barbarian invasions that followed, further contributed to the cultural impoverishment. As ancient texts vanished or were lost, the great studies of Greek physicians were no longer accessible to the learned clerics of the High Middle Ages.

Only to the East—more precisely, in Persia—was a tradition of medical care and teaching able to be passed down to new generations, thanks to doctors within the "Nestorian" dispensation of the Christian Church. Persian medicine was then perpetuated by the revelation of Muhammad, and the extraordinary Arab hegemony that followed. Thanks to the unity imposed by empire, religion, and, above all, the widespread diffusion of the Arab language, a long period of cultural and medical development began, spreading from the Middle East and the south of the Mediterranean basin all the way to Spain.

In medicine, two heroes would bear aloft the torch of the knowledge of past centuries: Avicenna, prince of physicians, whose *Canon* would inform not only Arab doctors, but also those of the Christian world, at least until the Renaissance; and the aforementioned great and unavoidable Galen, whose encyclopedic knowledge would form a staple reference for the Catholic Church.

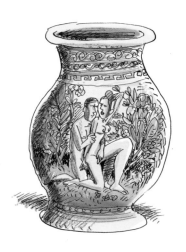

PERSIAN AND ARABIC MEDICINE

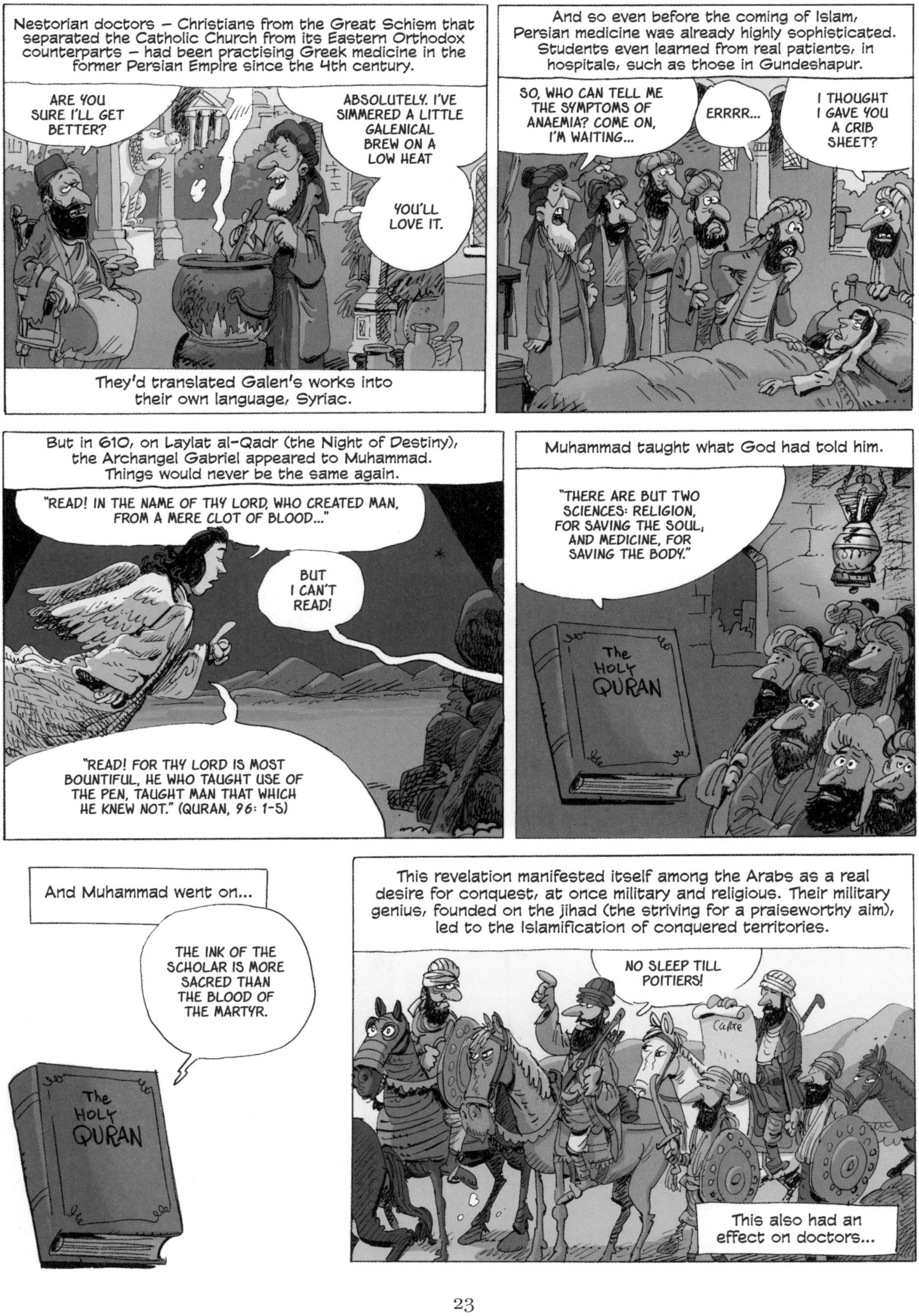
Nestorian doctors – Christians from the Great Schism that separated the Catholic Church from its Eastern Orthodox counterparts – had been practising Greek medicine in the former Persian Empire since the 4th century.
ARE YOU SURE I'LL GET BETTER?
ABSOLUTELY. I'VE SIMMERED A LITTLE GALENICAL BREW ON A LOW HEAT
YOU'LL LOVE IT.
They'd translated Galen's works into their own language, Syriac.
And so even before the coming of Islam, Persian medicine was already highly sophisticated. Students even learned from real patients, in hospitals, such as those in Gundeshapur.
SO, WHO CAN TELL ME THE SYMPTOMS OF ANAEMIA? COME ON, I'M WAITING...
ERRRR...
I THOUGHT I GAVE YOU A CRIB SHEET?
But in 610, on Laylat al-Qadr (the Night of Destiny), the Archangel Gabriel appeared to Muhammad. Things would never be the same again.
"READ! IN THE NAME OF THY LORD, WHO CREATED MAN, FROM A MERE CLOT OF BLOOD..."
BUT I CAN'T READ!
"READ! FOR THY LORD IS MOST BOUNTIFUL, HE WHO TAUGHT USE OF THE PEN, TAUGHT MAN THAT WHICH HE KNEW NOT." (QURAN, 96: 1-5)
Muhammad taught what God had told him.
"THERE ARE BUT TWO SCIENCES: RELIGION, FOR SAVING THE SOUL; AND MEDICINE, FOR SAVING THE BODY."
The HOLY QURAN
And Muhammad went on...
THE INK OF THE SCHOLAR IS MORE SACRED THAN THE BLOOD OF THE MARTYR.
The HOLY QURAN
This revelation manifested itself among the Arabs as a real desire for conquest, at once military and religious. Their military genius, founded on the jihad (the striving for a praiseworthy aim), led to the Islamification of conquered territories.
NO SLEEP TILL POITIERS!
CARTE
This also had an effect on doctors...

The year 710 saw the conquest of Northern Africa. Then the Muslims headed west into Spain, and east into India and China.
Atlantic Ocean
Europe
Asia
WAHOO!
Africa
Indian Ocean
These conquests were made possible by highly efficient administrations that respected local authorities.
The Caliph was assisted by the vizier and military governors known as emirs. Doctors were especially respected – but that didn't prevent a series of internal power struggles.
I WANT TO BE CALIPH INSTEAD OF THE CALIPH!
IT'S NO GOOD, DOCTOR...
The Arab advance was only stopped in its tracks by the Christian forces at Constantinople, and by the Franks under Charles Martel at Poitiers in 732.
OKAY, BOYS! THE BUCK STOPS HERE!
FRANCE FOR THE FRANKS!
POIT
Destabilized at first by the Arab invasion, Persian medicine quickly recovered. Books were translated into Arabic to save them from destruction.
SO, FIRST TRANSLATE ALL OF HIPPOCRATES INTO ARABIC, AND THEN YOU CAN DO ARISTOTLE AND GALEN.
SURE YOU DON'T WANT ME TO START WITH ERASISTRATUS?
All expert disciplines were gathered into Houses of Wisdom.
WE MAKE PAPER THE CHINESE WAY.
WE DO ALGEBRA THE INDIAN WAY.
Rhazes (854–925) was an Iranian scholar, a doctor at the hospital in Baghdad, and a great experimental specialist in medication.
THE MAIN PRINCIPLES OF MY LIFE: RELAX, DON'T OVEREAT, AVOID LIVING IN A SLUM, AND STAY ACTIVE!
EASY, RIGHT?

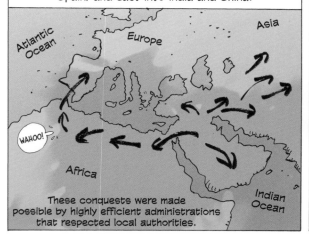

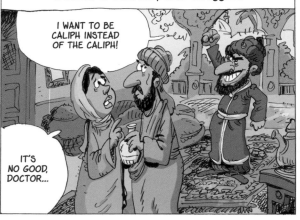

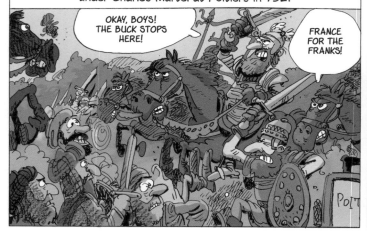

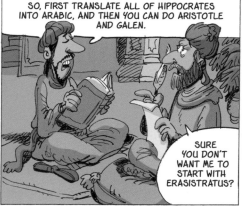

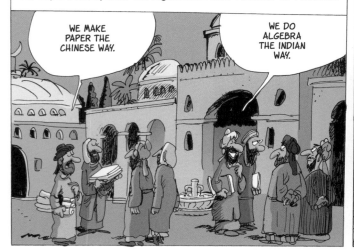

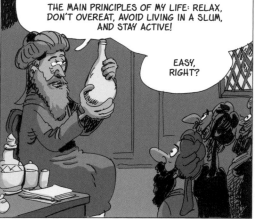

He worked at the hospital, which he reorganized, and was a great clinician who advocated vegetarianism.

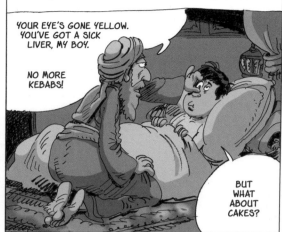

YOUR EYE'S GONE YELLOW. YOU'VE GOT A SICK LIVER, MY BOY.

NO MORE KEBABS!

BUT WHAT ABOUT CAKES?

Rhazes also categorized the various eruptive fevers.

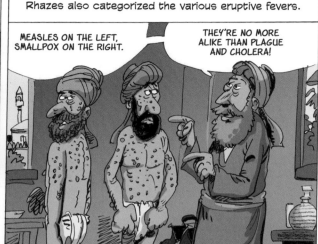

MEASLES ON THE LEFT, SMALLPOX ON THE RIGHT.

THEY'RE NO MORE ALIKE THAN PLAGUE AND CHOLERA!

Another star of the era was Avicenna (980–1037), without doubt the greatest influence on the centuries to come due to his authoritative *Canon of Medicine*, perhaps the central textbook until the Renaissance.

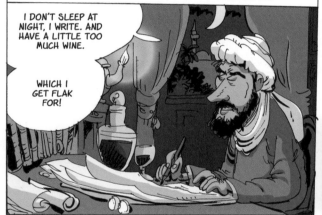

I DON'T SLEEP AT NIGHT, I WRITE. AND HAVE A LITTLE TOO MUCH WINE.

WHICH I GET FLAK FOR!

His life story resembled some sort of adventure novel.

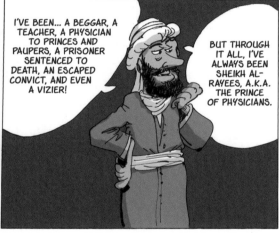

I'VE BEEN... A BEGGAR, A TEACHER, A PHYSICIAN TO PRINCES AND PAUPERS, A PRISONER SENTENCED TO DEATH, AN ESCAPED CONVICT, AND EVEN A VIZIER!

BUT THROUGH IT ALL, I'VE ALWAYS BEEN SHEIKH AL-RAYEES, A.K.A. THE PRINCE OF PHYSICIANS.

His knowledge was encyclopedic.

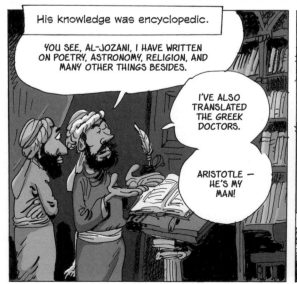

YOU SEE, AL-JOZANI, I HAVE WRITTEN ON POETRY, ASTRONOMY, RELIGION, AND MANY OTHER THINGS BESIDES.

I'VE ALSO TRANSLATED THE GREEK DOCTORS.

ARISTOTLE — HE'S MY MAN!

Arab domination led to a period of intense medical and intellectual activity.

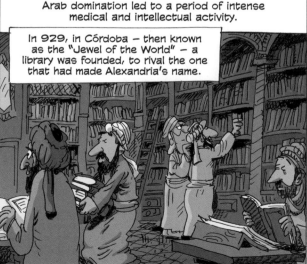

In 929, in Córdoba — then known as the "Jewel of the World" — a library was founded, to rival the one that had made Alexandria's name.

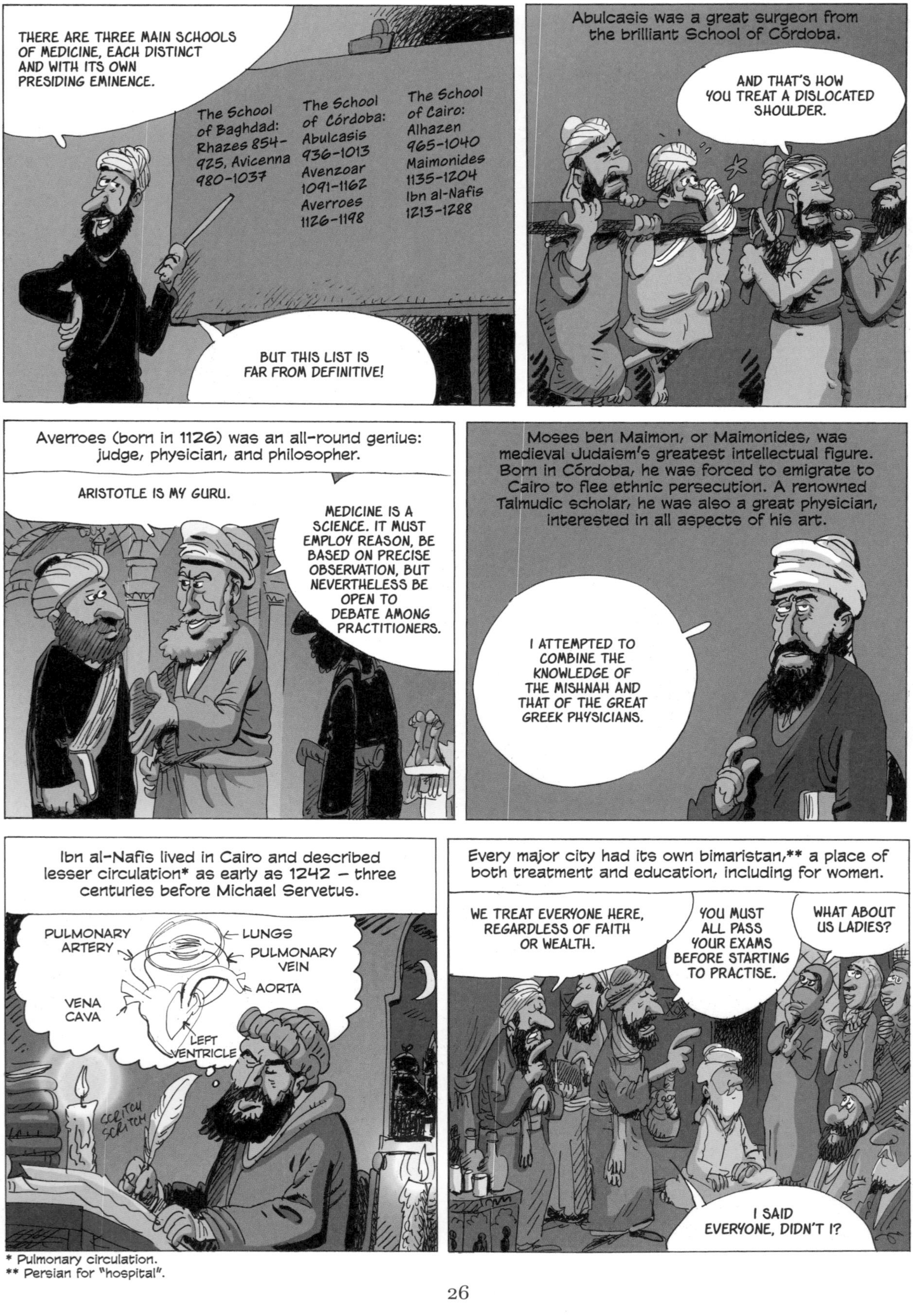

THERE ARE THREE MAIN SCHOOLS OF MEDICINE, EACH DISTINCT AND WITH ITS OWN PRESIDING EMINENCE.
The School of Baghdad: Rhazes 854-925, Avicenna 980-1037
The School of Córdoba: Abulcasis 936-1013 Avenzoar 1091-1162 Averroes 1126-1198
The School of Cairo: Alhazen 965-1040 Maimonides 1135-1204 Ibn al-Nafis 1213-1288
BUT THIS LIST IS FAR FROM DEFINITIVE!
Abulcasis was a great surgeon from the brilliant School of Córdoba.
AND THAT'S HOW YOU TREAT A DISLOCATED SHOULDER.
Averroes (born in 1126) was an all-round genius: judge, physician, and philosopher.
ARISTOTLE IS MY GURU.
MEDICINE IS A SCIENCE. IT MUST EMPLOY REASON, BE BASED ON PRECISE OBSERVATION, BUT NEVERTHELESS BE OPEN TO DEBATE AMONG PRACTITIONERS.
Moses ben Maimon, or Maimonides, was medieval Judaism's greatest intellectual figure. Born in Córdoba, he was forced to emigrate to Cairo to flee ethnic persecution. A renowned Talmudic scholar, he was also a great physician, interested in all aspects of his art.
I ATTEMPTED TO COMBINE THE KNOWLEDGE OF THE MISHNAH AND THAT OF THE GREAT GREEK PHYSICIANS.
Ibn al-Nafis lived in Cairo and described lesser circulation* as early as 1242 – three centuries before Michael Servetus.
PULMONARY ARTERY
LUNGS
PULMONARY VEIN
AORTA
VENA CAVA
LEFT VENTRICLE
SCRITCH SCRITCH
Every major city had its own bimaristan,** a place of both treatment and education, including for women.
WE TREAT EVERYONE HERE, REGARDLESS OF FAITH OR WEALTH.
YOU MUST ALL PASS YOUR EXAMS BEFORE STARTING TO PRACTISE.
WHAT ABOUT US LADIES?
I SAID EVERYONE, DIDN'T I?

* Pulmonary circulation.
** Persian for "hospital".

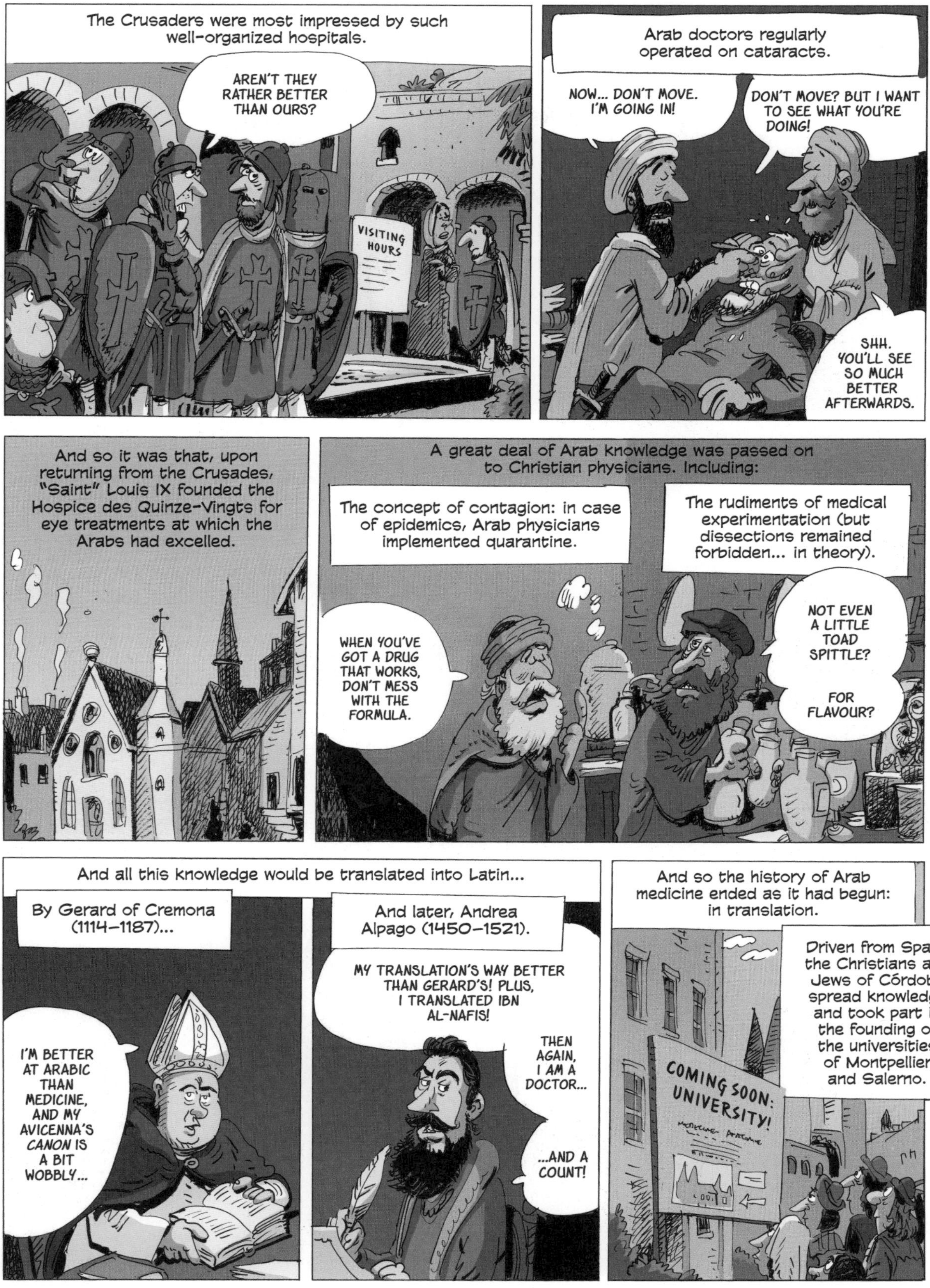
The Crusaders were most impressed by such well-organized hospitals.
AREN'T THEY RATHER BETTER THAN OURS?
VISITING HOURS
Arab doctors regularly operated on cataracts.
NOW... DON'T MOVE. I'M GOING IN!
DON'T MOVE? BUT I WANT TO SEE WHAT YOU'RE DOING!
SHH. YOU'LL SEE SO MUCH BETTER AFTERWARDS.
And so it was that, upon returning from the Crusades, "Saint" Louis IX founded the Hospice des Quinze-Vingts for eye treatments at which the Arabs had excelled.
A great deal of Arab knowledge was passed on to Christian physicians. Including:
The concept of contagion: in case of epidemics, Arab physicians implemented quarantine.
The rudiments of medical experimentation (but dissections remained forbidden... in theory).
WHEN YOU'VE GOT A DRUG THAT WORKS, DON'T MESS WITH THE FORMULA.
NOT EVEN A LITTLE TOAD SPITTLE?
FOR FLAVOUR?
And all this knowledge would be translated into Latin...
By Gerard of Cremona (1114–1187)...
I'M BETTER AT ARABIC THAN MEDICINE, AND MY AVICENNA'S *CANON* IS A BIT WOBBLY...
And later, Andrea Alpago (1450–1521).
MY TRANSLATION'S WAY BETTER THAN GERARD'S! PLUS, I TRANSLATED IBN AL-NAFIS!
THEN AGAIN, I AM A DOCTOR...
...AND A COUNT!
And so the history of Arab medicine ended as it had begun: in translation.
Driven from Spain, the Christians and Jews of Córdoba spread knowledge and took part in the founding of the universities of Montpellier and Salerno.
COMING SOON: UNIVERSITY!

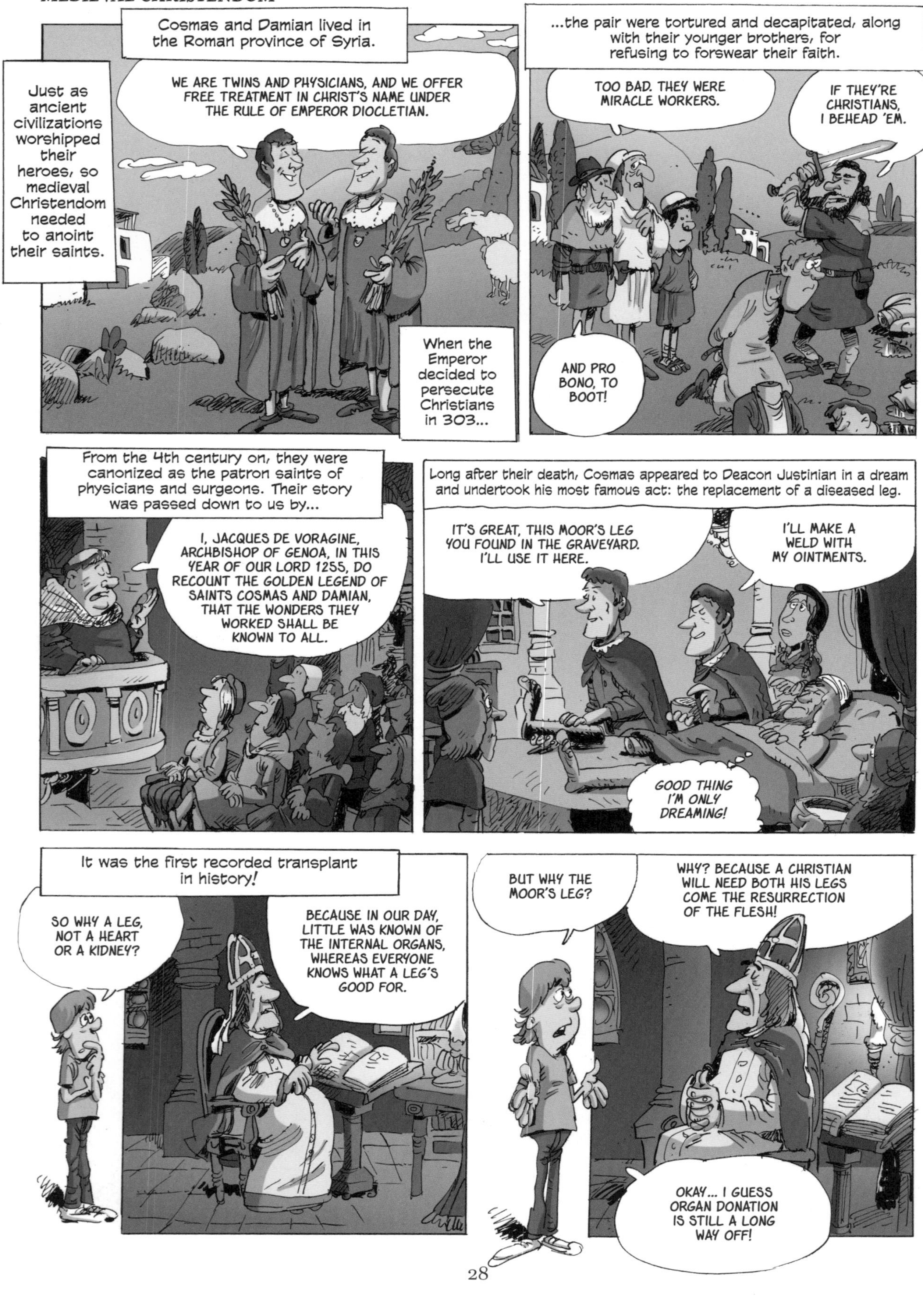
Just as ancient civilizations worshipped their heroes, so medieval Christendom needed to anoint their saints.
Cosmas and Damian lived in the Roman province of Syria.
WE ARE TWINS AND PHYSICIANS, AND WE OFFER FREE TREATMENT IN CHRIST'S NAME UNDER THE RULE OF EMPEROR DIOCLETIAN.
When the Emperor decided to persecute Christians in 303...
...the pair were tortured and decapitated, along with their younger brothers, for refusing to forswear their faith.
TOO BAD. THEY WERE MIRACLE WORKERS.
IF THEY'RE CHRISTIANS, I BEHEAD 'EM.
AND PRO BONO, TO BOOT!
From the 4th century on, they were canonized as the patron saints of physicians and surgeons. Their story was passed down to us by...
I, JACQUES DE VORAGINE, ARCHBISHOP OF GENOA, IN THIS YEAR OF OUR LORD 1255, DO RECOUNT THE GOLDEN LEGEND OF SAINTS COSMAS AND DAMIAN, THAT THE WONDERS THEY WORKED SHALL BE KNOWN TO ALL.
Long after their death, Cosmas appeared to Deacon Justinian in a dream and undertook his most famous act: the replacement of a diseased leg.
IT'S GREAT, THIS MOOR'S LEG YOU FOUND IN THE GRAVEYARD. I'LL USE IT HERE.
I'LL MAKE A WELD WITH MY OINTMENTS.
GOOD THING I'M ONLY DREAMING!
It was the first recorded transplant in history!
SO WHY A LEG, NOT A HEART OR A KIDNEY?
BECAUSE IN OUR DAY, LITTLE WAS KNOWN OF THE INTERNAL ORGANS, WHEREAS EVERYONE KNOWS WHAT A LEG'S GOOD FOR.
BUT WHY THE MOOR'S LEG?
WHY? BECAUSE A CHRISTIAN WILL NEED BOTH HIS LEGS COME THE RESURRECTION OF THE FLESH!
OKAY... I GUESS ORGAN DONATION IS STILL A LONG WAY OFF!

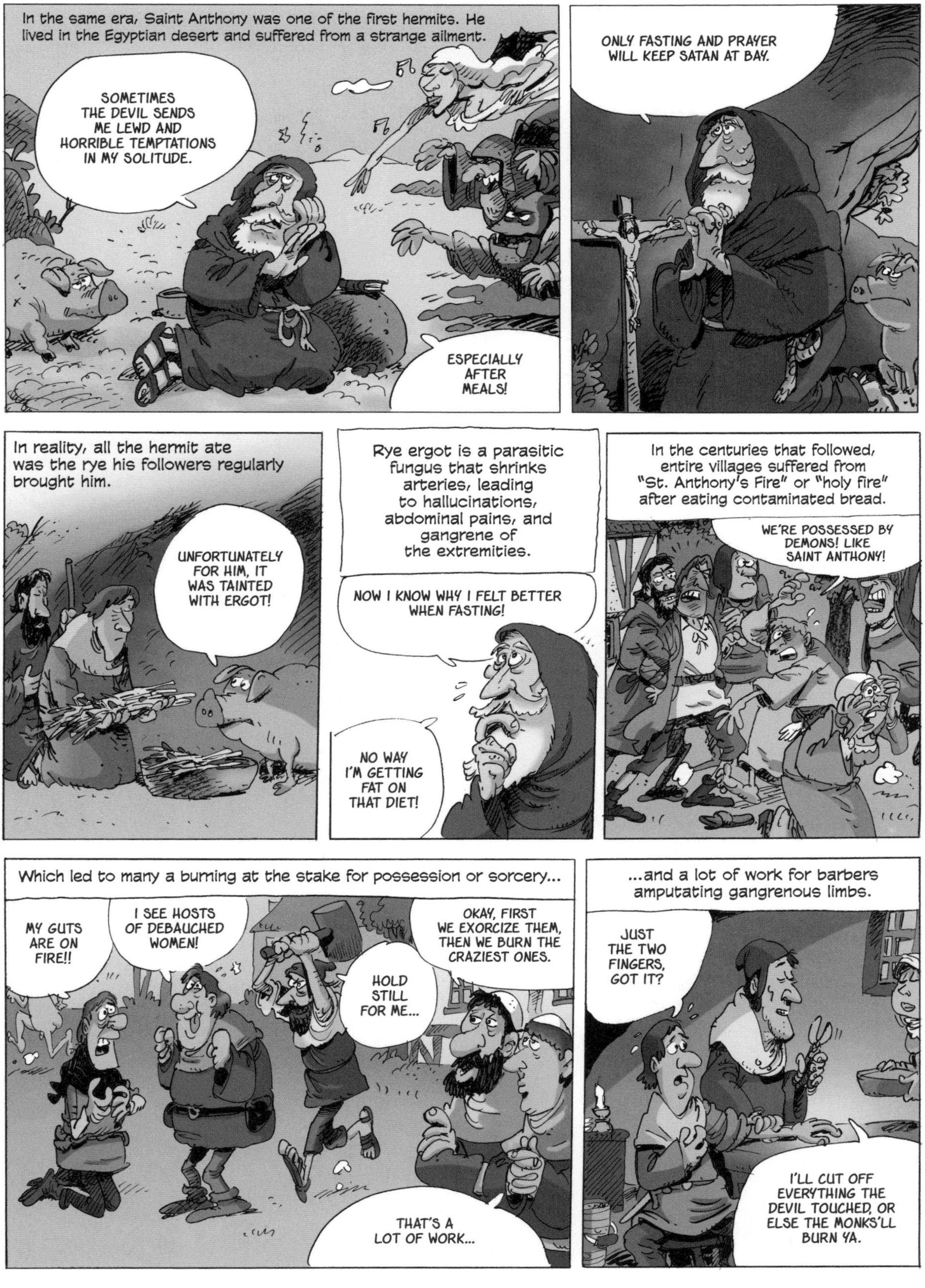
In the same era, Saint Anthony was one of the first hermits. He lived in the Egyptian desert and suffered from a strange ailment.
SOMETIMES THE DEVIL SENDS ME LEWD AND HORRIBLE TEMPTATIONS IN MY SOLITUDE.
ESPECIALLY AFTER MEALS!
ONLY FASTING AND PRAYER WILL KEEP SATAN AT BAY.
In reality, all the hermit ate was the rye his followers regularly brought him.
UNFORTUNATELY FOR HIM, IT WAS TAINTED WITH ERGOT!
Rye ergot is a parasitic fungus that shrinks arteries, leading to hallucinations, abdominal pains, and gangrene of the extremities.
NOW I KNOW WHY I FELT BETTER WHEN FASTING!
NO WAY I'M GETTING FAT ON THAT DIET!
In the centuries that followed, entire villages suffered from "St. Anthony's Fire" or "holy fire" after eating contaminated bread.
WE'RE POSSESSED BY DEMONS! LIKE SAINT ANTHONY!
Which led to many a burning at the stake for possession or sorcery...
MY GUTS ARE ON FIRE!!
I SEE HOSTS OF DEBAUCHED WOMEN!
HOLD STILL FOR ME...
OKAY, FIRST WE EXORCIZE THEM, THEN WE BURN THE CRAZIEST ONES.
THAT'S A LOT OF WORK...
...and a lot of work for barbers amputating gangrenous limbs.
JUST THE TWO FINGERS, GOT IT?
I'LL CUT OFF EVERYTHING THE DEVIL TOUCHED, OR ELSE THE MONKS'LL BURN YA.

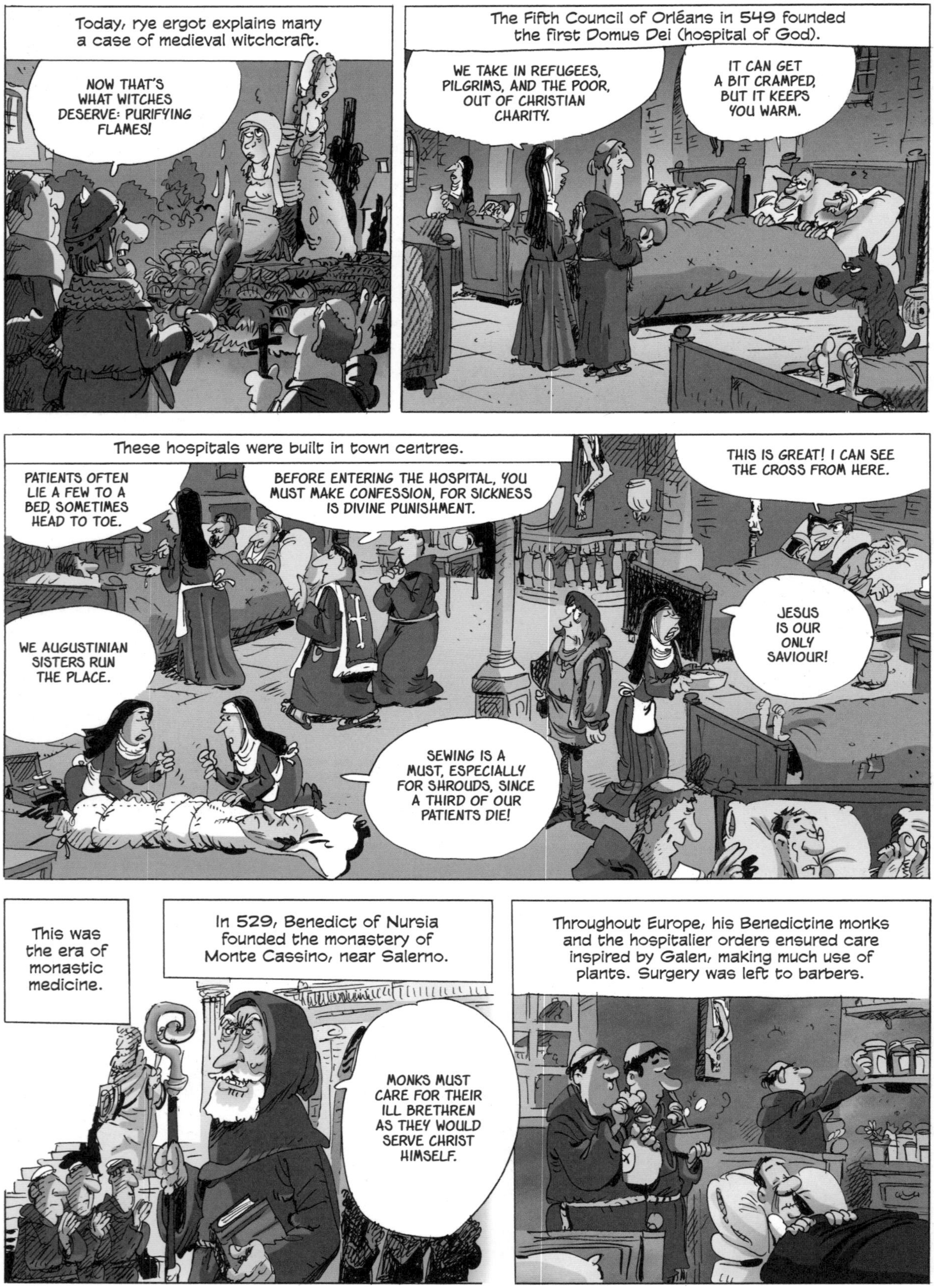
Today, rye ergot explains many a case of medieval witchcraft.
NOW THAT'S WHAT WITCHES DESERVE: PURIFYING FLAMES!
The Fifth Council of Orléans in 549 founded the first Domus Dei (hospital of God).
WE TAKE IN REFUGEES, PILGRIMS, AND THE POOR, OUT OF CHRISTIAN CHARITY.
IT CAN GET A BIT CRAMPED, BUT IT KEEPS YOU WARM.
These hospitals were built in town centres.
PATIENTS OFTEN LIE A FEW TO A BED, SOMETIMES HEAD TO TOE.
BEFORE ENTERING THE HOSPITAL, YOU MUST MAKE CONFESSION, FOR SICKNESS IS DIVINE PUNISHMENT.
THIS IS GREAT! I CAN SEE THE CROSS FROM HERE.
WE AUGUSTINIAN SISTERS RUN THE PLACE.
JESUS IS OUR ONLY SAVIOUR!
SEWING IS A MUST, ESPECIALLY FOR SHROUDS, SINCE A THIRD OF OUR PATIENTS DIE!
This was the era of monastic medicine.
In 529, Benedict of Nursia founded the monastery of Monte Cassino, near Salerno.
MONKS MUST CARE FOR THEIR ILL BRETHREN AS THEY WOULD SERVE CHRIST HIMSELF.
Throughout Europe, his Benedictine monks and the hospitalier orders ensured care inspired by Galen, making much use of plants. Surgery was left to barbers.

But between the years 1000 and 1300, the population tripled. Insufficient crops led to famine in the countryside, poverty and begging in the cities. On top of that, with sweeping epidemics there was an influx of extremely ill people, desperate for care. The sick and the poor necessarily flocked to the hospices. Which led to further problems...

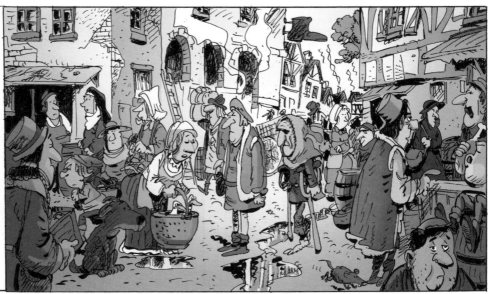

OUR CITIES ARE OVERRUN BY VAGRANT BEGGARS AND CRIPPLES.

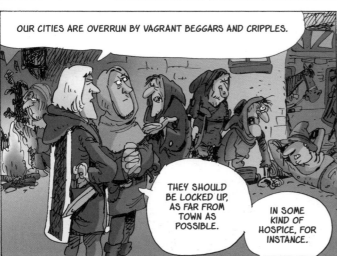

THEY SHOULD BE LOCKED UP, AS FAR FROM TOWN AS POSSIBLE.

IN SOME KIND OF HOSPICE, FOR INSTANCE.

To escort these nuisances by force, "beggar-drivers" were created.

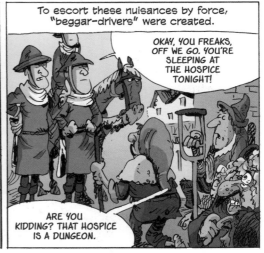

OKAY, YOU FREAKS, OFF WE GO. YOU'RE SLEEPING AT THE HOSPICE TONIGHT!

ARE YOU KIDDING? THAT HOSPICE IS A DUNGEON.

Pursuing this policy, Louis XIV signed a royal edict on 27 April 1656 to found a "general hospital for the confinement of Paris' poor".

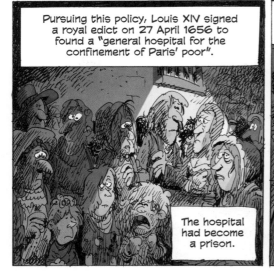

The hospital had become a prison.

But let's go back to the second half of the Middle Ages. A revival of medicine took place at the same time as the founding of universities: the monastic became scholastic.

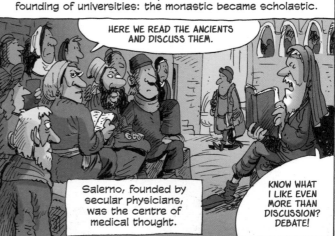

HERE WE READ THE ANCIENTS AND DISCUSS THEM.

Salerno, founded by secular physicians, was the centre of medical thought.

KNOW WHAT I LIKE EVEN MORE THAN DISCUSSION? DEBATE!

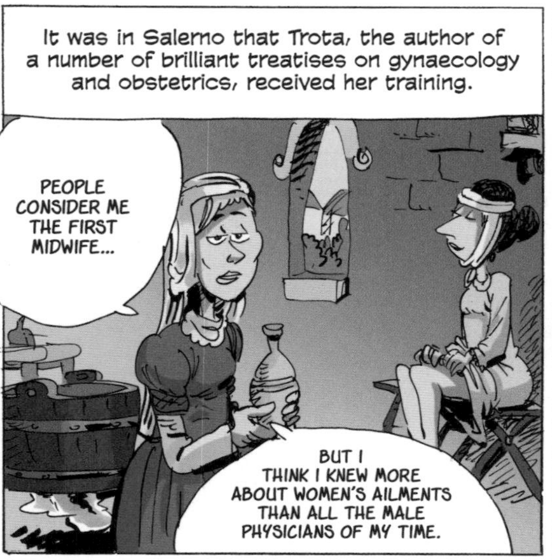
It was in Salerno that Trota, the author of a number of brilliant treatises on gynaecology and obstetrics, received her training.
PEOPLE CONSIDER ME THE FIRST MIDWIFE...
BUT I THINK I KNEW MORE ABOUT WOMEN'S AILMENTS THAN ALL THE MALE PHYSICIANS OF MY TIME.

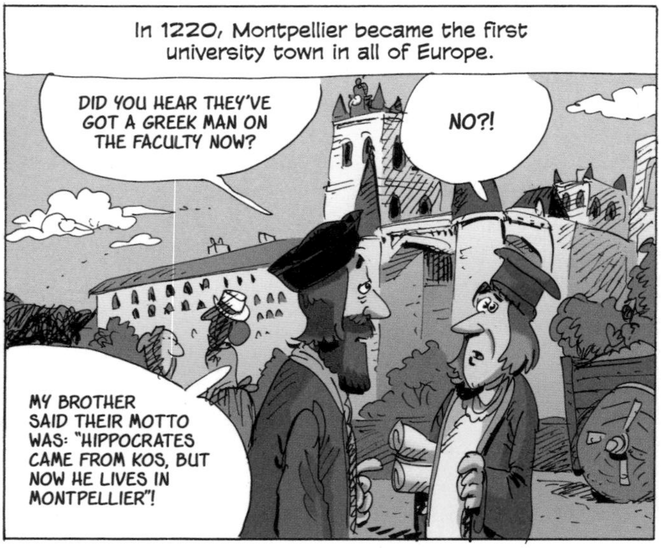
In 1220, Montpellier became the first university town in all of Europe.
DID YOU HEAR THEY'VE GOT A GREEK MAN ON THE FACULTY NOW?
NO?!
MY BROTHER SAID THEIR MOTTO WAS: "HIPPOCRATES CAME FROM KOS, BUT NOW HE LIVES IN MONTPELLIER"!

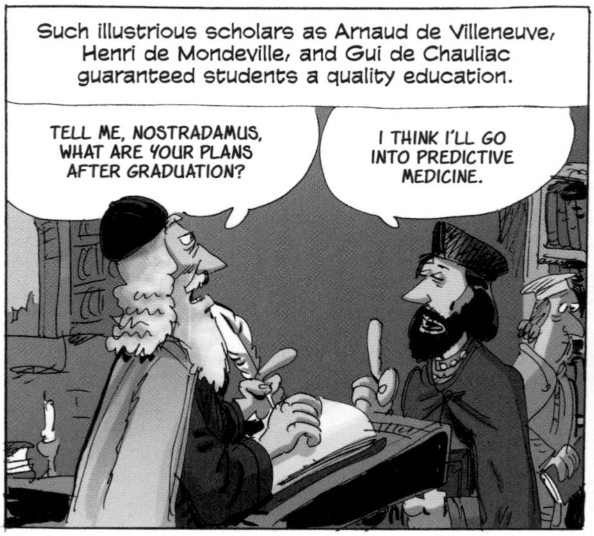
Such illustrious scholars as Arnaud de Villeneuve, Henri de Mondeville, and Gui de Chauliac guaranteed students a quality education.
TELL ME, NOSTRADAMUS, WHAT ARE YOUR PLANS AFTER GRADUATION?
I THINK I'LL GO INTO PREDICTIVE MEDICINE.

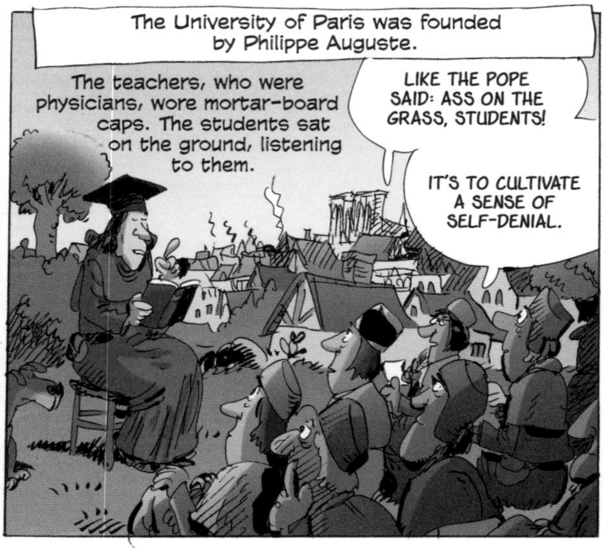
The University of Paris was founded by Philippe Auguste.
The teachers, who were physicians, wore mortar-board caps. The students sat on the ground, listening to them.
LIKE THE POPE SAID: ASS ON THE GRASS, STUDENTS!
IT'S TO CULTIVATE A SENSE OF SELF-DENIAL.

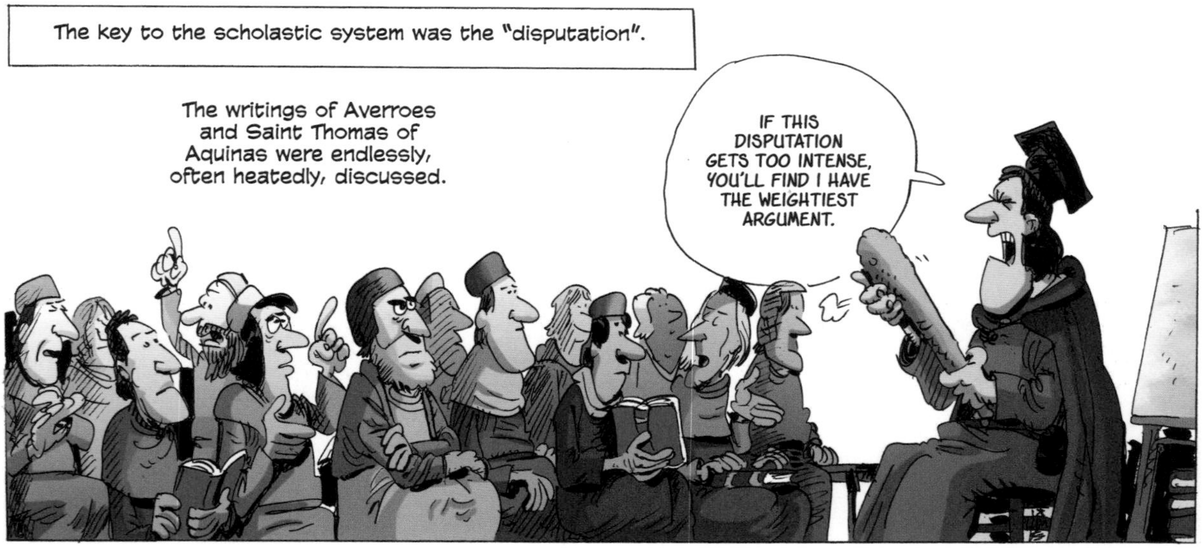
The key to the scholastic system was the "disputation".
The writings of Averroes and Saint Thomas of Aquinas were endlessly, often heatedly, discussed.
IF THIS DISPUTATION GETS TOO INTENSE, YOU'LL FIND I HAVE THE WEIGHTIEST ARGUMENT.

CHAPTER 3

FROM BARBERS TO SURGEONS

In the High Middle Ages, medicine was essentially practised by the regular clergy, according to the wishes of Saint Benedict of Nursia. However, in an attempt to redirect the monks' efforts towards saving souls, the Church repeatedly cleaved to the position that it "abhorred blood"—at the Councils of Clermont in 1130, Reims in 1131, and above all at Tours in 1163 and the Fourth Lateran Council in 1215. This effectively forbade the clergy—that is, the educated classes—from performing surgery.

As barbers were the only regular citizens to possess bladed instruments, they rushed in to fill the gap, carrying out the few documented operations from this time.

This situation gave rise to a lasting schism between medicine, which was the prerogative of scholars, and surgery, which was left to uncultivated journeymen who were illiterate in Latin and ignorant of Aristotle.

It took several centuries, and many a struggle, for surgeons to be seen, once again, as "operating physicians".

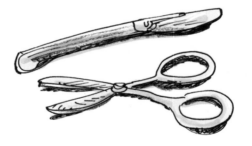

WHY BARBERS?

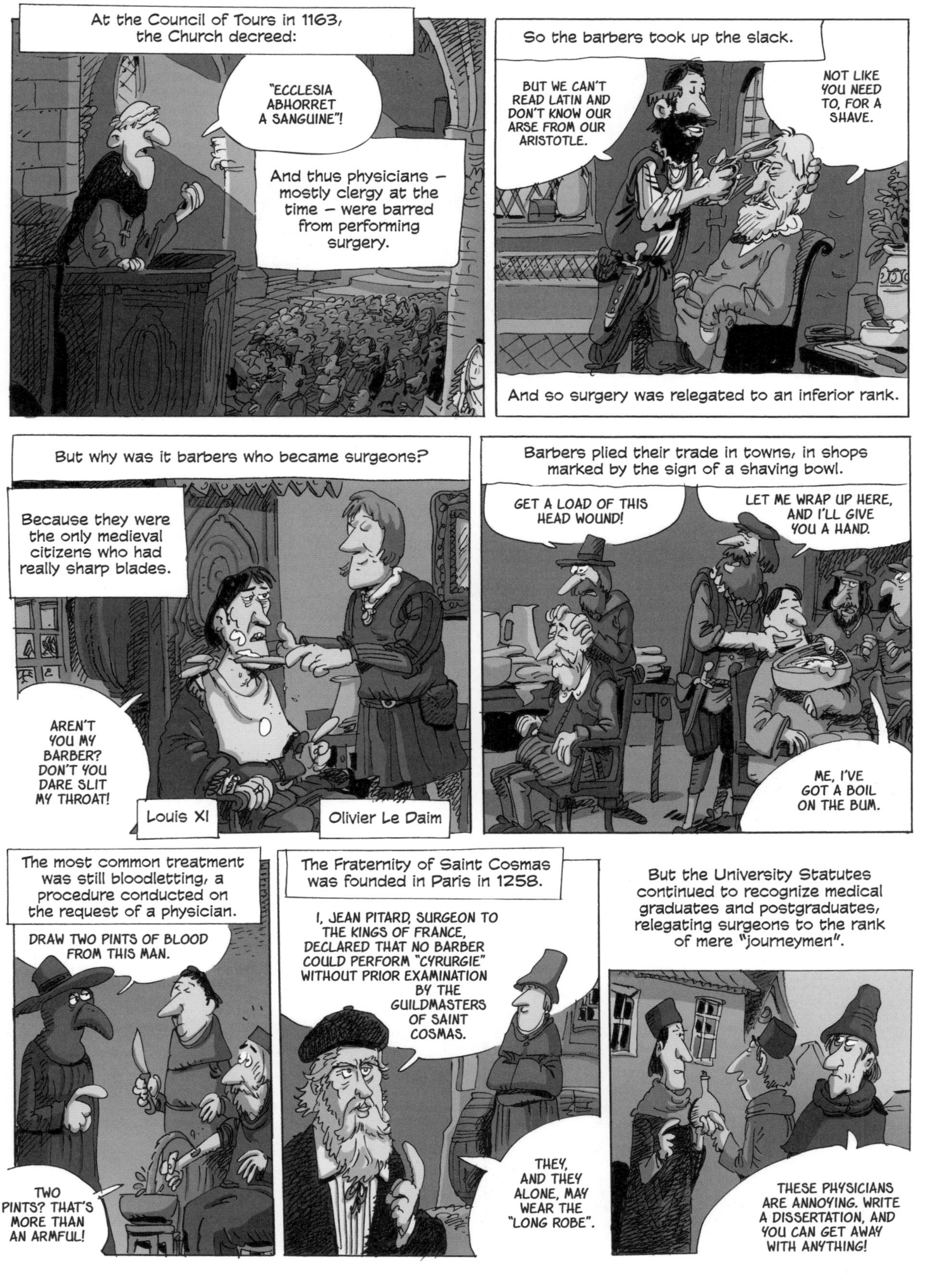
At the Council of Tours in 1163, the Church decreed:
"ECCLESIA ABHORRET A SANGUINE"!
And thus physicians – mostly clergy at the time – were barred from performing surgery.
So the barbers took up the slack.
BUT WE CAN'T READ LATIN AND DON'T KNOW OUR ARSE FROM OUR ARISTOTLE.
NOT LIKE YOU NEED TO, FOR A SHAVE.
And so surgery was relegated to an inferior rank.
But why was it barbers who became surgeons?
Because they were the only medieval citizens who had really sharp blades.
AREN'T YOU MY BARBER? DON'T YOU DARE SLIT MY THROAT!
Louis XI
Olivier Le Daim
Barbers plied their trade in towns, in shops marked by the sign of a shaving bowl.
GET A LOAD OF THIS HEAD WOUND!
LET ME WRAP UP HERE, AND I'LL GIVE YOU A HAND.
ME, I'VE GOT A BOIL ON THE BUM.
The most common treatment was still bloodletting, a procedure conducted on the request of a physician.
DRAW TWO PINTS OF BLOOD FROM THIS MAN.
TWO PINTS? THAT'S MORE THAN AN ARMFUL!
The Fraternity of Saint Cosmas was founded in Paris in 1258.
I, JEAN PITARD, SURGEON TO THE KINGS OF FRANCE, DECLARED THAT NO BARBER COULD PERFORM "CYRURGIE" WITHOUT PRIOR EXAMINATION BY THE GUILDMASTERS OF SAINT COSMAS.
THEY, AND THEY ALONE, MAY WEAR THE "LONG ROBE".
But the University Statutes continued to recognize medical graduates and postgraduates, relegating surgeons to the rank of mere "journeymen".
THESE PHYSICIANS ARE ANNOYING. WRITE A DISSERTATION, AND YOU CAN GET AWAY WITH ANYTHING!

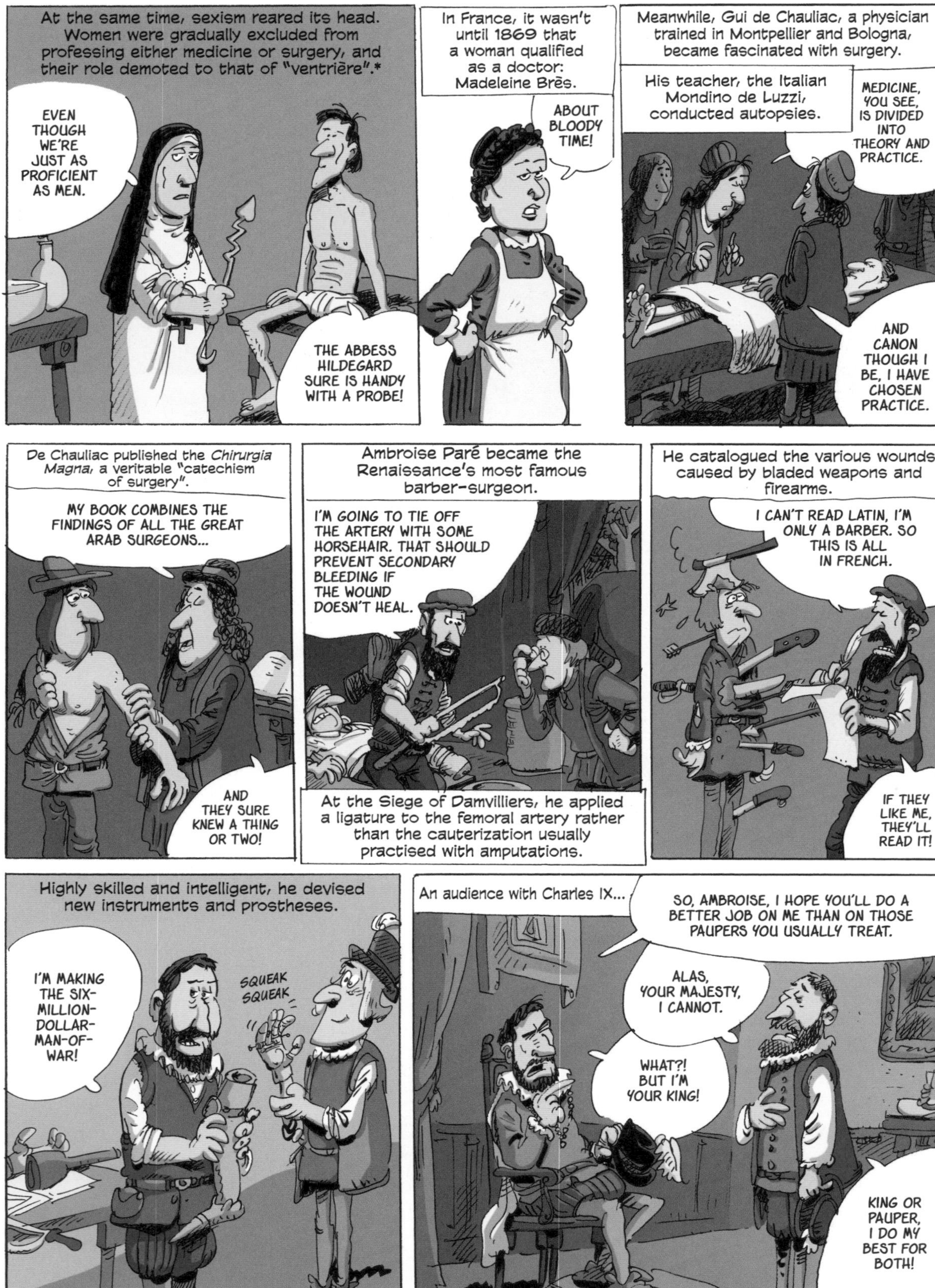
At the same time, sexism reared its head. Women were gradually excluded from professing either medicine or surgery, and their role demoted to that of "ventrière".*
EVEN THOUGH WE'RE JUST AS PROFICIENT AS MEN.
THE ABBESS HILDEGARD SURE IS HANDY WITH A PROBE!
In France, it wasn't until 1869 that a woman qualified as a doctor: Madeleine Brès.
ABOUT BLOODY TIME!
Meanwhile, Gui de Chauliac, a physician trained in Montpellier and Bologna, became fascinated with surgery.
His teacher, the Italian Mondino de Luzzi, conducted autopsies.
MEDICINE, YOU SEE, IS DIVIDED INTO THEORY AND PRACTICE.
AND CANON THOUGH I BE, I HAVE CHOSEN PRACTICE.
De Chauliac published the *Chirurgia Magna*, a veritable "catechism of surgery".
MY BOOK COMBINES THE FINDINGS OF ALL THE GREAT ARAB SURGEONS...
AND THEY SURE KNEW A THING OR TWO!
Ambroise Paré became the Renaissance's most famous barber-surgeon.
I'M GOING TO TIE OFF THE ARTERY WITH SOME HORSEHAIR. THAT SHOULD PREVENT SECONDARY BLEEDING IF THE WOUND DOESN'T HEAL.
At the Siege of Damvilliers, he applied a ligature to the femoral artery rather than the cauterization usually practised with amputations.
He catalogued the various wounds caused by bladed weapons and firearms.
I CAN'T READ LATIN, I'M ONLY A BARBER. SO THIS IS ALL IN FRENCH.
IF THEY LIKE ME, THEY'LL READ IT!
Highly skilled and intelligent, he devised new instruments and prostheses.
I'M MAKING THE SIX-MILLION-DOLLAR-MAN-OF-WAR!
SQUEAK SQUEAK
An audience with Charles IX...
SO, AMBROISE, I HOPE YOU'LL DO A BETTER JOB ON ME THAN ON THOSE PAUPERS YOU USUALLY TREAT.
ALAS, YOUR MAJESTY, I CANNOT.
WHAT?! BUT I'M YOUR KING!
KING OR PAUPER, I DO MY BEST FOR BOTH!

* Ventrière: the Old French word for "nurse" (which later came to mean a "sling").

FÉLIX AND THE CASE OF LOUIS XIV'S FISTULA

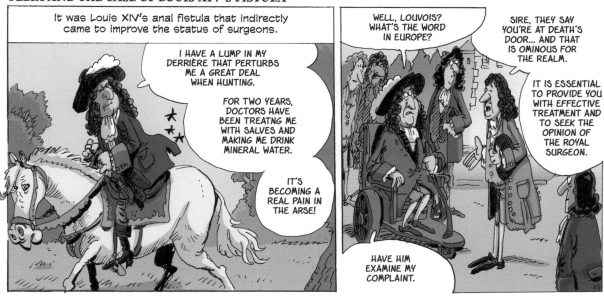

It was Louis XIV's anal fistula that indirectly came to improve the status of surgeons.

I HAVE A LUMP IN MY DERRIÈRE THAT PERTURBS ME A GREAT DEAL WHEN HUNTING.

FOR TWO YEARS, DOCTORS HAVE BEEN TREATNG ME WITH SALVES AND MAKING ME DRINK MINERAL WATER.

IT'S BECOMING A REAL PAIN IN THE ARSE!

WELL, LOUVOIS? WHAT'S THE WORD IN EUROPE?

SIRE, THEY SAY YOU'RE AT DEATH'S DOOR... AND THAT IS OMINOUS FOR THE REALM.

IT IS ESSENTIAL TO PROVIDE YOU WITH EFFECTIVE TREATMENT AND TO SEEK THE OPINION OF THE ROYAL SURGEON.

HAVE HIM EXAMINE MY COMPLAINT.

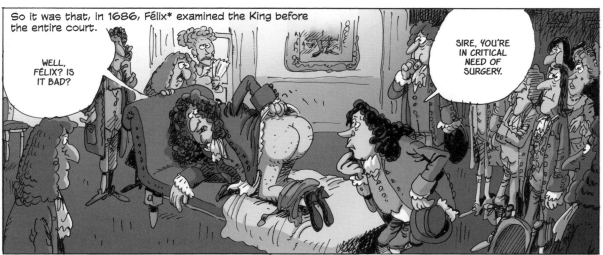

So it was that, in 1686, Félix* examined the King before the entire court.

WELL, FÉLIX? IS IT BAD?

SIRE, YOU'RE IN CRITICAL NEED OF SURGERY.

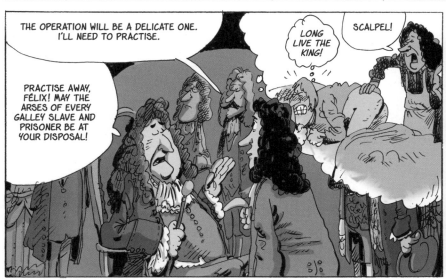

THE OPERATION WILL BE A DELICATE ONE. I'LL NEED TO PRACTISE.

PRACTISE AWAY, FÉLIX! MAY THE ARSES OF EVERY GALLEY SLAVE AND PRISONER BE AT YOUR DISPOSAL!

LONG LIVE THE KING!

SCALPEL!

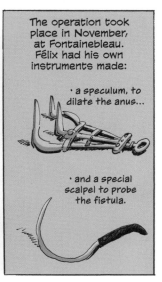

The operation took place in November, at Fontainebleau. Félix had his own instruments made:

• a speculum, to dilate the anus...

• and a special scalpel to probe the fistula.

* Barber-in-Chief to Louis XIV.

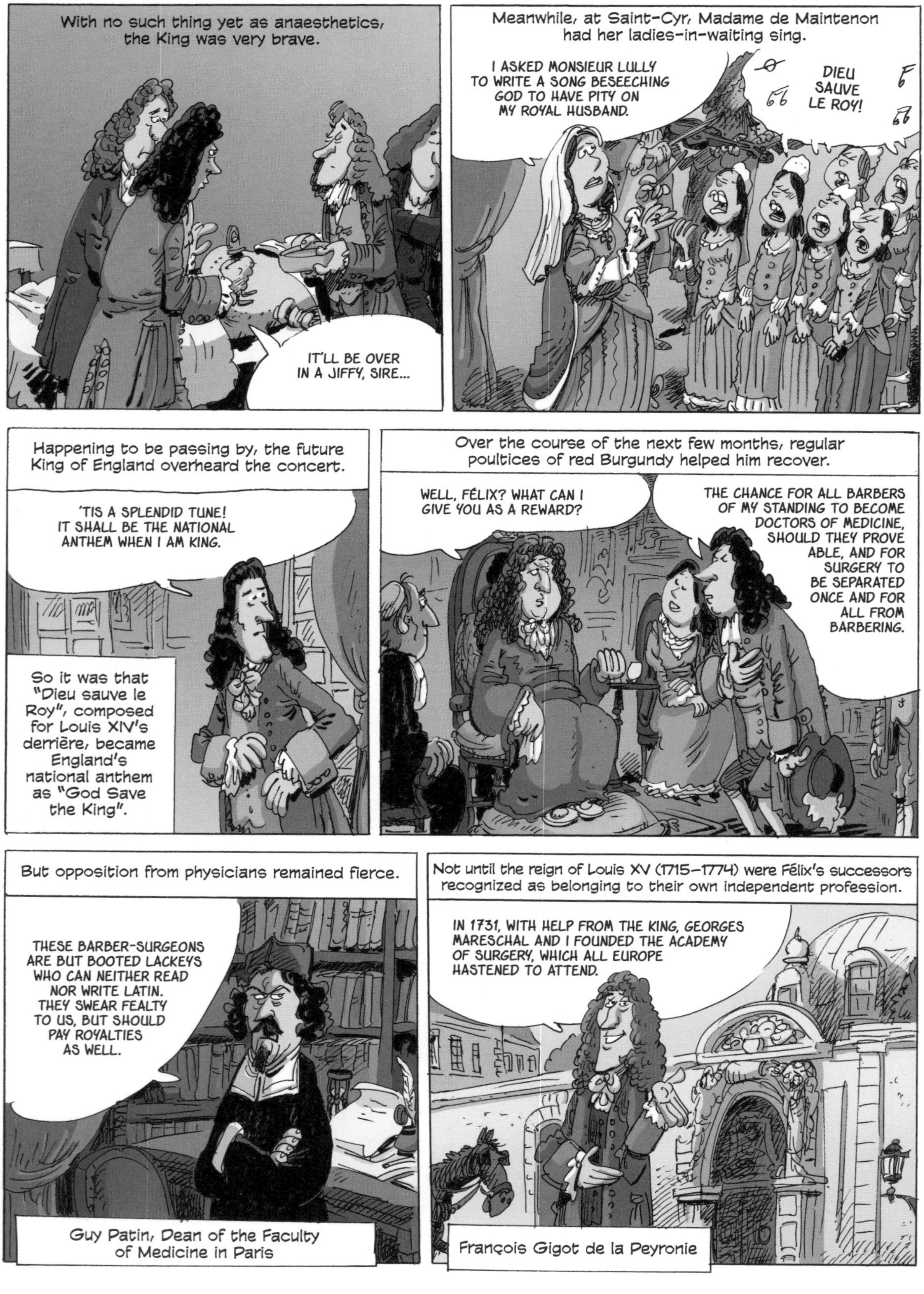
With no such thing yet as anaesthetics, the King was very brave.
IT'LL BE OVER IN A JIFFY, SIRE...
Meanwhile, at Saint-Cyr, Madame de Maintenon had her ladies-in-waiting sing.
I ASKED MONSIEUR LULLY TO WRITE A SONG BESEECHING GOD TO HAVE PITY ON MY ROYAL HUSBAND.
DIEU SAUVE LE ROY!
Happening to be passing by, the future King of England overheard the concert.
'TIS A SPLENDID TUNE! IT SHALL BE THE NATIONAL ANTHEM WHEN I AM KING.
So it was that "Dieu sauve le Roy", composed for Louis XIV's derrière, became England's national anthem as "God Save the King".
Over the course of the next few months, regular poultices of red Burgundy helped him recover.
WELL, FÉLIX? WHAT CAN I GIVE YOU AS A REWARD?
THE CHANCE FOR ALL BARBERS OF MY STANDING TO BECOME DOCTORS OF MEDICINE, SHOULD THEY PROVE ABLE, AND FOR SURGERY TO BE SEPARATED ONCE AND FOR ALL FROM BARBERING.
But opposition from physicians remained fierce.
THESE BARBER-SURGEONS ARE BUT BOOTED LACKEYS WHO CAN NEITHER READ NOR WRITE LATIN. THEY SWEAR FEALTY TO US, BUT SHOULD PAY ROYALTIES AS WELL.
Guy Patin, Dean of the Faculty of Medicine in Paris
Not until the reign of Louis XV (1715–1774) were Félix's successors recognized as belonging to their own independent profession.
IN 1731, WITH HELP FROM THE KING, GEORGES MARESCHAL AND I FOUNDED THE ACADEMY OF SURGERY, WHICH ALL EUROPE HASTENED TO ATTEND.
François Gigot de la Peyronie

CHAPTER 4

THE GREAT EPIDEMICS

From the Neolithic period onwards, one of the consequences of population concentration was the spread of epidemics.

Poorly diagnosed (for a long time, all eruptive fevers were dubbed "the plague") and without effective treatment (since no one had yet grasped the concept of contagion), epidemics took a considerable toll in mortality for centuries.

Not until Jenner in the 18th century, and above all Pasteur and Koch in the 19th, were effective treatments implemented.

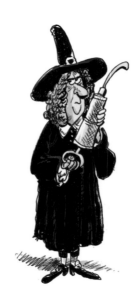

SMALLPOX, OR VARIOLA: the great killer of humankind

It may have killed more people than all wars combined.

Smallpox has been around since the Neolithic Era, but did not become an epidemic until the concentration of population (3000 BCE).

As certain Egyptian mummies will testify.

THEY FINALLY DIAGNOSED ME WITH THE POX (THE SMALL ONE)!

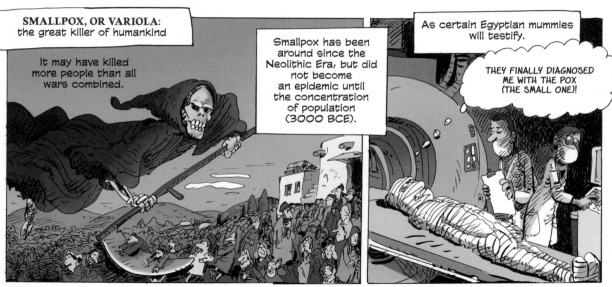

Some of Antiquity's great plagues were in fact smallpox epidemics.

The Antonine Plague in Rome (166) is credited with hastening the Empire's fall.

ET TU, BRUTE?

It took at least 5 million lives.

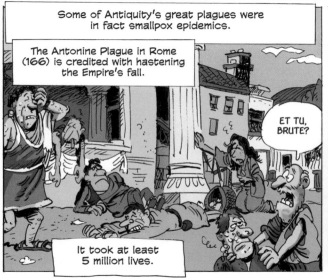

Actually, for a long time, all epidemics of eruptive fevers were called "the plague".

I FEEL HOT AND I'M BREAKING OUT. THEY SAY IT'S THE PLAGUE...

WHATEVER IT IS, IT DOESN'T LOOK GOOD!

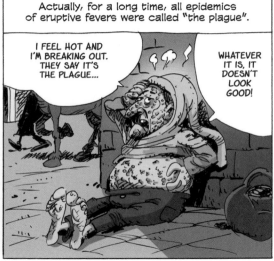

The Persian physician Rhazes sought order in chaos and distinguished smallpox from the measles.*

THEY'RE JUST NOT THE SAME THING!

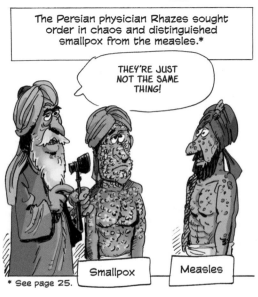

Smallpox

Measles

* See page 25.

When Cortés reached Mexico in 1518, there were 25 million Aztecs.

WE'VE ALSO GOT A SECRET WEAPON...

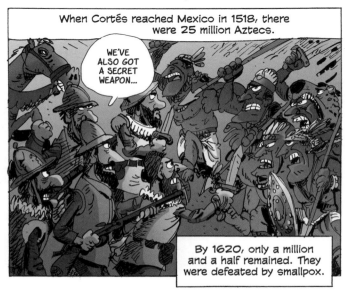

By 1620, only a million and a half remained. They were defeated by smallpox.

During the 18th century, a terrible smallpox epidemic raged in France and England.

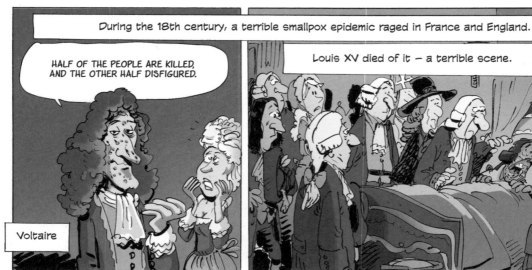

HALF OF THE PEOPLE ARE KILLED, AND THE OTHER HALF DISFIGURED.

Voltaire

Louis XV died of it – a terrible scene.

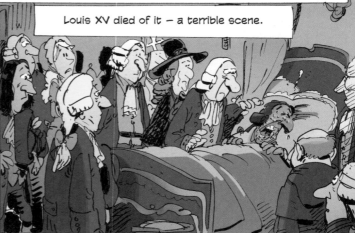

Since ancient times, people had tried to immunize themselves using smallpox blisters as a defensive measure.

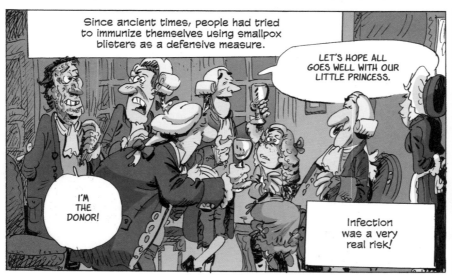

LET'S HOPE ALL GOES WELL WITH OUR LITTLE PRINCESS.

I'M THE DONOR!

Infection was a very real risk!

It was then that Edward Jenner, an English physician...

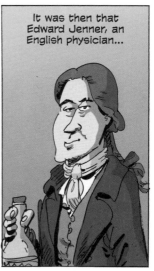

...noticed that milkmaids never came down with smallpox.

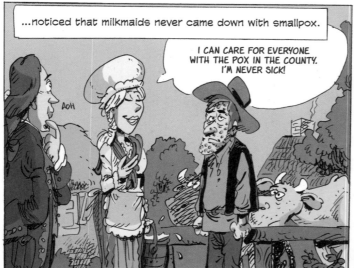

I CAN CARE FOR EVERYONE WITH THE POX IN THE COUNTY. I'M NEVER SICK!

From contact with cows that had cowpox (*Variolae vaccinae*), they developed an illness that only affected their arms.

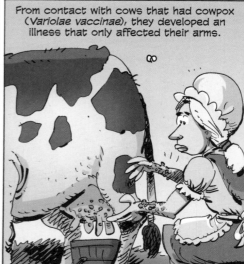

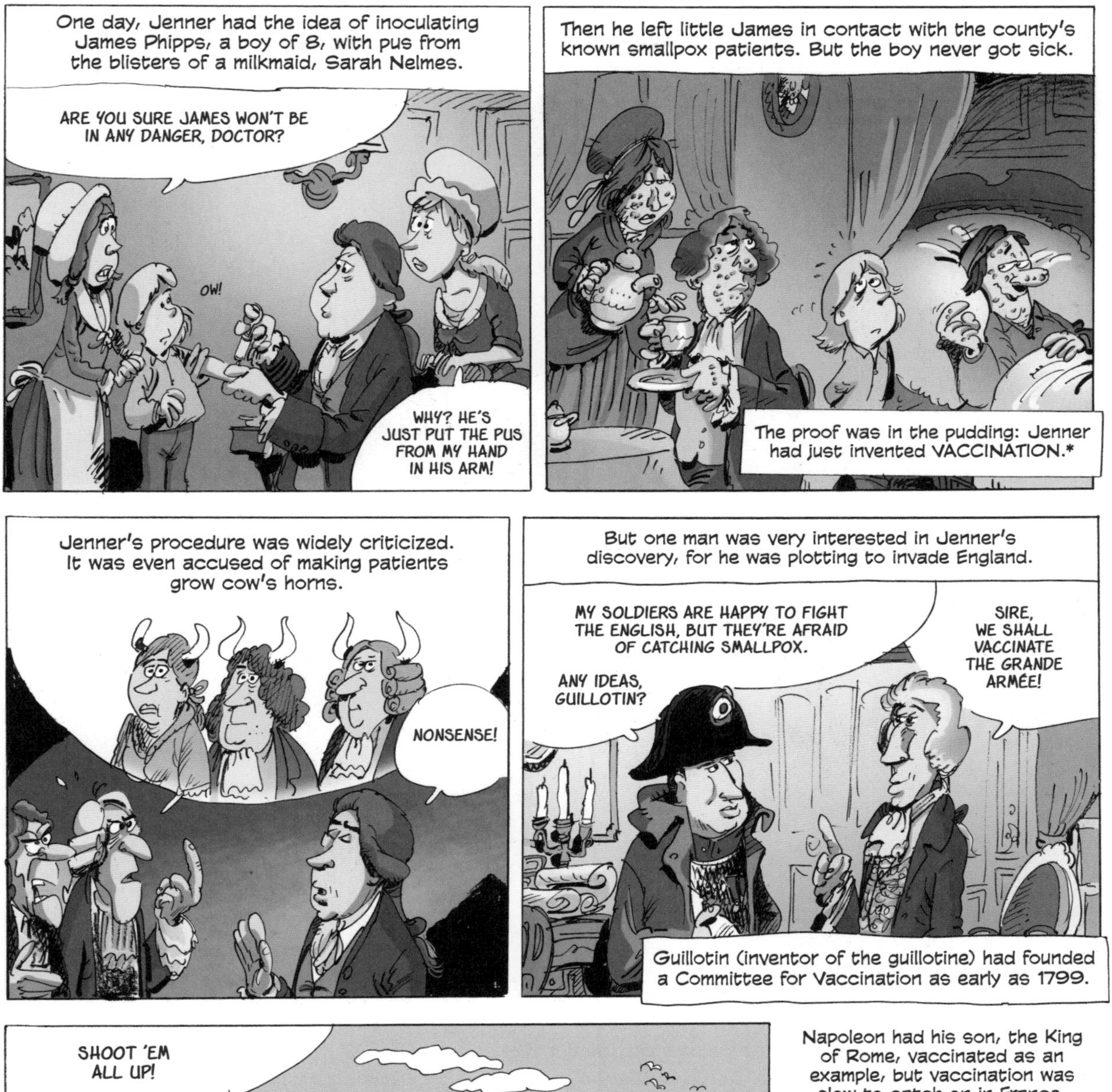
One day, Jenner had the idea of inoculating James Phipps, a boy of 8, with pus from the blisters of a milkmaid, Sarah Nelmes.
ARE YOU SURE JAMES WON'T BE IN ANY DANGER, DOCTOR?
OW!
WHY? HE'S JUST PUT THE PUS FROM MY HAND IN HIS ARM!
Then he left little James in contact with the county's known smallpox patients. But the boy never got sick.
The proof was in the pudding: Jenner had just invented VACCINATION.*
Jenner's procedure was widely criticized. It was even accused of making patients grow cow's horns.
NONSENSE!
But one man was very interested in Jenner's discovery, for he was plotting to invade England.
MY SOLDIERS ARE HAPPY TO FIGHT THE ENGLISH, BUT THEY'RE AFRAID OF CATCHING SMALLPOX.
ANY IDEAS, GUILLOTIN?
SIRE, WE SHALL VACCINATE THE GRANDE ARMÉE!
Guillotin (inventor of the guillotine) had founded a Committee for Vaccination as early as 1799.
SHOOT 'EM ALL UP!
Napoleon had his son, the King of Rome, vaccinated as an example, but vaccination was slow to catch on in France.
THE PAIN'S ONLY JUST BEGINNING.

* The word "vaccination" comes from the Latin "vacca", meaning "cow".

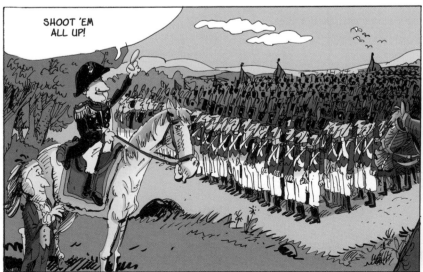

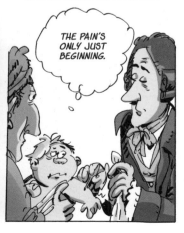

Despite vaccination, smallpox was still endemic to Africa and Asia in 1960, when the W.H.O. decided to eradicate the disease.

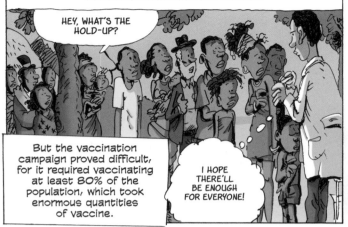

HEY, WHAT'S THE HOLD-UP?

But the vaccination campaign proved difficult, for it required vaccinating at least 80% of the population, which took enormous quantities of vaccine.

I HOPE THERE'LL BE ENOUGH FOR EVERYONE!

One W.H.O. doctor, William Foege, came up with a strategy: "ring vaccination".

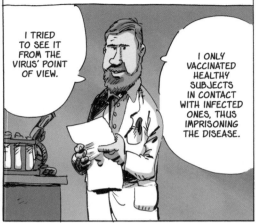

I TRIED TO SEE IT FROM THE VIRUS' POINT OF VIEW.

I ONLY VACCINATED HEALTHY SUBJECTS IN CONTACT WITH INFECTED ONES, THUS IMPRISONING THE DISEASE.

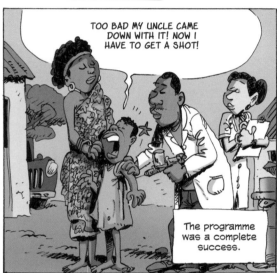

TOO BAD MY UNCLE CAME DOWN WITH IT! NOW I HAVE TO GET A SHOT!

The programme was a complete success.

In 1980, Foege declared that the disease had been wiped out all over the world.

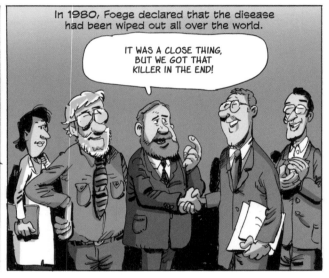

IT WAS A CLOSE THING, BUT WE GOT THAT KILLER IN THE END!

All remaining reserves of the virus were destroyed in labs...

...unless, that is, some was secretly set aside as a biological weapon for a terrorist attack.

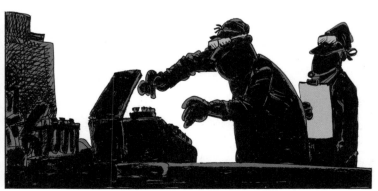

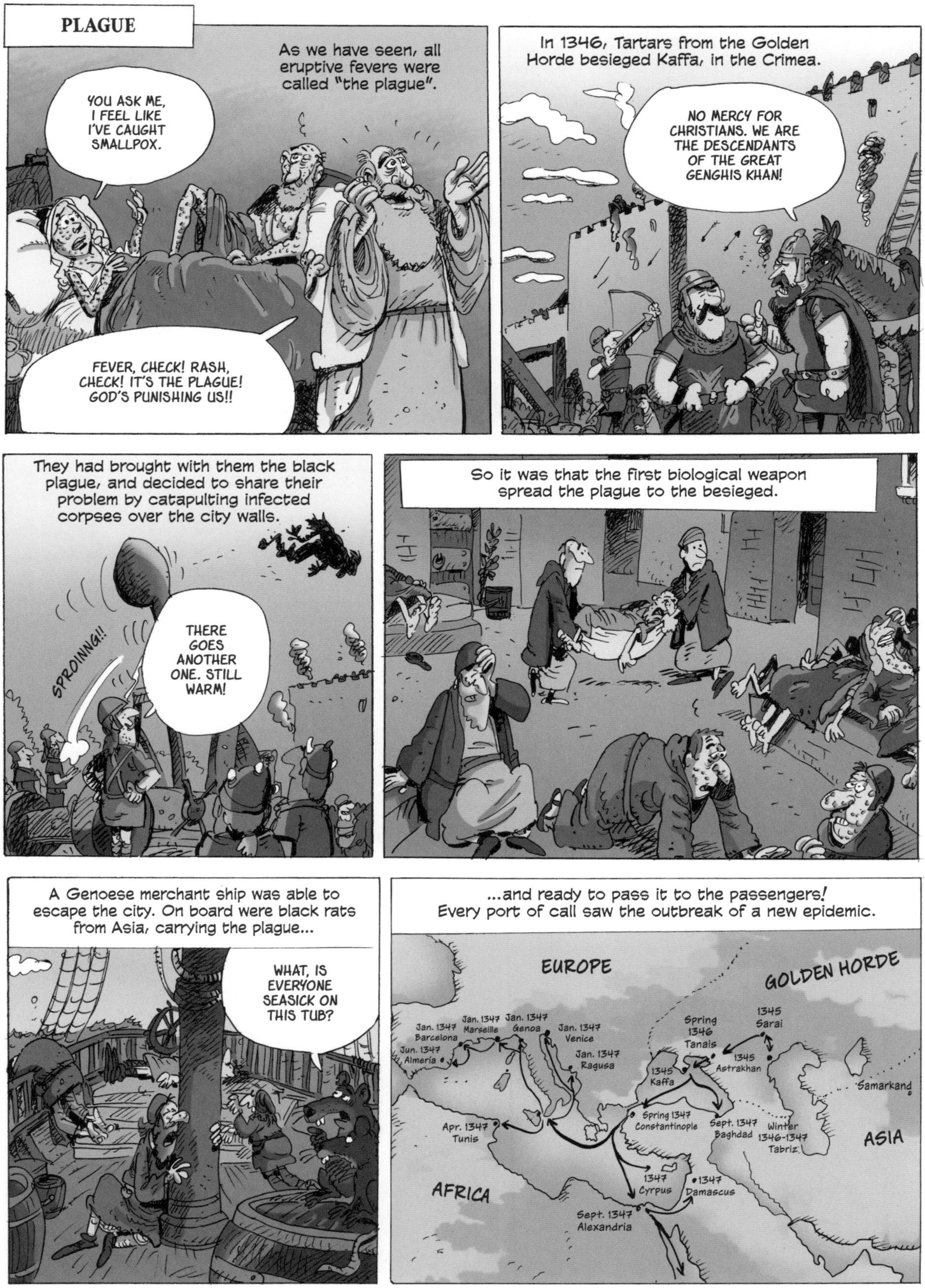
PLAGUE
As we have seen, all eruptive fevers were called "the plague".
YOU ASK ME, I FEEL LIKE I'VE CAUGHT SMALLPOX.
FEVER, CHECK! RASH, CHECK! IT'S THE PLAGUE! GOD'S PUNISHING US!!
In 1346, Tartars from the Golden Horde besieged Kaffa, in the Crimea.
NO MERCY FOR CHRISTIANS. WE ARE THE DESCENDANTS OF THE GREAT GENGHIS KHAN!
They had brought with them the black plague, and decided to share their problem by catapulting infected corpses over the city walls.
SPROING!!
THERE GOES ANOTHER ONE. STILL WARM!
So it was that the first biological weapon spread the plague to the besieged.
A Genoese merchant ship was able to escape the city. On board were black rats from Asia, carrying the plague...
WHAT, IS EVERYONE SEASICK ON THIS TUB?
...and ready to pass it to the passengers! Every port of call saw the outbreak of a new epidemic.
EUROPE
GOLDEN HORDE
1345 Sarai
Spring 1346 Tanais
1345 Astrakhan
1345 Kaffa
Jan. 1347 Barcelona
Jan. 1347 Marseille
Jan. 1347 Genoa
Jan. 1347 Venice
Jun. 1347 Almeria
Jan. 1347 Ragusa
Samarkand
Spring 1347 Constantinople
Sept. 1347 Baghdad
Winter 1346-1347 Tabriz
Apr. 1347 Tunis
ASIA
AFRICA
1347 Cyprus
1347 Damascus
Sept. 1347 Alexandria

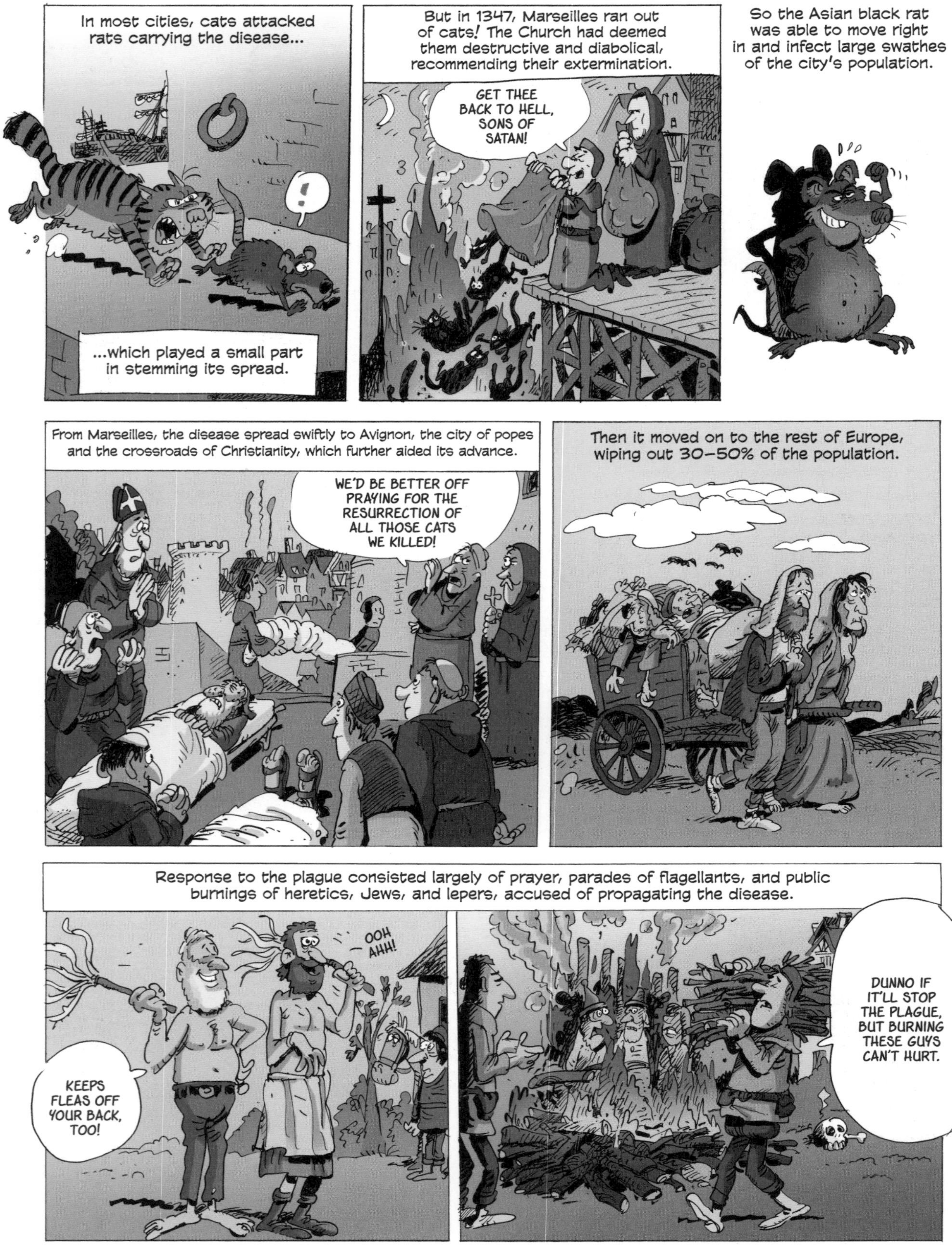
In most cities, cats attacked rats carrying the disease...
!
...which played a small part in stemming its spread.
But in 1347, Marseilles ran out of cats! The Church had deemed them destructive and diabolical, recommending their extermination.
GET THEE BACK TO HELL, SONS OF SATAN!
So the Asian black rat was able to move right in and infect large swathes of the city's population.
From Marseilles, the disease spread swiftly to Avignon, the city of popes and the crossroads of Christianity, which further aided its advance.
WE'D BE BETTER OFF PRAYING FOR THE RESURRECTION OF ALL THOSE CATS WE KILLED!
Then it moved on to the rest of Europe, wiping out 30–50% of the population.
Response to the plague consisted largely of prayer, parades of flagellants, and public burnings of heretics, Jews, and lepers, accused of propagating the disease.
— OOH — AHH!
KEEPS FLEAS OFF YOUR BACK, TOO!
DUNNO IF IT'LL STOP THE PLAGUE, BUT BURNING THESE GUYS CAN'T HURT.

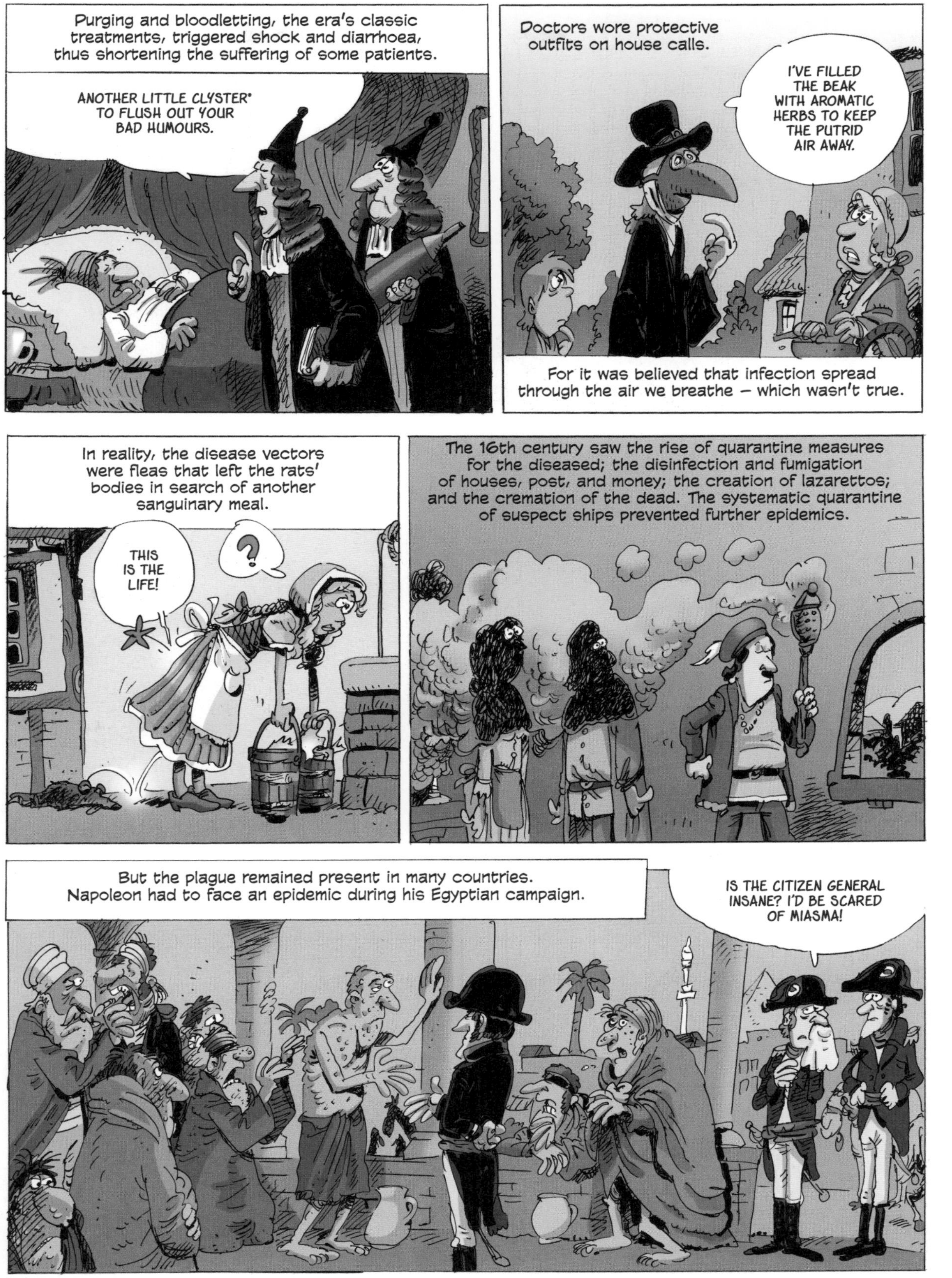
Purging and bloodletting, the era's classic treatments, triggered shock and diarrhoea, thus shortening the suffering of some patients.
ANOTHER LITTLE CLYSTER* TO FLUSH OUT YOUR BAD HUMOURS.
Doctors wore protective outfits on house calls.
I'VE FILLED THE BEAK WITH AROMATIC HERBS TO KEEP THE PUTRID AIR AWAY.
For it was believed that infection spread through the air we breathe – which wasn't true.
In reality, the disease vectors were fleas that left the rats' bodies in search of another sanguinary meal.
THIS IS THE LIFE!
?
The 16th century saw the rise of quarantine measures for the diseased; the disinfection and fumigation of houses, post, and money; the creation of lazarettos; and the cremation of the dead. The systematic quarantine of suspect ships prevented further epidemics.
But the plague remained present in many countries. Napoleon had to face an epidemic during his Egyptian campaign.
IS THE CITIZEN GENERAL INSANE? I'D BE SCARED OF MIASMA!

* Enema.

In 1894, Alexandre Yersin, a student of Pasteur's, left for Hong Kong, where an epidemic was raging, to seek the origin of the plague.

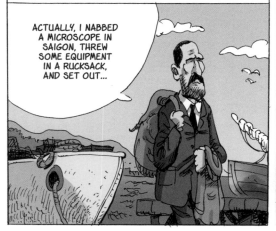

ACTUALLY, I NABBED A MICROSCOPE IN SAIGON, THREW SOME EQUIPMENT IN A RUCKSACK, AND SET OUT...

But upon arrival, he found a team of Japanese scientists already studying the disease. Yersin was deliberately barred from the hospital.

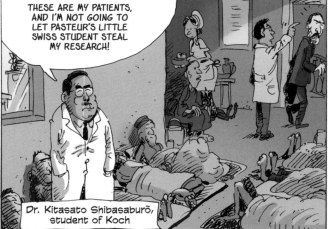

THESE ARE MY PATIENTS, AND I'M NOT GOING TO LET PASTEUR'S LITTLE SWISS STUDENT STEAL MY RESEARCH!

Dr. Kitasato Shibasaburō, student of Koch

Kitasato hadn't reckoned with Yersin's obstinacy. Rejected by the authorities, he built himself a hut beside the hospital and set up his lab.

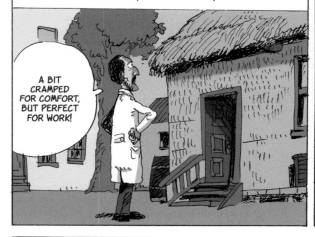

A BIT CRAMPED FOR COMFORT, BUT PERFECT FOR WORK!

Bribing the sailors who buried the bodies, he gained access to the morgue, where he took samples from buboes back to his lab.

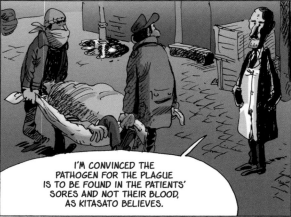

I'M CONVINCED THE PATHOGEN FOR THE PLAGUE IS TO BE FOUND IN THE PATIENTS' SORES AND NOT THEIR BLOOD, AS KITASATO BELIEVES.

I PREPARED A FILM FOR MY MICROSCOPE. AT FIRST GLANCE, I SAW BUT A MASS OF BACILLI, ALL IDENTICAL: VERY SMALL RODS, THICK WITH ROUNDED ENDS AND LIGHTLY COLOURED.

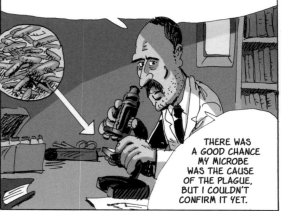

THERE WAS A GOOD CHANCE MY MICROBE WAS THE CAUSE OF THE PLAGUE, BUT I COULDN'T CONFIRM IT YET.

The swellings, or buboes, in fact comprised an inflammation of the lymph nodes.

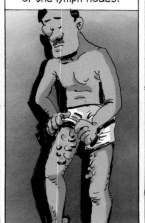

Yersin sent an exact description of the bacillus to the French Academy of Sciences, where it was read on 30 July 1894.

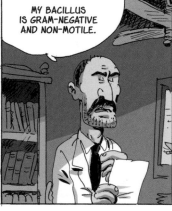

MY BACILLUS IS GRAM-NEGATIVE AND NON-MOTILE.

For his part, Kitasato published his discovery of a bacillus (found in the blood) in *The Lancet* on 25 August 1894.

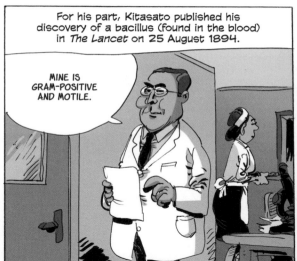

MINE IS GRAM-POSITIVE AND MOTILE.

Actually, Kitasato's "bacillus" resembled a pneumococcus.

Yersin had succeeded in isolating the "real" bacterium behind the plague — and the millions of deaths it had caused throughout history.

Yet he failed to grasp the role that the rat played in infecting humans.

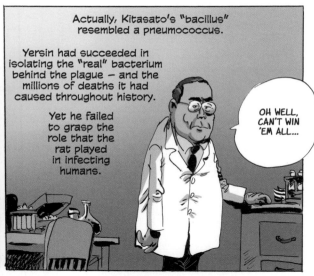

OH WELL, CAN'T WIN 'EM ALL...

The cycle of transmission was discovered in 1898 by another of Pasteur's students, Paul-Louis Simond.

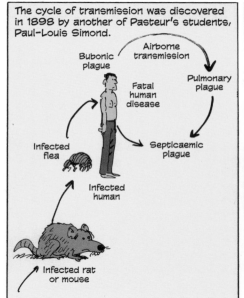

Bubonic plague

Airborne transmission

Pulmonary plague

Fatal human disease

Septicaemic plague

Infected flea

Infected human

Infected rat or mouse

But still no cure had been found. Then, in 1913, a new epidemic of the plague broke out in Madagascar.

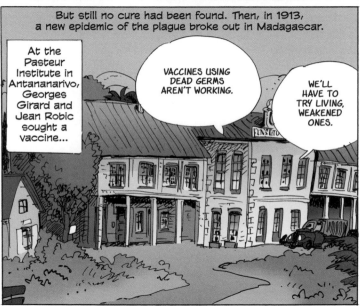

At the Pasteur Institute in Antananarivo, Georges Girard and Jean Robic sought a vaccine...

VACCINES USING DEAD GERMS AREN'T WORKING.

WE'LL HAVE TO TRY LIVING, WEAKENED ONES.

In 1932, the two scientists ran the first successful tests... on themselves!

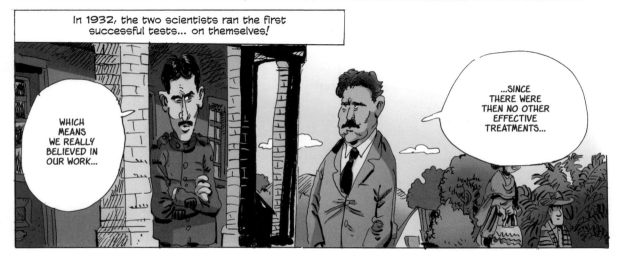

WHICH MEANS WE REALLY BELIEVED IN OUR WORK...

...SINCE THERE WERE THEN NO OTHER EFFECTIVE TREATMENTS...

CHOLERA

Cholera, caused by a bacterially produced toxin, can lead to death in a matter of days as a result of dehydration due to diarrhoea and vomiting.

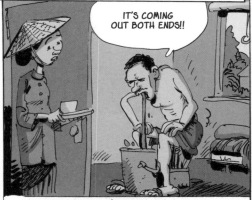

IT'S COMING OUT BOTH ENDS!!

The disease's breeding ground was Asia and the Middle East.

The first European to describe the disease was an officer of Vasco da Gama's, in 1503. In India, he witnessed an epidemic of calamitous diarrhoea that swiftly proved fatal.

I MUST SAY, THAT RIVER THOSE PEOPLE ARE BATHING IN IS MORE LIKE A SEWER.

In the 19th century, six major cholera pandemics shook the world, all spread by new forms of transport.

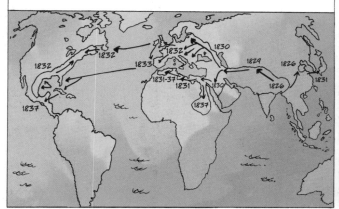

The 1832 epidemic in Paris claimed around 100,000 lives.

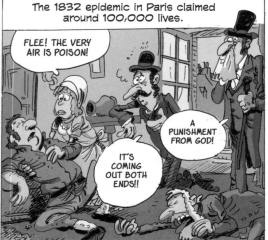

FLEE! THE VERY AIR IS POISON!

A PUNISHMENT FROM GOD!

IT'S COMING OUT BOTH ENDS!!

That same year, in Edinburgh, surgeon Thomas Latta had an idea: rehydrating patients with saline injected into the colon.

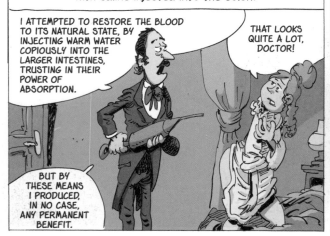

I ATTEMPTED TO RESTORE THE BLOOD TO ITS NATURAL STATE, BY INJECTING WARM WATER COPIOUSLY INTO THE LARGER INTESTINES, TRUSTING IN THEIR POWER OF ABSORPTION.

THAT LOOKS QUITE A LOT, DOCTOR!

BUT BY THESE MEANS I PRODUCED, IN NO CASE, ANY PERMANENT BENEFIT.

Faced with this initial setback, he tried gradually injecting six pints of (non-sterilized) saline into the arm via a goosefeather quill.

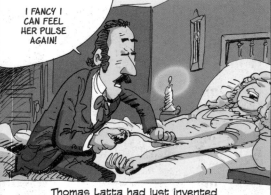

I FANCY I CAN FEEL HER PULSE AGAIN!

Thomas Latta had just invented the intravenous catheter.

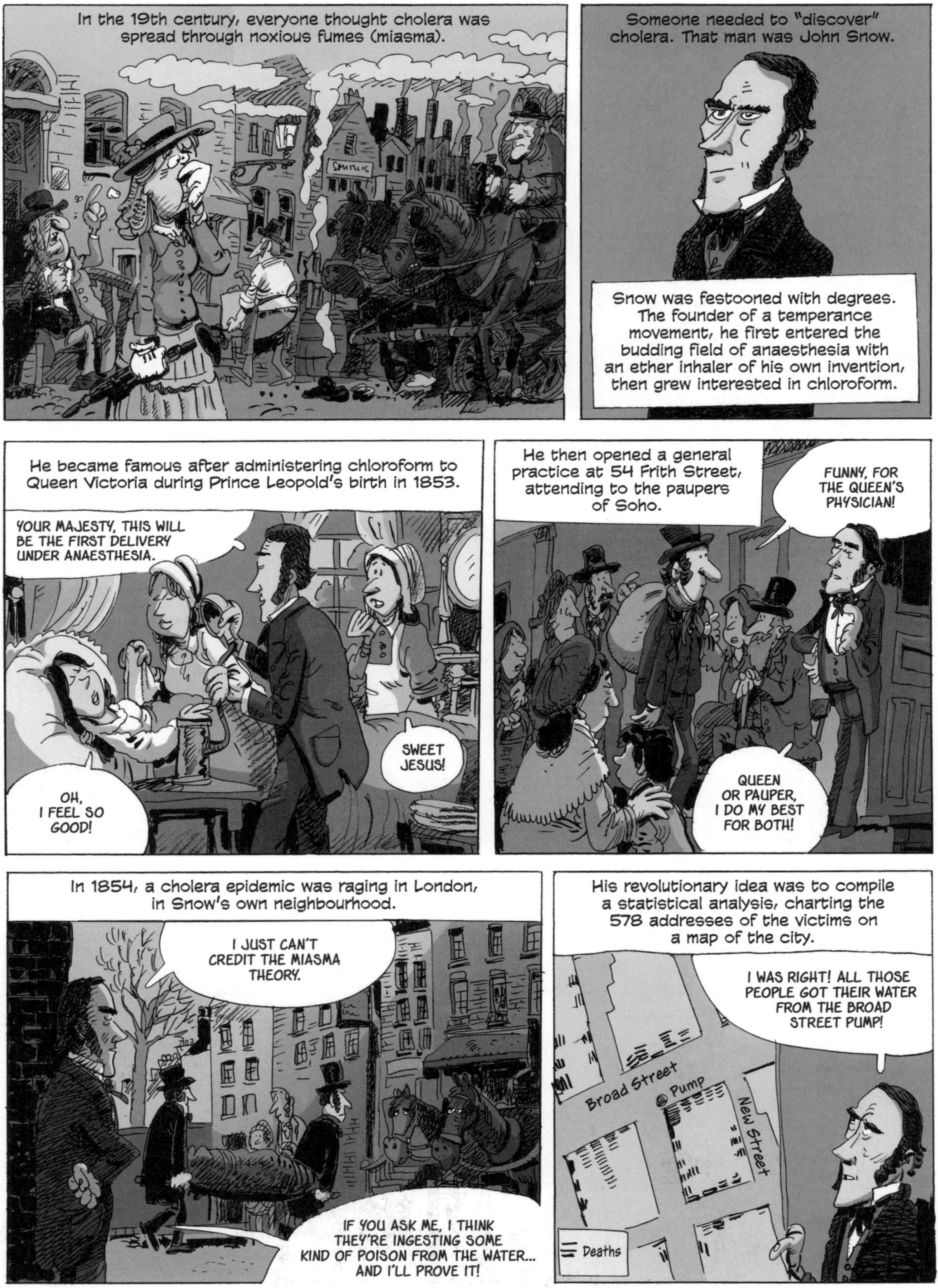
In the 19th century, everyone thought cholera was spread through noxious fumes (miasma).
Someone needed to "discover" cholera. That man was John Snow.
Snow was festooned with degrees. The founder of a temperance movement, he first entered the budding field of anaesthesia with an ether inhaler of his own invention, then grew interested in chloroform.
He became famous after administering chloroform to Queen Victoria during Prince Leopold's birth in 1853.
YOUR MAJESTY, THIS WILL BE THE FIRST DELIVERY UNDER ANAESTHESIA.
SWEET JESUS!
OH, I FEEL SO GOOD!
He then opened a general practice at 54 Frith Street, attending to the paupers of Soho.
FUNNY, FOR THE QUEEN'S PHYSICIAN!
QUEEN OR PAUPER, I DO MY BEST FOR BOTH!
In 1854, a cholera epidemic was raging in London, in Snow's own neighbourhood.
I JUST CAN'T CREDIT THE MIASMA THEORY.
IF YOU ASK ME, I THINK THEY'RE INGESTING SOME KIND OF POISON FROM THE WATER... AND I'LL PROVE IT!
His revolutionary idea was to compile a statistical analysis, charting the 578 addresses of the victims on a map of the city.
I WAS RIGHT! ALL THOSE PEOPLE GOT THEIR WATER FROM THE BROAD STREET PUMP!
Broad Street
Pump
New Street
Deaths

After initial resistance, he succeeded in having the Broad Street pump closed. And the epidemic stopped.

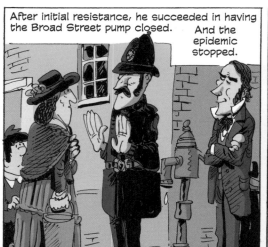

Believers in miasma remained sceptical, however.

WOT'S SNOW ON ABOUT, THEN? CAN'T SEE NUFFINK IN THIS WATER!

OUT OF USE

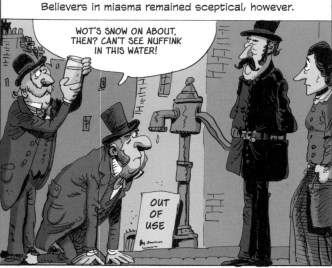

The Reverend Henry Whitehead sought to prove Snow wrong, but his investigations had the opposite effect.

SNOW WAS RIGHT!

THE PUMP DRILLS DOWN LESS THAN A YARD AWAY FROM A DRAIN WHERE DIRTY WATER WAS THROWN AFTER CLEANING A BABY'S NAPPIES — AND THAT BABY HAD CHOLERA!

Back kitchen
Front kitchen
Level
A
Well
B
Sewer
C

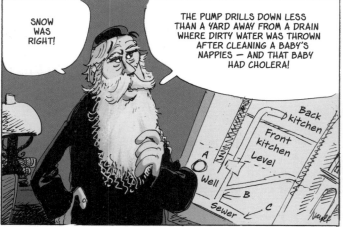

Snow had demonstrated that water was the cause of the epidemic. He further proposed that an "animalcule",* once ingested, developed in the intestine before being evacuated via excreta.

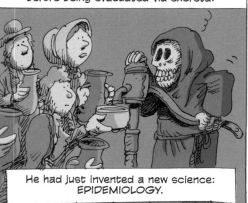

He had just invented a new science: EPIDEMIOLOGY.

In 1883, a fresh epidemic was raging in Egypt.

The Germans and the French dispatched missions to study it. They met with failure.

Pasteur's colleague Louis Thuillier contracted cholera and died.

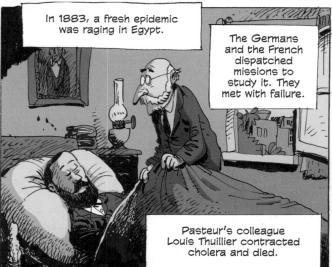

The following year, Robert Koch discovered the bacillus in Calcutta.

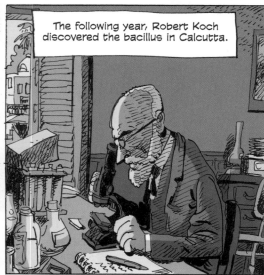

* The word means "tiny animal", since microbes were yet to be defined.

The cholera vibrion was a wormlike bacterium that Koch named "Komma bacillus" (*vibrio comma*) after its comma-like shape.

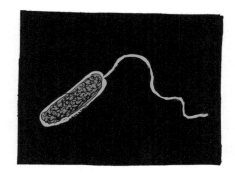

In fact, Filippo Pacini had already described the germ in 1854!

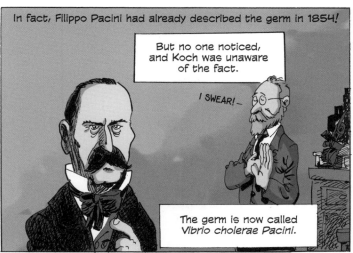

But no one noticed, and Koch was unaware of the fact.

I SWEAR!—

The germ is now called *Vibrio cholerae Pacini*.

The Catalan doctor Jaume Ferran was the man behind the first cholera vaccine, in 1885.

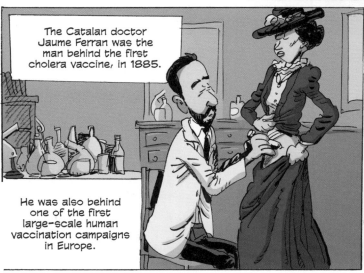

He was also behind one of the first large-scale human vaccination campaigns in Europe.

In the 1950s, Sambhu Nath De and N.K. Dutta showed that the cholera vibrion produced a powerful exotoxin responsible for diarrhoea.

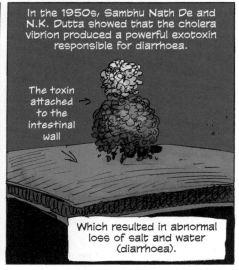

The toxin attached to the intestinal wall →

Which resulted in abnormal loss of salt and water (diarrhoea).

Today, an oral vaccine is available.

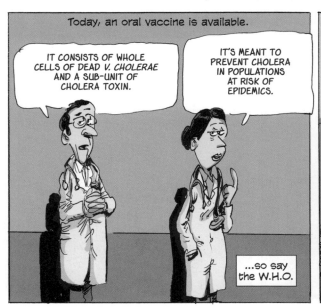

IT CONSISTS OF WHOLE CELLS OF DEAD *V. CHOLERAE* AND A SUB-UNIT OF CHOLERA TOXIN.

IT'S MEANT TO PREVENT CHOLERA IN POPULATIONS AT RISK OF EPIDEMICS.

...so say the W.H.O.

But despite all this, the disease remains widespread.

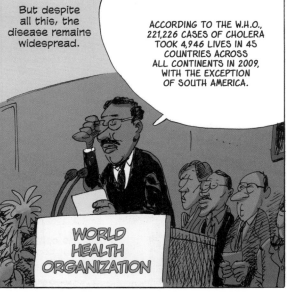

ACCORDING TO THE W.H.O., 221,226 CASES OF CHOLERA TOOK 4,946 LIVES IN 45 COUNTRIES ACROSS ALL CONTINENTS IN 2009, WITH THE EXCEPTION OF SOUTH AMERICA.

WORLD HEALTH ORGANIZATION

SYPHILIS, OR THE POX

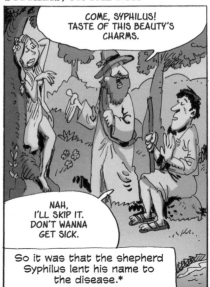

COME, SYPHILUS! TASTE OF THIS BEAUTY'S CHARMS.

NAH, I'LL SKIP IT. DON'T WANNA GET SICK.

So it was that the shepherd Syphilus lent his name to the disease.*

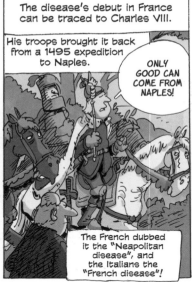

The disease's debut in France can be traced to Charles VIII.

His troops brought it back from a 1495 expedition to Naples.

ONLY GOOD CAN COME FROM NAPLES!

The French dubbed it the "Neapolitan disease", and the Italians the "French disease"!

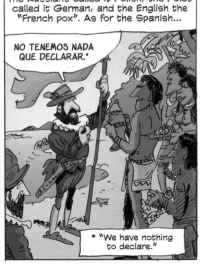

It was always someone else's disease. The Russians called it Polish, the Poles called it German, and the English the "French pox". As for the Spanish...

NO TENEMOS NADA QUE DECLARAR.*

* "We have nothing to declare."

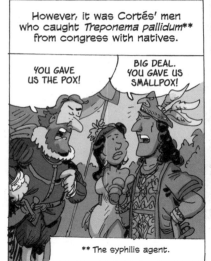

However, it was Cortés' men who caught *Treponema pallidum*** from congress with natives.

YOU GAVE US THE POX!

BIG DEAL. YOU GAVE US SMALLPOX!

** The syphilis agent.

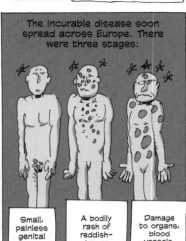

The incurable disease soon spread across Europe. There were three stages:

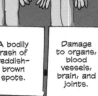

Small, painless genital sores.

A bodily rash of reddish-brown spots.

Damage to organs, blood vessels, brain, and joints.

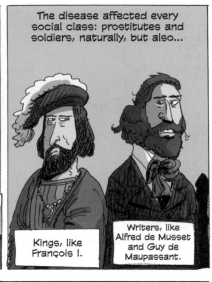

The disease affected every social class: prostitutes and soldiers, naturally, but also...

Kings, like François I.

Writers, like Alfred de Musset and Guy de Maupassant.

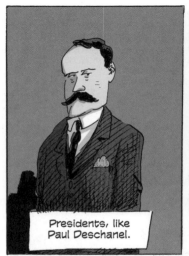

Presidents, like Paul Deschanel.

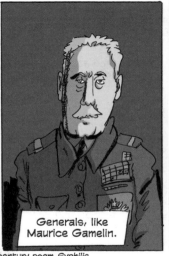

Generals, like Maurice Gamelin.

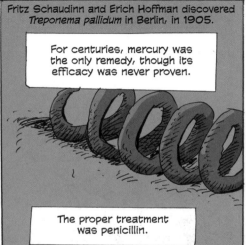

Fritz Schaudinn and Erich Hoffman discovered *Treponema pallidum* in Berlin, in 1905.

For centuries, mercury was the only remedy, though its efficacy was never proven.

The proper treatment was penicillin.

* From Italian Girolamo Fracastoro's 16th-century poem *Syphilis sive morbus gallicus* ("Syphilis or The French Disease").

54

LEPROSY

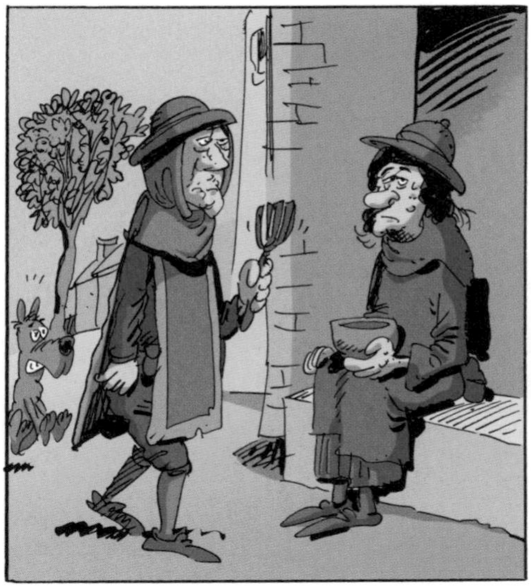

Discovered by Norwegian Gerhard Hansen, the bacillus that causes the infectious disease leprosy is endemic to tropical regions, though not very contagious.

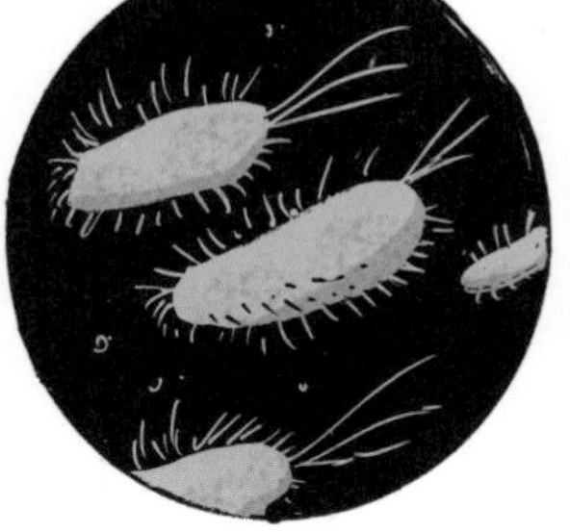

Leprosy bacillus

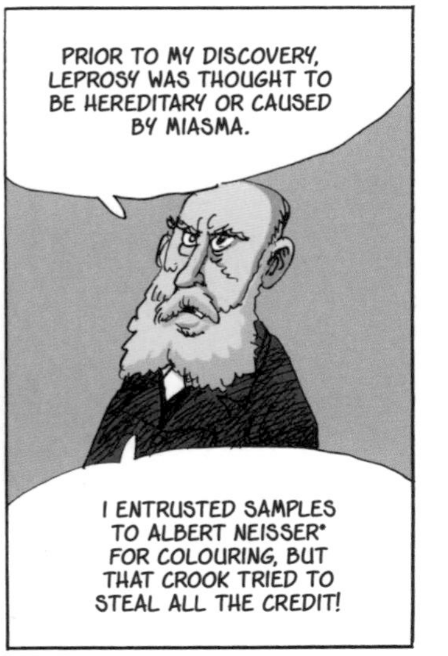
PRIOR TO MY DISCOVERY, LEPROSY WAS THOUGHT TO BE HEREDITARY OR CAUSED BY MIASMA.
I ENTRUSTED SAMPLES TO ALBERT NEISSER* FOR COLOURING, BUT THAT CROOK TRIED TO STEAL ALL THE CREDIT!

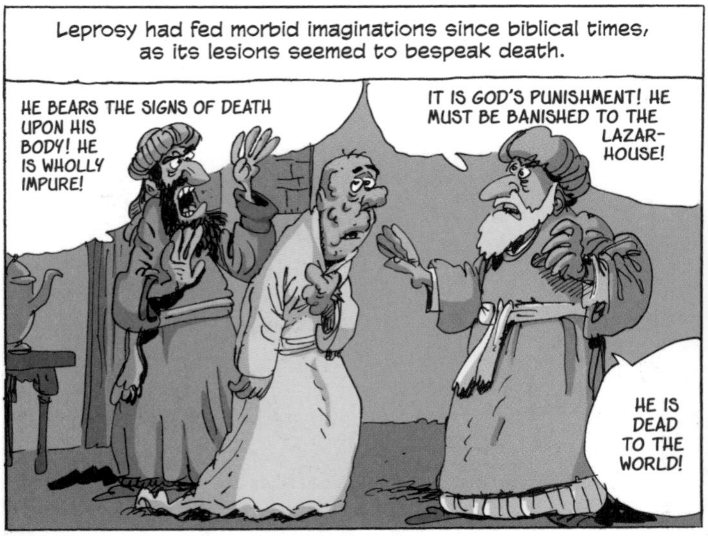
Leprosy had fed morbid imaginations since biblical times, as its lesions seemed to bespeak death.
HE BEARS THE SIGNS OF DEATH UPON HIS BODY! HE IS WHOLLY IMPURE!
IT IS GOD'S PUNISHMENT! HE MUST BE BANISHED TO THE LAZAR-HOUSE!
HE IS DEAD TO THE WORLD!

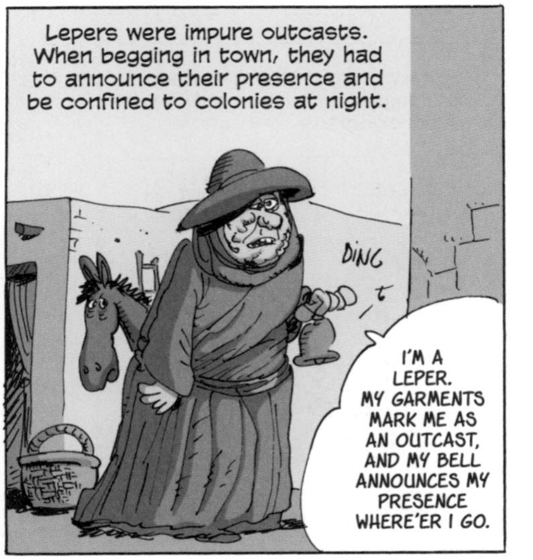
Lepers were impure outcasts. When begging in town, they had to announce their presence and be confined to colonies at night.
DING
I'M A LEPER. MY GARMENTS MARK ME AS AN OUTCAST, AND MY BELL ANNOUNCES MY PRESENCE WHERE'ER I GO.

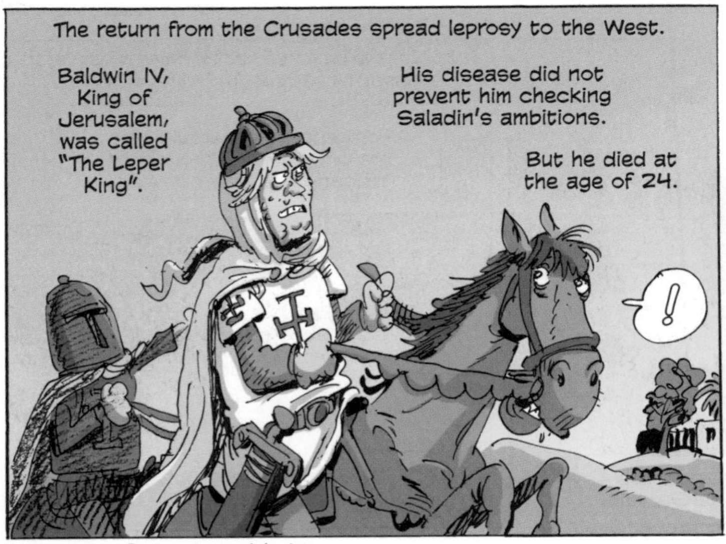
The return from the Crusades spread leprosy to the West.
Baldwin IV, King of Jerusalem, was called "The Leper King".
His disease did not prevent him checking Saladin's ambitions.
But he died at the age of 24.
!

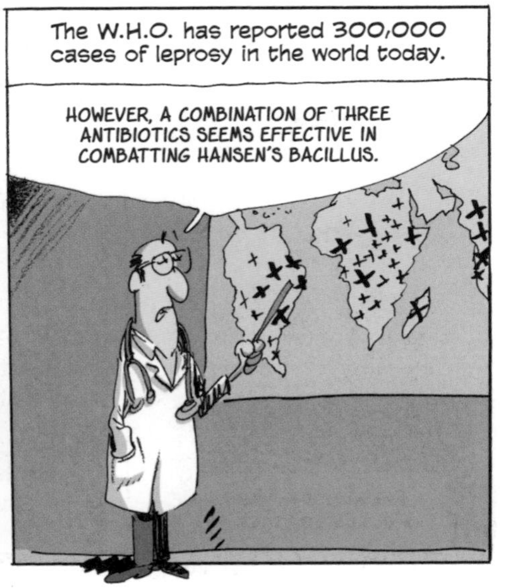
The W.H.O. has reported 300,000 cases of leprosy in the world today.
HOWEVER, A COMBINATION OF THREE ANTIBIOTICS SEEMS EFFECTIVE IN COMBATTING HANSEN'S BACILLUS.

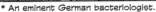

* An eminent German bacteriologist.

CHAPTER 5

THE CIRCULATION OF BLOOD

The Renaissance saw a systematic questioning of Church doctrine, as enforced by the long arm of its law, the fearsome Inquisition, which absolutely forbade the dissection of corpses and any opposition to the theories of Galen.

Doctors faced a time of constant battle to overturn these two prohibitions. And so the first major step forward (at long last!) was an accurate description of human anatomy.

From this knowledge arose an understanding of the true role of the heart, and the notion of a circulatory system.

All this, in an atmosphere of religious struggle, human tragedy, scientific theft, war, and intense passion.

In short: the Renaissance.

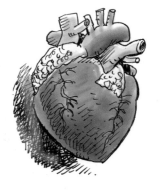

One day in December 1924, Muhyo,* an Egyptian student working on his thesis, made a strange discovery in the great Prussian State Library in Berlin.

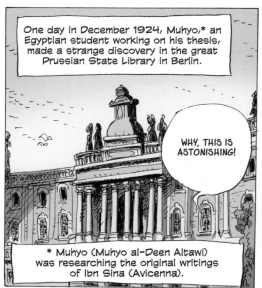

WHY, THIS IS ASTONISHING!

* Muhyo (Muhyo al-Deen Altawi) was researching the original writings of Ibn Sina (Avicenna).

Fritz, the library assistant, had just accidentally given him an unknown text that perfectly described blood circulation three centuries before Servetus in 1553.

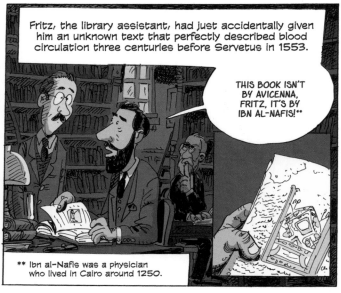

THIS BOOK ISN'T BY AVICENNA, FRITZ, IT'S BY IBN AL-NAFIS!**

** Ibn al-Nafis was a physician who lived in Cairo around 1250.

As part of his thesis, Muhyo translated Ibn al-Nafis' work into German.

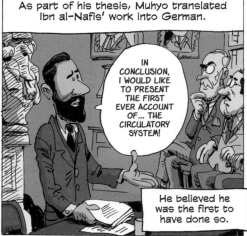

IN CONCLUSION, I WOULD LIKE TO PRESENT THE FIRST EVER ACCOUNT OF... THE CIRCULATORY SYSTEM!

He believed he was the first to have done so.

However, Max Meyerhof, an eminent German medical historian then working in Egypt, informed him that the work had been translated into Latin in the 1500s.

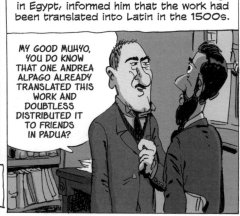

MY GOOD MUHYO, YOU DO KNOW THAT ONE ANDREA ALPAGO ALREADY TRANSLATED THIS WORK AND DOUBTLESS DISTRIBUTED IT TO FRIENDS IN PADUA?

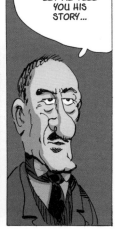

LET ME TELL YOU HIS STORY...

ANDREA ALPAGO, COUNT OF BELLUNO, WAS A DOCTOR AT THE FAMOUS FACULTY IN PADUA. THE DOGE OF VENICE SENT HIM TO DAMASCUS AS PHYSICIAN TO THE VENETIAN DELEGATION BECAUSE OF HIS PERFECT COMMAND OF ARABIC.

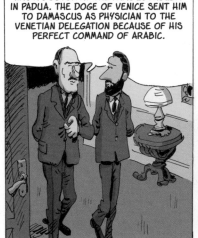

There he was presented to the Viceroy as part of Consul Malpiero's entourage in 1487. In fact, he was the Doge's spy.

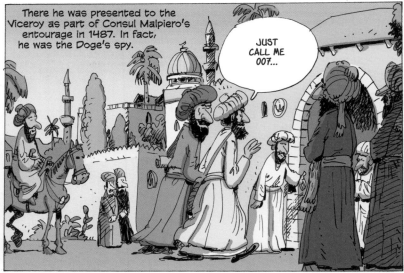

JUST CALL ME 007...

Augustin Barbarigo, Doge of La Serenissima, had given him a mission.
YOUR OBJECTIVE IS TO OBSERVE THE OTTOMANS, THE PERSIANS, AND THE MAMELUKES TO SEE WHERE OUR INTERESTS LIE.
BUT YOU NEED A COVER: YOU'LL CONTINUE THE WORK OF YOUR PREDECESSOR RAMUSIO, WHO TRANSLATED THE ARAB PHYSICIANS.
So it was that, like you, Alpago discovered Ibn al-Nafis' text.
When he realized Ibn al-Nafis' work cast doubt on Galen's theories, he decided not to publish the text in question, for fear of the INQUISITION.
IF I DIE, I CHARGE MY NEPHEW PAOLO WITH DISTRIBUTING THIS MESSAGE, FULL OF NEW FINDINGS, TO THOSE, AND ONLY THOSE, WHO ARE WORTHY.
It should be said that Galen's model of circulation had no basis in reality. Here, the liver, and not the heart, was the reservoir of human blood, emptying itself twice daily.
Useful nutrients were transported to the liver, where they underwent coction, which turned them into venous blood.
PART OF THE BLOOD PASSES THROUGH THE VENA CAVA IN THE RIGHT HALF OF THE HEART, AND FROM THERE, A PORTION TRAVELS ALONG THE PULMONARY ARTERY TO THE LUNGS, WHERE IT IS "CONSUMED".
LUNGS
VENOUS BLOOD
VENOUS ARTERY (AIR)
ARTERIAL BLOOD
CONSUMPTION
HEART
AORTA ARTERIES
(COCTION)
LIVER (COCTION)
FAECES URINE
CLEAR BLOOD ENRICHED IN VITAL HEAT
BLOOD FROM FOOD
PERIPHERAL TISSUES
(CONSUMPTION)
PERSPIRATION
ANOTHER PORTION OF THE BLOOD SEEPS THROUGH PORES IN THE INTERVENTRICULAR WALL IN THE HEART'S LEFT HALF, THE SEAT OF INNATE HEAT.
THERE IT BECOMES RED AND FOAMING, AND IS MIXED WITH AIR FROM THE LUNGS VIA THE PULMONARY ARTERY.
LUNGS
HEART
LEFT
RIGHT
BLOOD
FOODSTUFF
VEINS
ARTERIES
BLOOD IS CONSUMED IN THE PERIPHERY
TODAY, GALEN'S THEORY SEEMS NOT ONLY INCONCEIVABLE BUT UNNECESSARILY COMPLICATED.
HE PILES ON ERROR AFTER ERROR: A CIRCULATORY SYSTEM CENTRED ON THE LIVER. THE LUNGS CONSUMING BLOOD, BUT FROM THERE, WHO KNOWS. PORES IN THE INTERVENTRICULAR WALL — WRONG! TWO-WAY CIRCULATION IN THE LEFT VENTRICLE. THE MIXING OF BLOOD AND AIR IN THE VENTRICLE...

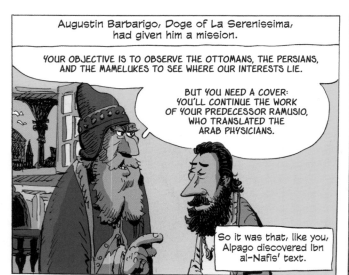

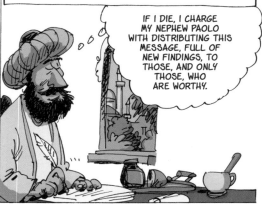

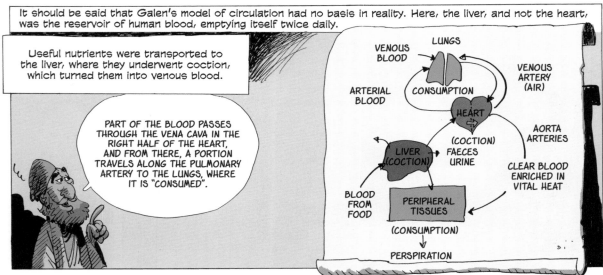

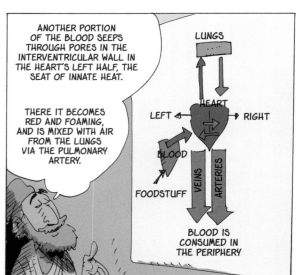

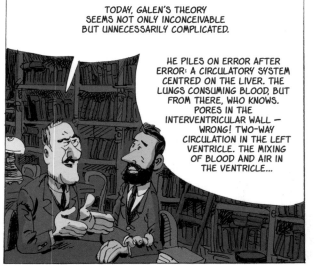

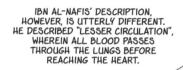

IBN AL-NAFIS' DESCRIPTION, HOWEVER, IS UTTERLY DIFFERENT. HE DESCRIBED "LESSER CIRCULATION", WHEREIN ALL BLOOD PASSES THROUGH THE LUNGS BEFORE REACHING THE HEART.

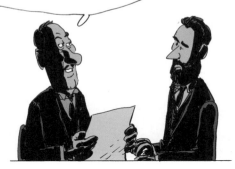

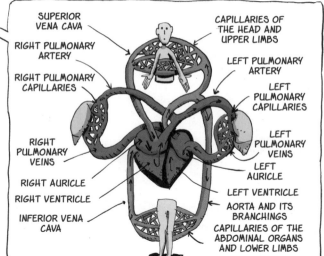

SUPERIOR VENA CAVA

RIGHT PULMONARY ARTERY

RIGHT PULMONARY CAPILLARIES

RIGHT PULMONARY VEINS

RIGHT AURICLE

RIGHT VENTRICLE

INFERIOR VENA CAVA

CAPILLARIES OF THE HEAD AND UPPER LIMBS

LEFT PULMONARY ARTERY

LEFT PULMONARY CAPILLARIES

LEFT PULMONARY VEINS

LEFT AURICLE

LEFT VENTRICLE

AORTA AND ITS BRANCHINGS

CAPILLARIES OF THE ABDOMINAL ORGANS AND LOWER LIMBS

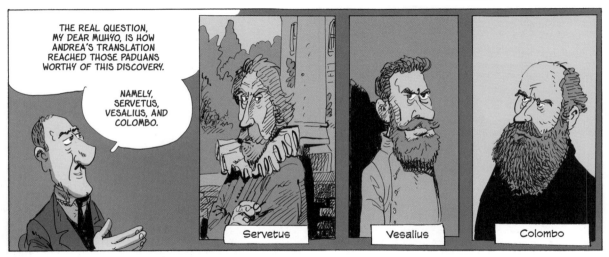

THE REAL QUESTION, MY DEAR MUHYO, IS HOW ANDREA'S TRANSLATION REACHED THOSE PADUANS WORTHY OF THIS DISCOVERY.

NAMELY, SERVETUS, VESALIUS, AND COLOMBO.

Servetus

Vesalius

Colombo

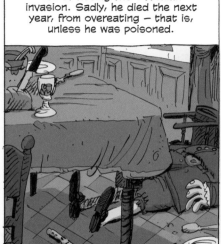

Andrea returned to Padua in 1520, fleeing the Ottoman invasion. Sadly, he died the next year, from overeating — that is, unless he was poisoned.

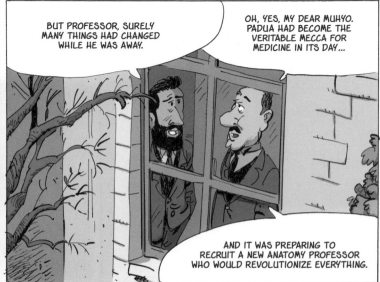

BUT PROFESSOR, SURELY MANY THINGS HAD CHANGED WHILE HE WAS AWAY.

OH, YES, MY DEAR MUHYO. PADUA HAD BECOME THE VERITABLE MECCA FOR MEDICINE IN ITS DAY...

AND IT WAS PREPARING TO RECRUIT A NEW ANATOMY PROFESSOR WHO WOULD REVOLUTIONIZE EVERYTHING.

VESALIUS, OR THE DISCOVERY OF THE HUMAN BODY

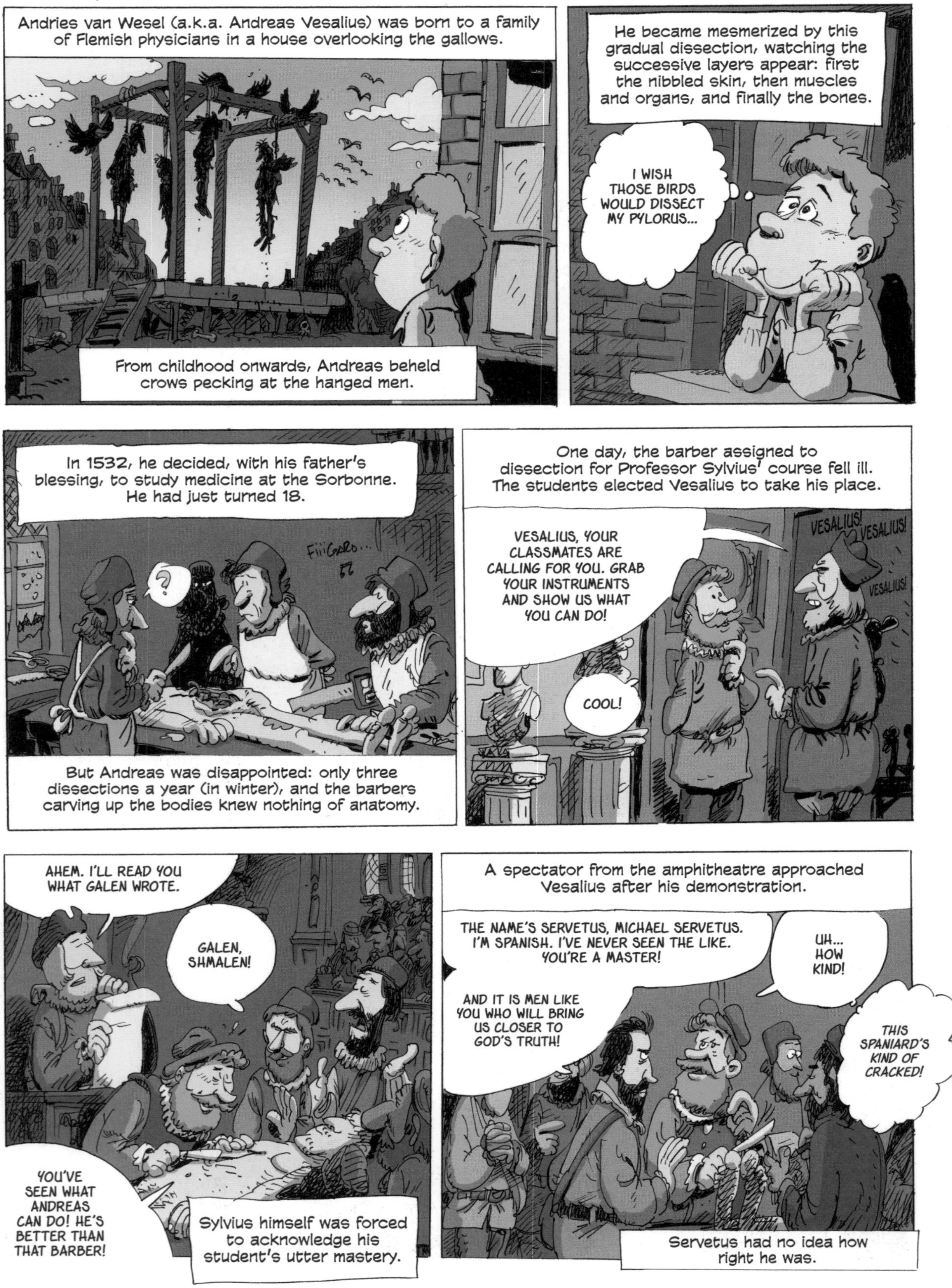
Andries van Wesel (a.k.a. Andreas Vesalius) was born to a family of Flemish physicians in a house overlooking the gallows.
From childhood onwards, Andreas beheld crows pecking at the hanged men.
He became mesmerized by this gradual dissection, watching the successive layers appear: first the nibbled skin, then muscles and organs, and finally the bones.
I WISH THOSE BIRDS WOULD DISSECT MY PYLORUS...
In 1532, he decided, with his father's blessing, to study medicine at the Sorbonne. He had just turned 18.
?
FIIIGARO...
But Andreas was disappointed: only three dissections a year (in winter), and the barbers carving up the bodies knew nothing of anatomy.
One day, the barber assigned to dissection for Professor Sylvius' course fell ill. The students elected Vesalius to take his place.
VESALIUS! VESALIUS!
VESALIUS!
VESALIUS, YOUR CLASSMATES ARE CALLING FOR YOU. GRAB YOUR INSTRUMENTS AND SHOW US WHAT YOU CAN DO!
COOL!
AHEM. I'LL READ YOU WHAT GALEN WROTE.
GALEN, SHMALEN!
YOU'VE SEEN WHAT ANDREAS CAN DO! HE'S BETTER THAN THAT BARBER!
Sylvius himself was forced to acknowledge his student's utter mastery.
A spectator from the amphitheatre approached Vesalius after his demonstration.
THE NAME'S SERVETUS, MICHAEL SERVETUS. I'M SPANISH. I'VE NEVER SEEN THE LIKE. YOU'RE A MASTER!
UH... HOW KIND!
AND IT IS MEN LIKE YOU WHO WILL BRING US CLOSER TO GOD'S TRUTH!
THIS SPANIARD'S KIND OF CRACKED!
Servetus had no idea how right he was.

In 1537, the University of Padua appointed Andreas Professor of Anatomy. Upon his arrival, the Podestà, or governor, greeted him.

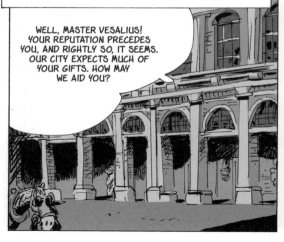

WELL, MASTER VESALIUS! YOUR REPUTATION PRECEDES YOU, AND RIGHTLY SO, IT SEEMS. OUR CITY EXPECTS MUCH OF YOUR GIFTS. HOW MAY WE AID YOU?

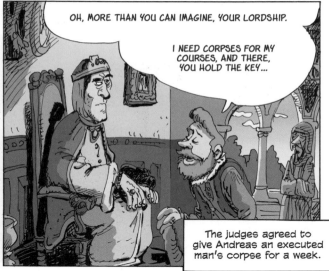

OH, MORE THAN YOU CAN IMAGINE, YOUR LORDSHIP.

I NEED CORPSES FOR MY COURSES, AND THERE, YOU HOLD THE KEY...

The judges agreed to give Andreas an executed man's corpse for a week.

Vesalius got to work. He alone stayed behind after class to complete his dissections, for he was planning a lavish tome wherein he could express the truth, often contrary to received ideas.

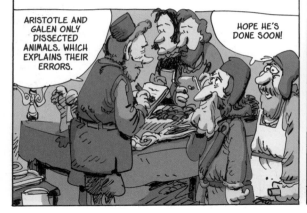

ARISTOTLE AND GALEN ONLY DISSECTED ANIMALS. WHICH EXPLAINS THEIR ERRORS.

HOPE HE'S DONE SOON!

He met Jan van Calcar, a student of Titian's, in a tavern.

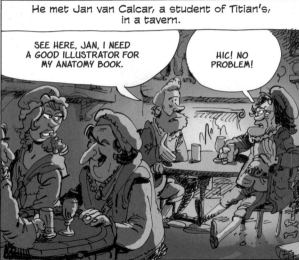

SEE HERE, JAN, I NEED A GOOD ILLUSTRATOR FOR MY ANATOMY BOOK.

HIC! NO PROBLEM!

Van Calcar had a flair for anatomical diagrams "from life".

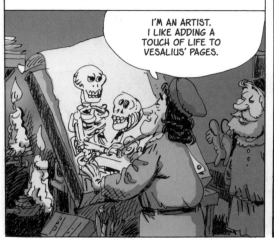

I'M AN ARTIST. I LIKE ADDING A TOUCH OF LIFE TO VESALIUS' PAGES.

He asked his master Titian to draw the frontispiece of Andreas' great tome: the *Fabrica*.

I'M NOT FOND OF DRAWING SUCH THINGS! PUTS ME OFF MY DINNER!

MAKES ME HUNGRY FOR MINE!

Up till then, anatomy primarily concerned the external parts of the human body, linking them to the signs of the zodiac.

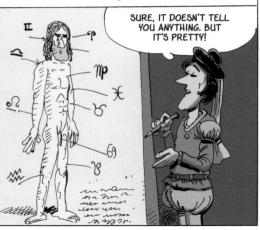

SURE, IT DOESN'T TELL YOU ANYTHING. BUT IT'S PRETTY!

The great Leonardo was Vesalius' contemporary, and wonderfully drew his own dissections.

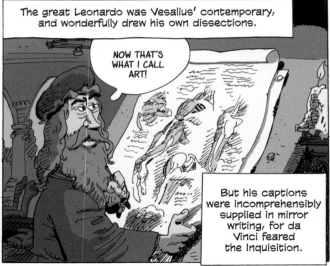

NOW THAT'S WHAT I CALL ART!

But his captions were incomprehensibly supplied in mirror writing, for da Vinci feared the Inquisition.

The *Fabrica** was the first ever book of scientific anatomy.

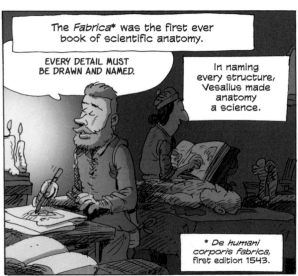

EVERY DETAIL MUST BE DRAWN AND NAMED.

In naming every structure, Vesalius made anatomy a science.

* *De humani corporis fabrica*, first edition 1543.

He and van Calcar also produced a popular edition aimed at students, with pages intended to be cut out and pasted on skeletons: the *Epitome*.

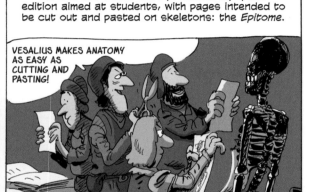

VESALIUS MAKES ANATOMY AS EASY AS CUTTING AND PASTING!

In the first edition, Vesalius corrected only a few of Galen's errors, and dared not (or didn't want to) go too far.

But his former teacher, Jacobus Sylvius, still strongly criticized him.

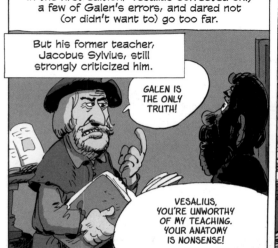

GALEN IS THE ONLY TRUTH!

VESALIUS, YOU'RE UNWORTHY OF MY TEACHING. YOUR ANATOMY IS NONSENSE!

In 1555, he published a second edition, in which his account of the circulatory system resembled that of Ibn al-Nafis.

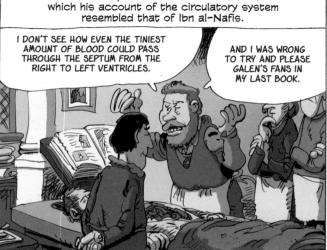

I DON'T SEE HOW EVEN THE TINIEST AMOUNT OF BLOOD COULD PASS THROUGH THE SEPTUM FROM THE RIGHT TO LEFT VENTRICLES.

AND I WAS WRONG TO TRY AND PLEASE GALEN'S FANS IN MY LAST BOOK.

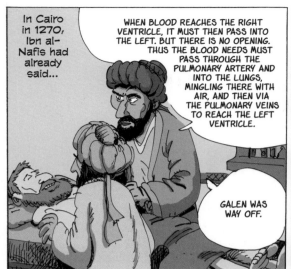

In Cairo in 1270, Ibn al-Nafis had already said...

WHEN BLOOD REACHES THE RIGHT VENTRICLE, IT MUST THEN PASS INTO THE LEFT. BUT THERE IS NO OPENING. THUS THE BLOOD NEEDS MUST PASS THROUGH THE PULMONARY ARTERY AND INTO THE LUNGS, MINGLING THERE WITH AIR, AND THEN VIA THE PULMONARY VEINS TO REACH THE LEFT VENTRICLE.

GALEN WAS WAY OFF.

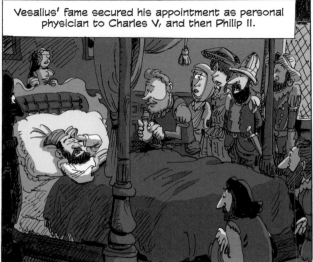

Vesalius' fame secured his appointment as personal physician to Charles V, and then Philip II.

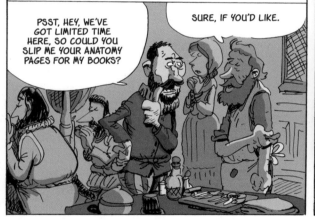

He was summoned to consult everywhere. So it was that when the French King Henri II died, Vesalius met Ambroise Paré, who begged a favour.

PSST, HEY, WE'VE GOT LIMITED TIME HERE, SO COULD YOU SLIP ME YOUR ANATOMY PAGES FOR MY BOOKS?

SURE, IF YOU'D LIKE.

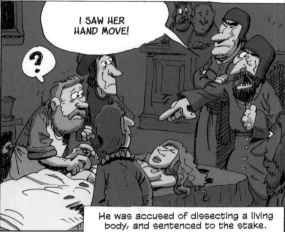

But the Inquisition was watching. One day, as he was dissecting a young woman who'd died in the night...

I SAW HER HAND MOVE!

He was accused of dissecting a living body, and sentenced to the stake.

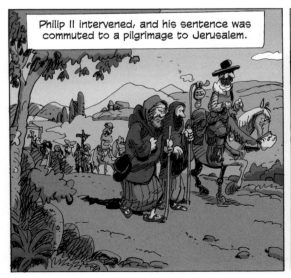

Philip II intervened, and his sentence was commuted to a pilgrimage to Jerusalem.

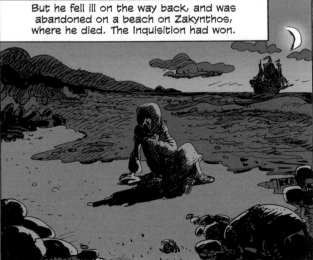

But he fell ill on the way back, and was abandoned on a beach on Zakynthos, where he died. The Inquisition had won.

MICHAEL SERVETUS, THE AGITATOR

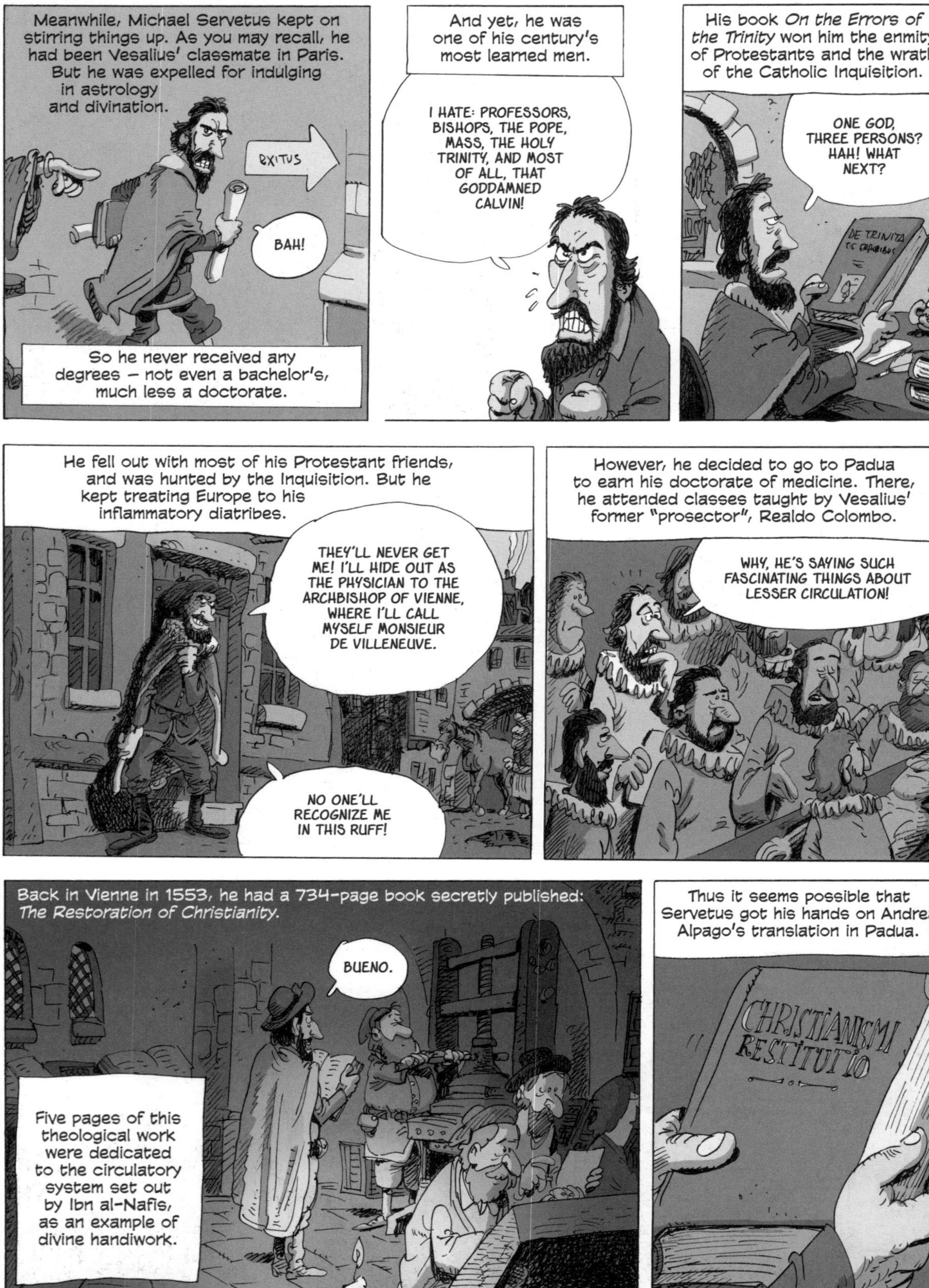

Meanwhile, Michael Servetus kept on stirring things up. As you may recall, he had been Vesalius' classmate in Paris. But he was expelled for indulging in astrology and divination.
EXITUS
BAH!
So he never received any degrees – not even a bachelor's, much less a doctorate.
And yet, he was one of his century's most learned men.
I HATE: PROFESSORS, BISHOPS, THE POPE, MASS, THE HOLY TRINITY, AND MOST OF ALL, THAT GODDAMNED CALVIN!
His book *On the Errors of the Trinity* won him the enmity of Protestants and the wrath of the Catholic Inquisition.
ONE GOD, THREE PERSONS? HAH! WHAT NEXT?
He fell out with most of his Protestant friends, and was hunted by the Inquisition. But he kept treating Europe to his inflammatory diatribes.
THEY'LL NEVER GET ME! I'LL HIDE OUT AS THE PHYSICIAN TO THE ARCHBISHOP OF VIENNE, WHERE I'LL CALL MYSELF MONSIEUR DE VILLENEUVE.
NO ONE'LL RECOGNIZE ME IN THIS RUFF!
However, he decided to go to Padua to earn his doctorate of medicine. There, he attended classes taught by Vesalius' former "prosector", Realdo Colombo.
WHY, HE'S SAYING SUCH FASCINATING THINGS ABOUT LESSER CIRCULATION!
Back in Vienne in 1553, he had a 734-page book secretly published: *The Restoration of Christianity*.
BUENO.
Five pages of this theological work were dedicated to the circulatory system set out by Ibn al-Nafis, as an example of divine handiwork.
Thus it seems possible that Servetus got his hands on Andrea Alpago's translation in Padua.
CHRISTIANISMI RESTITUTIO

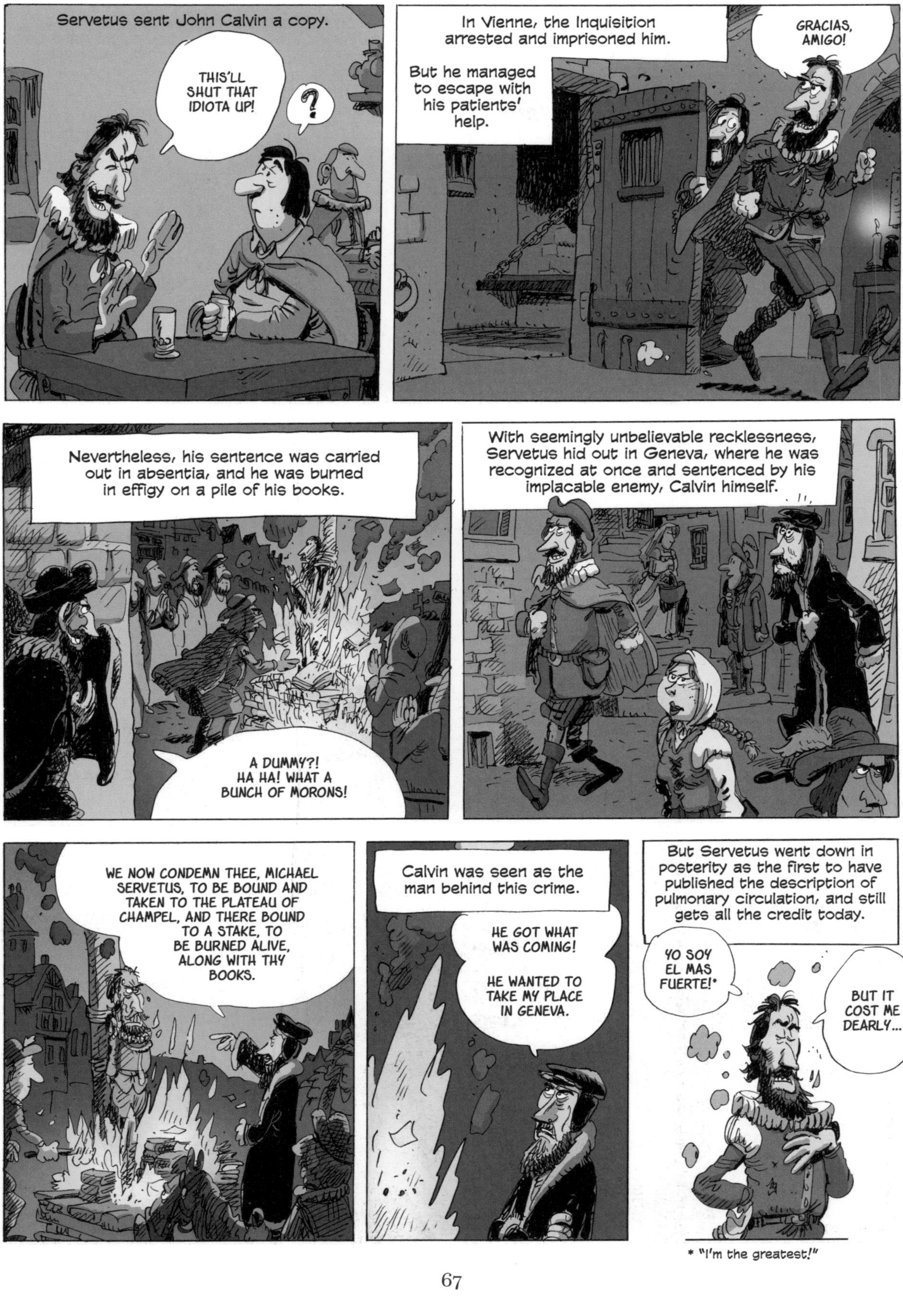
Servetus sent John Calvin a copy.
THIS'LL SHUT THAT IDIOTA UP!
?
In Vienne, the Inquisition arrested and imprisoned him.
But he managed to escape with his patients' help.
GRACIAS, AMIGO!
Nevertheless, his sentence was carried out in absentia, and he was burned in effigy on a pile of his books.
A DUMMY?! HA HA! WHAT A BUNCH OF MORONS!
With seemingly unbelievable recklessness, Servetus hid out in Geneva, where he was recognized at once and sentenced by his implacable enemy, Calvin himself.
WE NOW CONDEMN THEE, MICHAEL SERVETUS, TO BE BOUND AND TAKEN TO THE PLATEAU OF CHAMPEL, AND THERE BOUND TO A STAKE, TO BE BURNED ALIVE, ALONG WITH THY BOOKS.
Calvin was seen as the man behind this crime.
HE GOT WHAT WAS COMING!
HE WANTED TO TAKE MY PLACE IN GENEVA.
But Servetus went down in posterity as the first to have published the description of pulmonary circulation, and still gets all the credit today.
YO SOY EL MAS FUERTE!*
BUT IT COST ME DEARLY...

* "I'm the greatest!"

WILLIAM HARVEY, THE MAN WHO DISCOVERED CIRCULATION

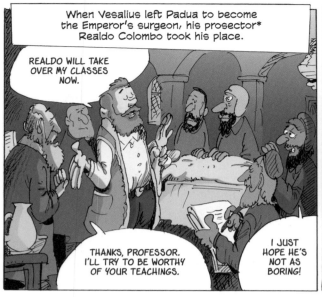

When Vesalius left Padua to become the Emperor's surgeon, his prosector* Realdo Colombo took his place.

REALDO WILL TAKE OVER MY CLASSES NOW.

THANKS, PROFESSOR. I'LL TRY TO BE WORTHY OF YOUR TEACHINGS.

I JUST HOPE HE'S NOT AS BORING!

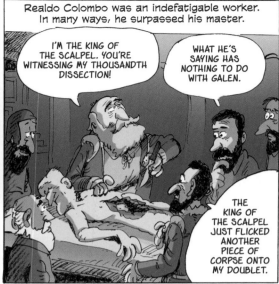

Realdo Colombo was an indefatigable worker. In many ways, he surpassed his master.

I'M THE KING OF THE SCALPEL. YOU'RE WITNESSING MY THOUSANDTH DISSECTION!

WHAT HE'S SAYING HAS NOTHING TO DO WITH GALEN.

THE KING OF THE SCALPEL JUST FLICKED ANOTHER PIECE OF CORPSE ONTO MY DOUBLET.

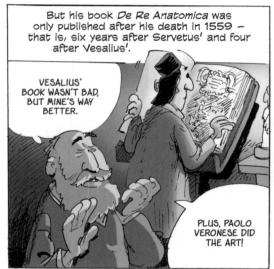

But his book *De Re Anatomica* was only published after his death in 1559 – that is, six years after Servetus' and four after Vesalius'.

VESALIUS' BOOK WASN'T BAD, BUT MINE'S WAY BETTER.

PLUS, PAOLO VERONESE DID THE ART!

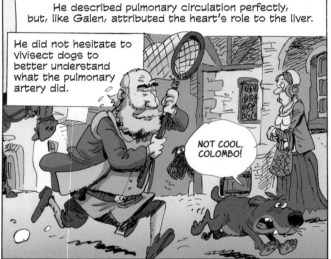

He described pulmonary circulation perfectly, but, like Galen, attributed the heart's role to the liver.

He did not hesitate to vivisect dogs to better understand what the pulmonary artery did.

NOT COOL, COLOMBO!

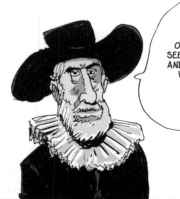

He was later appointed to Pisa, where he taught the brilliant Andrea Cisalpino.

I WAS THE FIRST TO SPEAK OF CIRCULATION, TO SEE VALVULES IN VEINS, AND TO BELIEVE THERE WERE CAPILLARIES BETWEEN VEINS AND ARTERIES!

Not bad, for a mere philosopher!

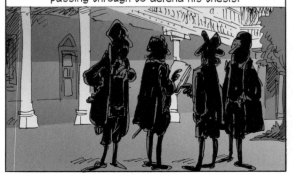

One important detail to help understand this sudden interest in lesser circulation: Andrea Alpago's nephew Paolo studied in Padua from 1527 to 1541, and showed Ibn al-Nafis' manuscript to his teachers – that is, Vesalius, Colombo, and more, including Servetus, who was passing through to defend his thesis.

---

* Assistant demonstrator to the Professor of Anatomy.

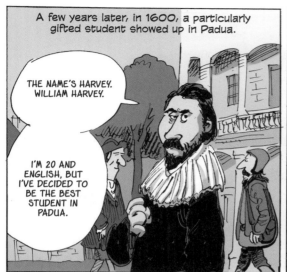

A few years later, in 1600, a particularly gifted student showed up in Padua.

THE NAME'S HARVEY. WILLIAM HARVEY.

I'M 20 AND ENGLISH, BUT I'VE DECIDED TO BE THE BEST STUDENT IN PADUA.

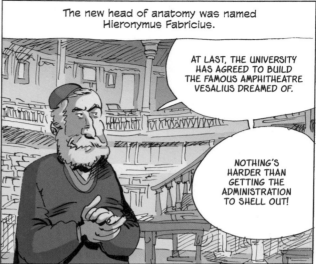

The new head of anatomy was named Hieronymus Fabricius.

AT LAST, THE UNIVERSITY HAS AGREED TO BUILD THE FAMOUS AMPHITHEATRE VESALIUS DREAMED OF.

NOTHING'S HARDER THAN GETTING THE ADMINISTRATION TO SHELL OUT!

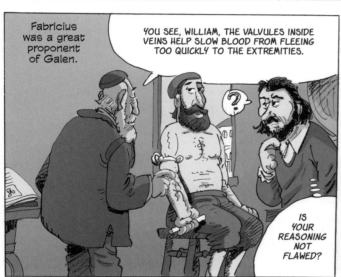

Fabricius was a great proponent of Galen.

YOU SEE, WILLIAM, THE VALVULES INSIDE VEINS HELP SLOW BLOOD FROM FLEEING TOO QUICKLY TO THE EXTREMITIES.

IS YOUR REASONING NOT FLAWED?

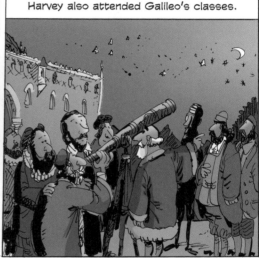

Harvey also attended Galileo's classes.

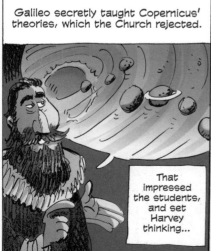

Galileo secretly taught Copernicus' theories, which the Church rejected.

That impressed the students, and set Harvey thinking...

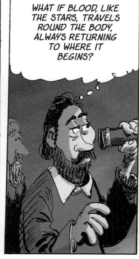

WHAT IF BLOOD, LIKE THE STARS, TRAVELS ROUND THE BODY, ALWAYS RETURNING TO WHERE IT BEGINS?

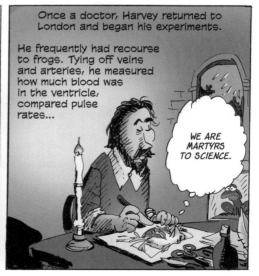

Once a doctor, Harvey returned to London and began his experiments.

He frequently had recourse to frogs. Tying off veins and arteries, he measured how much blood was in the ventricle, compared pulse rates...

WE ARE MARTYRS TO SCIENCE.

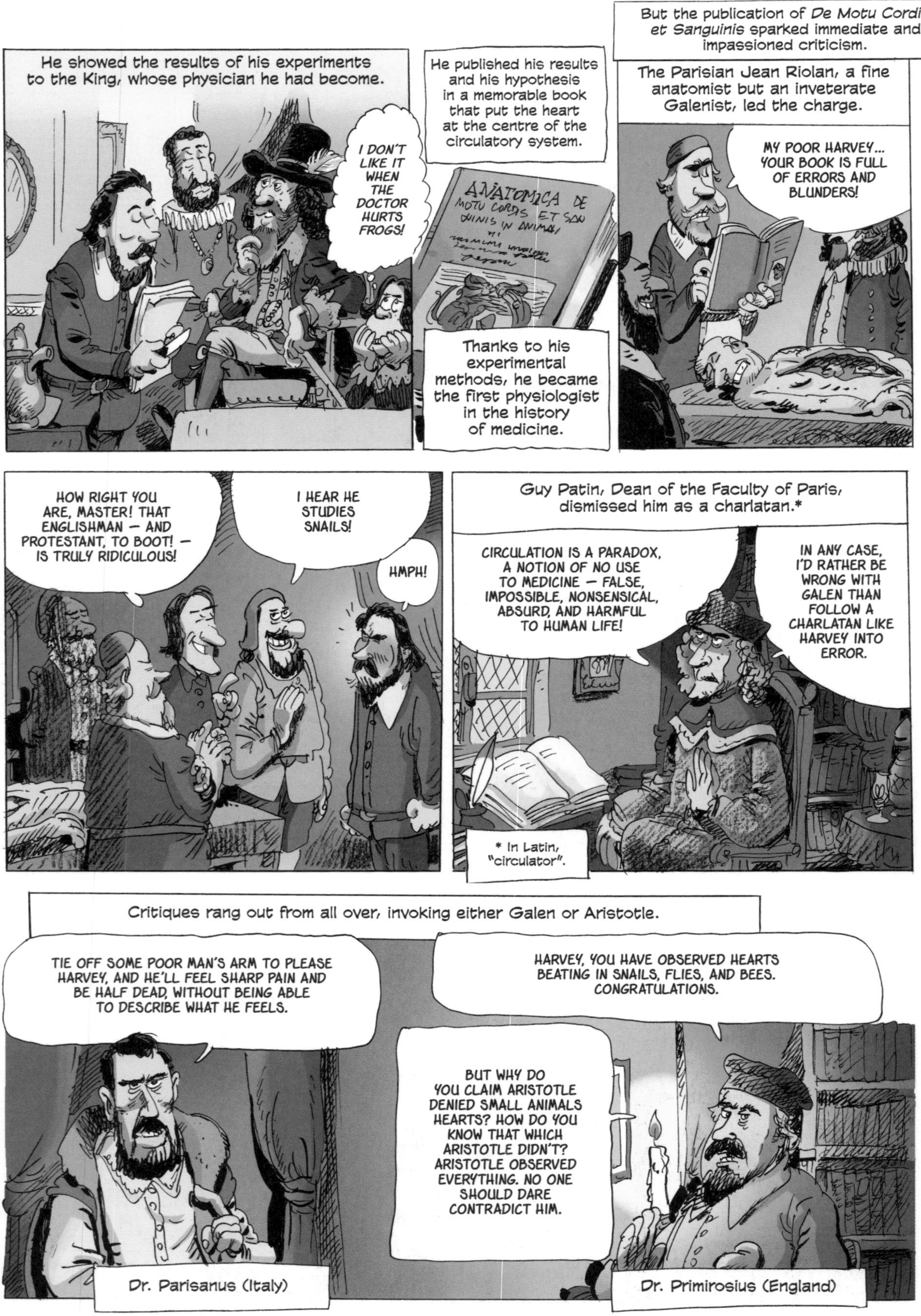

He showed the results of his experiments to the King, whose physician he had become.
I DON'T LIKE IT WHEN THE DOCTOR HURTS FROGS!
He published his results and his hypothesis in a memorable book that put the heart at the centre of the circulatory system.
Thanks to his experimental methods, he became the first physiologist in the history of medicine.
But the publication of *De Motu Cordis et Sanguinis* sparked immediate and impassioned criticism.
The Parisian Jean Riolan, a fine anatomist but an inveterate Galenist, led the charge.
MY POOR HARVEY... YOUR BOOK IS FULL OF ERRORS AND BLUNDERS!
HOW RIGHT YOU ARE, MASTER! THAT ENGLISHMAN — AND PROTESTANT, TO BOOT! — IS TRULY RIDICULOUS!
I HEAR HE STUDIES SNAILS!
HMPH!
Guy Patin, Dean of the Faculty of Paris, dismissed him as a charlatan.*
CIRCULATION IS A PARADOX, A NOTION OF NO USE TO MEDICINE — FALSE, IMPOSSIBLE, NONSENSICAL, ABSURD, AND HARMFUL TO HUMAN LIFE!
IN ANY CASE, I'D RATHER BE WRONG WITH GALEN THAN FOLLOW A CHARLATAN LIKE HARVEY INTO ERROR.
* In Latin, "circulator".
Critiques rang out from all over, invoking either Galen or Aristotle.
TIE OFF SOME POOR MAN'S ARM TO PLEASE HARVEY, AND HE'LL FEEL SHARP PAIN AND BE HALF DEAD, WITHOUT BEING ABLE TO DESCRIBE WHAT HE FEELS.
Dr. Parisanus (Italy)
HARVEY, YOU HAVE OBSERVED HEARTS BEATING IN SNAILS, FLIES, AND BEES. CONGRATULATIONS.
BUT WHY DO YOU CLAIM ARISTOTLE DENIED SMALL ANIMALS HEARTS? HOW DO YOU KNOW THAT WHICH ARISTOTLE DIDN'T? ARISTOTLE OBSERVED EVERYTHING. NO ONE SHOULD DARE CONTRADICT HIM.
Dr. Primirosius (England)

His supporters were few.

Descartes thought circulation fitted in well with his theory of "animal-machines".

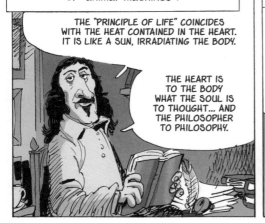

THE "PRINCIPLE OF LIFE" COINCIDES WITH THE HEAT CONTAINED IN THE HEART. IT IS LIKE A SUN, IRRADIATING THE BODY.

THE HEART IS TO THE BODY WHAT THE SOUL IS TO THOUGHT... AND THE PHILOSOPHER TO PHILOSOPHY.

Humorists were the next to rise to Harvey's defence. So it was that Boileau, in his *Ludicrous Judgement*, said...

THE COURT FORBIDS THE BLOOD TO BE ANY LONGER VAGABOND, WANDERING AND CIRCULATING ABOUT THE BODY, ON PAIN OF BEING WHOLLY GIVEN OVER TO THE FACULTY OF PARIS TO BE LET WITHOUT MEASURE.

La Fontaine had at it with a little verse.

TWO DOORS HAS THE HEART, A VALVE AND ITS MATE. BLOOD, LIFE'S SOURCE, BY ONE ENTERS INCREASINGLY. THE OTHER ALLOWS IT TO CIRCULATE FROM VEIN TO ARTERY UNCEASINGLY.

While Molière staged *The Imaginary Invalid*.

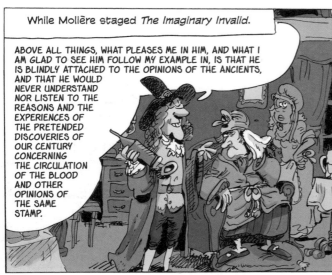

ABOVE ALL THINGS, WHAT PLEASES ME IN HIM, AND WHAT I AM GLAD TO SEE HIM FOLLOW MY EXAMPLE IN, IS THAT HE IS BLINDLY ATTACHED TO THE OPINIONS OF THE ANCIENTS, AND THAT HE WOULD NEVER UNDERSTAND NOR LISTEN TO THE REASONS AND THE EXPERIENCES OF THE PRETENDED DISCOVERIES OF OUR CENTURY CONCERNING THE CIRCULATION OF THE BLOOD AND OTHER OPINIONS OF THE SAME STAMP.

The matter needed settling. Dionis, the Queen's surgeon, pressed Louis XIV to give his opinion on circulation.

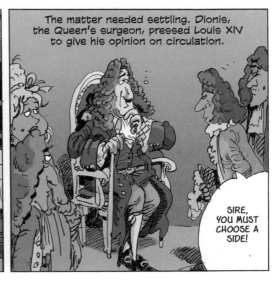

SIRE, YOU MUST CHOOSE A SIDE!

It took the King's authority to impose the teaching of circulation in France, against the advice of the Faculty of Medicine.

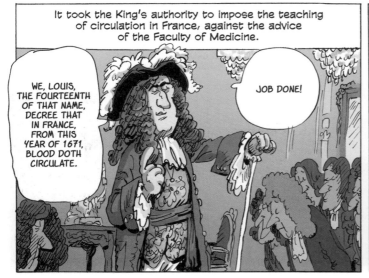

WE, LOUIS, THE FOURTEENTH OF THAT NAME, DECREE THAT IN FRANCE, FROM THIS YEAR OF 1671, BLOOD DOTH CIRCULATE.

JOB DONE!

Pierre Dionis du Séjour was made caretaker of the Jardin du Roy.*

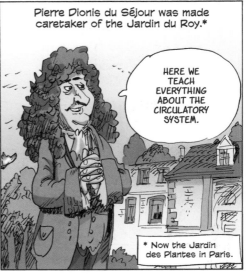

HERE WE TEACH EVERYTHING ABOUT THE CIRCULATORY SYSTEM.

* Now the Jardin des Plantes in Paris.

71

CHAPTER 6

THE INSTRUMENTS OF MEDICINE

More than any other science, medicine has needed instruments to identify signs and determine their scope, understand what could not be seen, and heal sickness.

The discoveries of these instruments were often the beginnings of whole swathes of knowledge.

So it was that the microscope allowed us to understand structures invisible to the naked eye, and the stethoscope to hear the sounds of the heart and lungs in order to describe and classify the main diseases.

As was often the case in medicine, the tireless research of a few brave souls, aided by good fortune, was the driving force behind these great leaps forward.

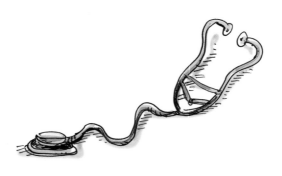

MEASURING TIME

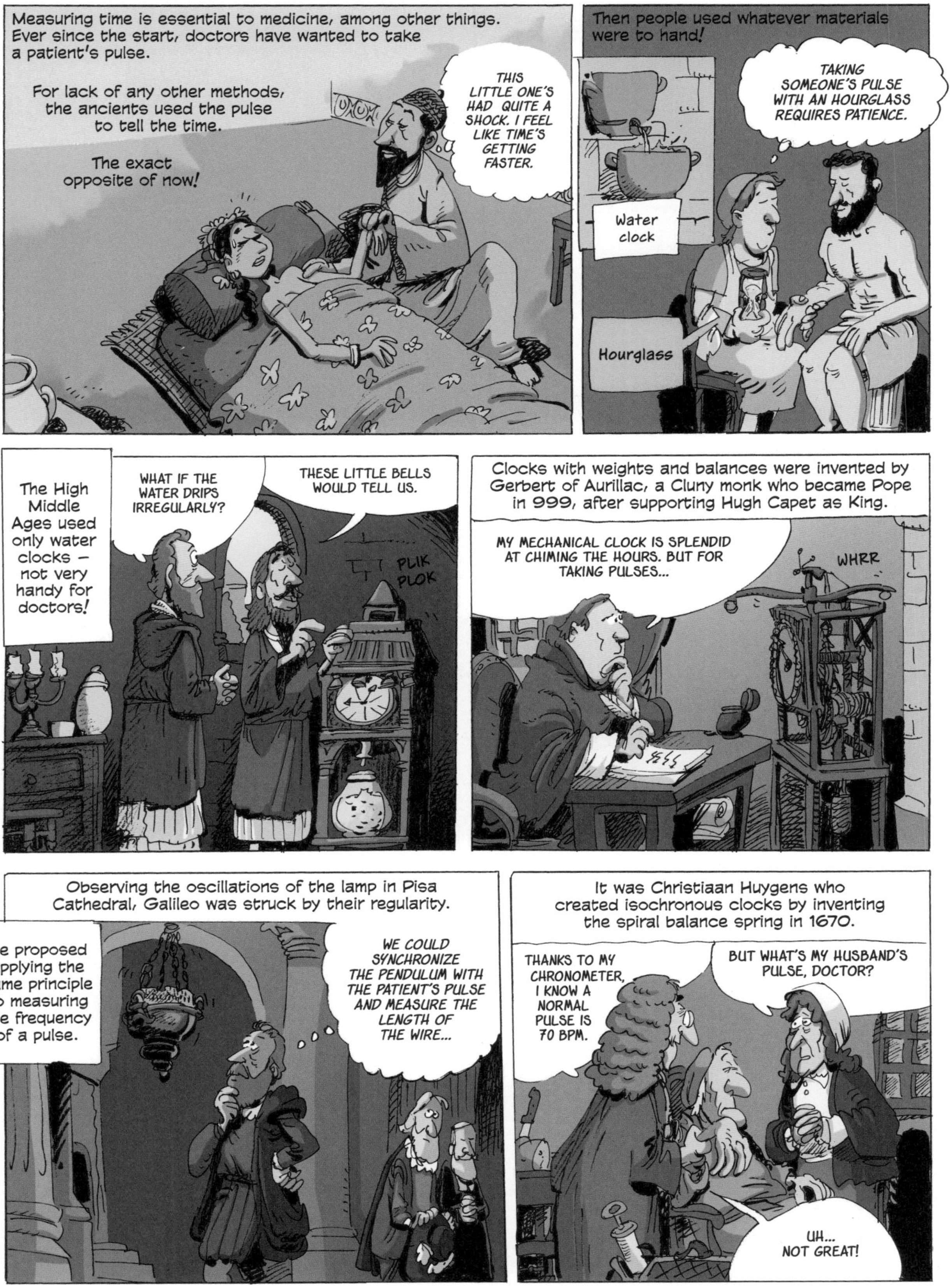
Measuring time is essential to medicine, among other things. Ever since the start, doctors have wanted to take a patient's pulse.
For lack of any other methods, the ancients used the pulse to tell the time.
The exact opposite of now!
THIS LITTLE ONE'S HAD QUITE A SHOCK. I FEEL LIKE TIME'S GETTING FASTER.
Then people used whatever materials were to hand!
TAKING SOMEONE'S PULSE WITH AN HOURGLASS REQUIRES PATIENCE.
Water clock
Hourglass
The High Middle Ages used only water clocks – not very handy for doctors!
WHAT IF THE WATER DRIPS IRREGULARLY?
THESE LITTLE BELLS WOULD TELL US.
PLIK PLOK
Clocks with weights and balances were invented by Gerbert of Aurillac, a Cluny monk who became Pope in 999, after supporting Hugh Capet as King.
MY MECHANICAL CLOCK IS SPLENDID AT CHIMING THE HOURS. BUT FOR TAKING PULSES...
WHRR
Observing the oscillations of the lamp in Pisa Cathedral, Galileo was struck by their regularity.
He proposed applying the same principle to measuring the frequency of a pulse.
WE COULD SYNCHRONIZE THE PENDULUM WITH THE PATIENT'S PULSE AND MEASURE THE LENGTH OF THE WIRE...
It was Christiaan Huygens who created isochronous clocks by inventing the spiral balance spring in 1670.
THANKS TO MY CHRONOMETER, I KNOW A NORMAL PULSE IS 70 BPM.
BUT WHAT'S MY HUSBAND'S PULSE, DOCTOR?
UH... NOT GREAT!

THE DISCOVERY OF BODILY SOUNDS

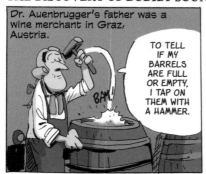

Dr. Auenbrugger's father was a wine merchant in Graz, Austria.

TO TELL IF MY BARRELS ARE FULL OR EMPTY, I TAP ON THEM WITH A HAMMER.

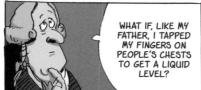

WHAT IF, LIKE MY FATHER, I TAPPED MY FINGERS ON PEOPLE'S CHESTS TO GET A LIQUID LEVEL?

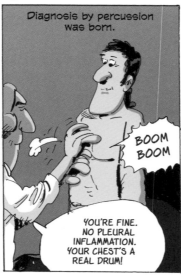

Diagnosis by percussion was born.

BOOM BOOM

YOU'RE FINE. NO PLEURAL INFLAMMATION. YOUR CHEST'S A REAL DRUM!

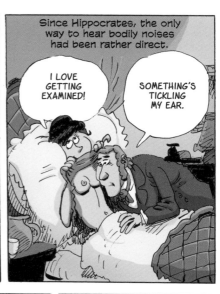

Since Hippocrates, the only way to hear bodily noises had been rather direct.

I LOVE GETTING EXAMINED!

SOMETHING'S TICKLING MY EAR.

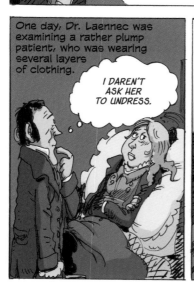

One day, Dr. Laennec was examining a rather plump patient, who was wearing several layers of clothing.

I DAREN'T ASK HER TO UNDRESS.

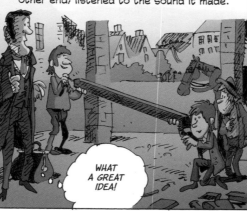

A solution was needed. He saw some children playing at the Louvre. One was scratching the end of a beam with a pin, while his friend, ear pressed against the other end, listened to the sound it made.

WHAT A GREAT IDEA!

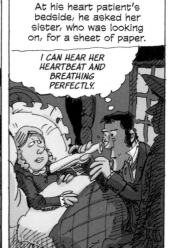

At his heart patient's bedside, he asked her sister, who was looking on, for a sheet of paper.

I CAN HEAR HER HEARTBEAT AND BREATHING PERFECTLY.

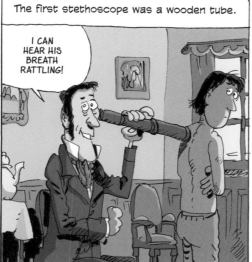

The first stethoscope was a wooden tube.

I CAN HEAR HIS BREATH RATTLING!

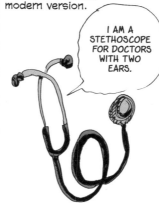

Then they gradually improved until the modern version.

I AM A STETHOSCOPE FOR DOCTORS WITH TWO EARS.

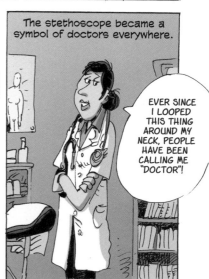

The stethoscope became a symbol of doctors everywhere.

EVER SINCE I LOOPED THIS THING AROUND MY NECK, PEOPLE HAVE BEEN CALLING ME "DOCTOR"!

BLOOD PRESSURE

Up until Harvey's work on the heart, arteries were believed to have their own pulsatility, independent of the heart's beating.

Stephen Hales, a pastor from Twickenham, showed that arteries were under pressure by sticking a pipe into his mare's artery.

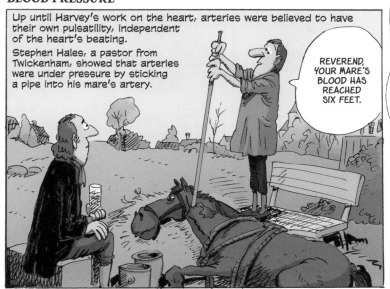

REVEREND, YOUR MARE'S BLOOD HAS REACHED SIX FEET.

But it was Étienne-Jules Marey who first measured blood pressure in 1844.

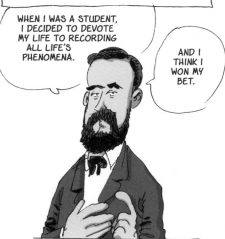

WHEN I WAS A STUDENT, I DECIDED TO DEVOTE MY LIFE TO RECORDING ALL LIFE'S PHENOMENA.

AND I THINK I WON MY BET.

With remarkable ingenuity, Marey designed a host of devices for measuring pressure, pulse, breathing, and all sorts of bodily movements.

He and veterinarian Auguste Chauveau were the first to record the heart's movements by catheterizing a horse.

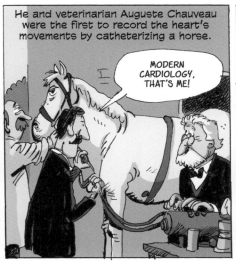

MODERN CARDIOLOGY, THAT'S ME!

In 1909, Pachon came out with an oscillometer that would measure systolic (maximum) and diastolic (minimum) pressure with a stethoscope.

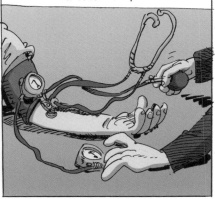

Carlo Matteucci's work had made the electric potential responsible for heartbeats known since 1842. But some way was needed to measure it.

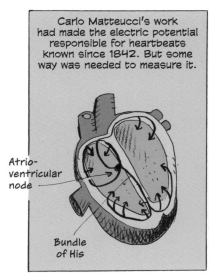

Atrio-ventricular node

Bundle of His

Thanks to Willem Einthoven's invention of the string galvanometer in 1895, cardiac activity could now be recorded and electrode positioning standardized.

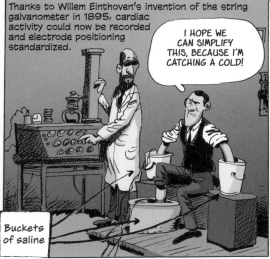

I HOPE WE CAN SIMPLIFY THIS, BECAUSE I'M CATCHING A COLD!

Buckets of saline

In 1924, he won the Nobel Prize for his work on electrocardiography.

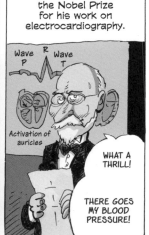

Wave P   R   Wave T

Activation of auricles

WHAT A THRILL!

THERE GOES MY BLOOD PRESSURE!

THE MICROSCOPE

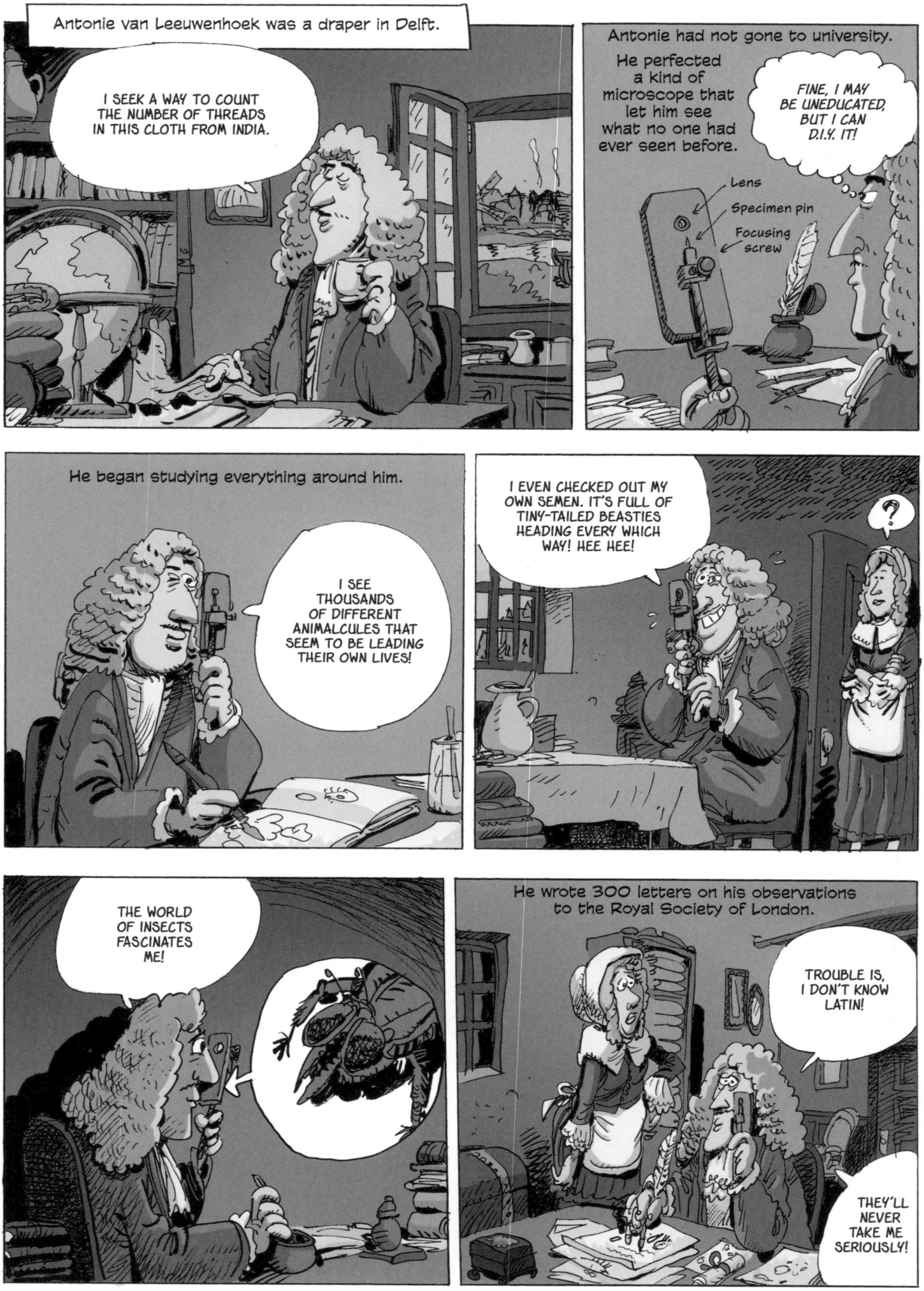
Antonie van Leeuwenhoek was a draper in Delft.
I SEEK A WAY TO COUNT THE NUMBER OF THREADS IN THIS CLOTH FROM INDIA.
Antonie had not gone to university.
He perfected a kind of microscope that let him see what no one had ever seen before.
FINE, I MAY BE UNEDUCATED, BUT I CAN D.I.Y. IT!
Lens
Specimen pin
Focusing screw
He began studying everything around him.
I SEE THOUSANDS OF DIFFERENT ANIMALCULES THAT SEEM TO BE LEADING THEIR OWN LIVES!
I EVEN CHECKED OUT MY OWN SEMEN. IT'S FULL OF TINY-TAILED BEASTIES HEADING EVERY WHICH WAY! HEE HEE!
?
THE WORLD OF INSECTS FASCINATES ME!
He wrote 300 letters on his observations to the Royal Society of London.
TROUBLE IS, I DON'T KNOW LATIN!
THEY'LL NEVER TAKE ME SERIOUSLY!

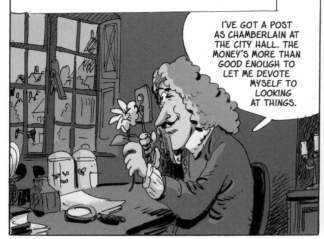

Obsessed by the infinitely minuscule, van Leeuwenhoek abandoned his trade.

I'VE GOT A POST AS CHAMBERLAIN AT THE CITY HALL. THE MONEY'S MORE THAN GOOD ENOUGH TO LET ME DEVOTE MYSELF TO LOOKING AT THINGS.

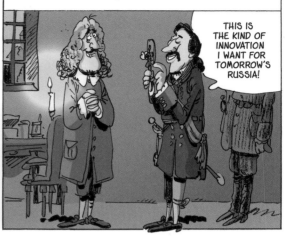

Bit by bit, his fame grew, and many notables paid him a visit, including Peter the Great of Russia.

THIS IS THE KIND OF INNOVATION I WANT FOR TOMORROW'S RUSSIA!

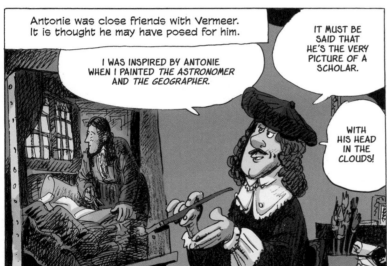

Antonie was close friends with Vermeer. It is thought he may have posed for him.

I WAS INSPIRED BY ANTONIE WHEN I PAINTED *THE ASTRONOMER* AND *THE GEOGRAPHER*.

IT MUST BE SAID THAT HE'S THE VERY PICTURE OF A SCHOLAR.

WITH HIS HEAD IN THE CLOUDS!

Other single-lens microscopes were later developed, but their magnification was not much more powerful than van Leeuwenhoek's (400x).

In the 18th century, for example, optician John Dollond corrected the flaws of Zacharias Janssen's compound microscope, which only magnified 10x.

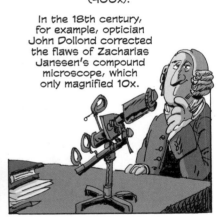

Not until 1932 did the German Ernst Ruska develop the electron microscope, capable of 5,000,000x magnification.

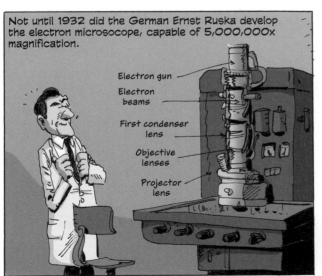

Electron gun
Electron beams
First condenser lens
Objective lenses
Projector lens

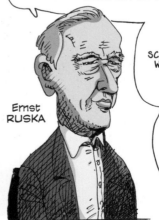

FOR THE FIRST TIME, WE COULD SEE VIRUSES. BUT MATTER'S INTERNAL STRUCTURE, LIKE MOLECULES, COULD NOT YET BE ANALYSED.

BINNIG AND ROHRER MADE THAT POSSIBLE WITH THE NEW SCANNING TUNNELLING MICROSCOPE, WHICH ALLOWED US TO DISCOVER THE D.N.A. MOLECULE.

Ernst RUSKA

TOGETHER, WE RECEIVED THE 1986 NOBEL PRIZE. ABOUT TIME — I WAS 85!

X-RAYS

In 1878, William Crookes, investigating the conduction of electricity in tubes of low pressure gas, showed that cathodes emitted light.

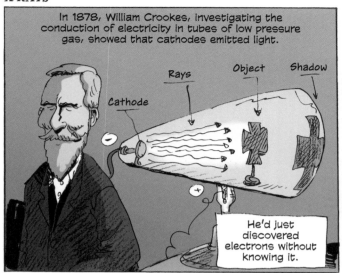

Cathode

Rays

Object

Shadow

He'd just discovered electrons without knowing it.

Later, one night in November 1895, German physicist Wilhelm Röntgen had a strange idea: to cover the Crookes tube with cardboard and observe the phenomenon in the dark.

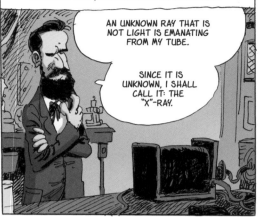

AN UNKNOWN RAY THAT IS NOT LIGHT IS EMANATING FROM MY TUBE.

SINCE IT IS UNKNOWN, I SHALL CALL IT: THE "X"-RAY.

But further surprises awaited Röntgen.

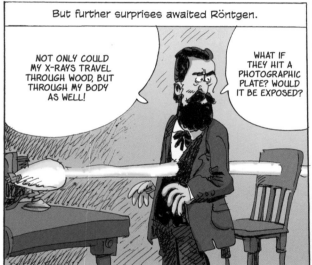

NOT ONLY COULD MY X-RAYS TRAVEL THROUGH WOOD, BUT THROUGH MY BODY AS WELL!

WHAT IF THEY HIT A PHOTOGRAPHIC PLATE? WOULD IT BE EXPOSED?

Röntgen asked his wife to lend a hand.

Frau Röntgen's hand was the first radiograph in history.

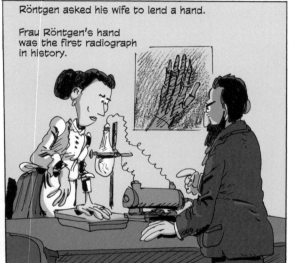

It opened a door to exploring the inside of the human body.

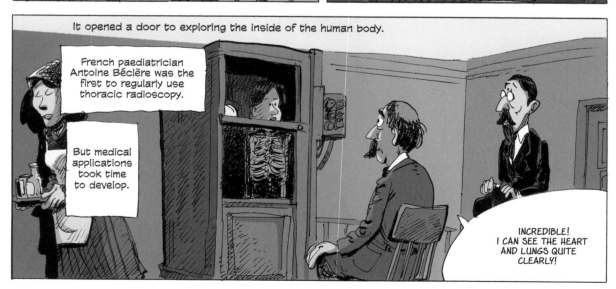

French paediatrician Antoine Béclère was the first to regularly use thoracic radioscopy.

But medical applications took time to develop.

INCREDIBLE! I CAN SEE THE HEART AND LUNGS QUITE CLEARLY!

RADIATION THERAPY

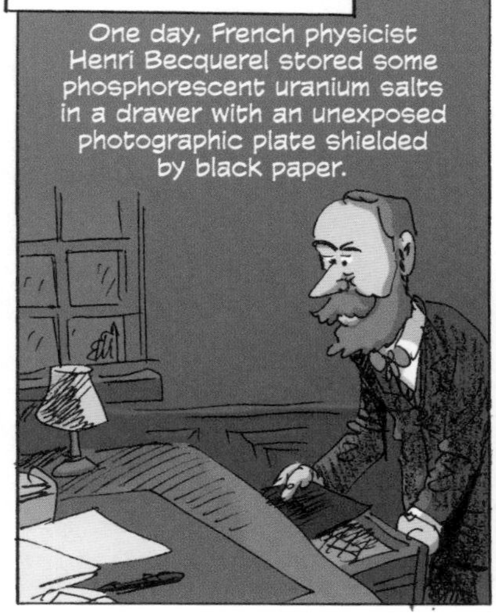
One day, French physicist Henri Becquerel stored some phosphorescent uranium salts in a drawer with an unexposed photographic plate shielded by black paper.

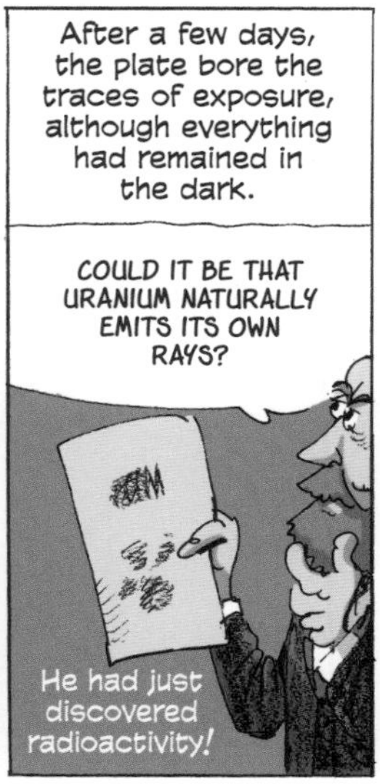
After a few days, the plate bore the traces of exposure, although everything had remained in the dark.
COULD IT BE THAT URANIUM NATURALLY EMITS ITS OWN RAYS?
He had just discovered radioactivity!

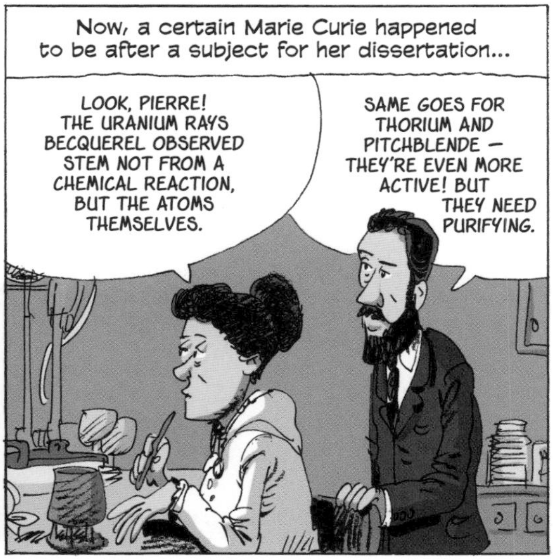
Now, a certain Marie Curie happened to be after a subject for her dissertation...
LOOK, PIERRE! THE URANIUM RAYS BECQUEREL OBSERVED STEM NOT FROM A CHEMICAL REACTION, BUT THE ATOMS THEMSELVES.
SAME GOES FOR THORIUM AND PITCHBLENDE — THEY'RE EVEN MORE ACTIVE! BUT THEY NEED PURIFYING.

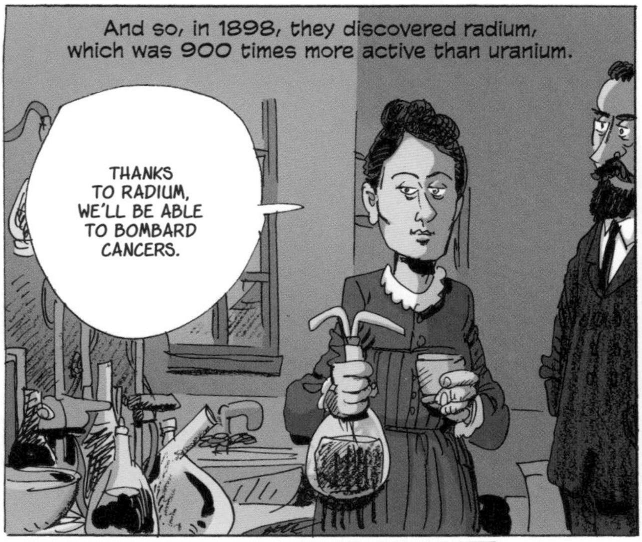
And so, in 1898, they discovered radium, which was 900 times more active than uranium.
THANKS TO RADIUM, WE'LL BE ABLE TO BOMBARD CANCERS.

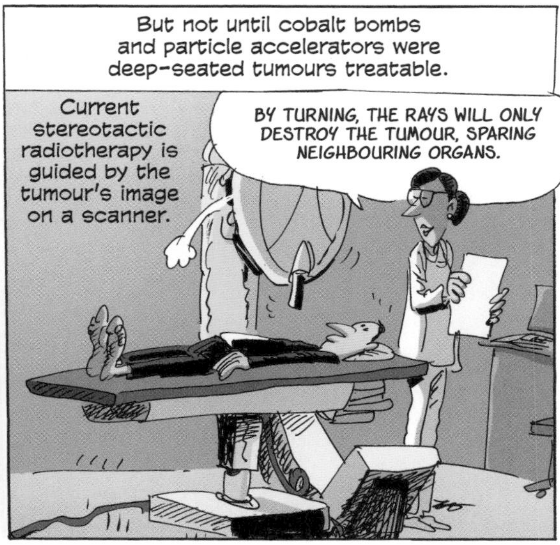
But not until cobalt bombs and particle accelerators were deep-seated tumours treatable.
Current stereotactic radiotherapy is guided by the tumour's image on a scanner.
BY TURNING, THE RAYS WILL ONLY DESTROY THE TUMOUR, SPARING NEIGHBOURING ORGANS.

MAGNETIC RESONANCE IMAGING

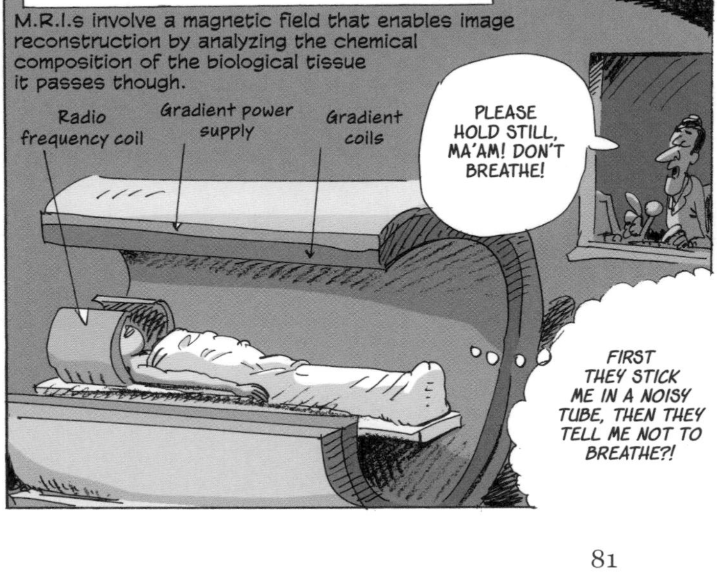
M.R.I.s involve a magnetic field that enables image reconstruction by analyzing the chemical composition of the biological tissue it passes though.
Radio frequency coil
Gradient power supply
Gradient coils
PLEASE HOLD STILL, MA'AM! DON'T BREATHE!
FIRST THEY STICK ME IN A NOISY TUBE, THEN THEY TELL ME NOT TO BREATHE?!

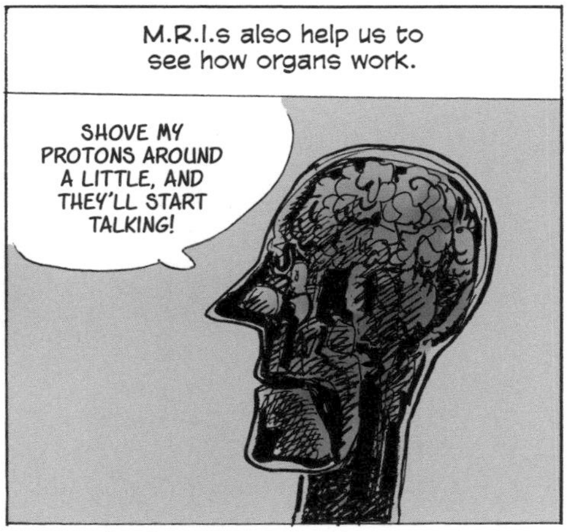
M.R.I.s also help us to see how organs work.
SHOVE MY PROTONS AROUND A LITTLE, AND THEY'LL START TALKING!

Its inventors, Paul Lauterbur and Peter Mansfield, received the Nobel Prize in 2003.

ULTRASOUND

Medical ultrasound derives from Paul Langevin's research on sonar (1917).

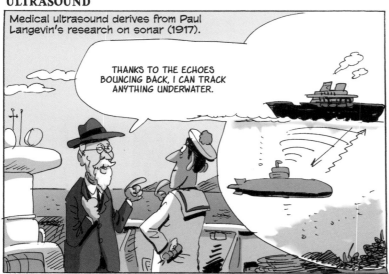

THANKS TO THE ECHOES BOUNCING BACK, I CAN TRACK ANYTHING UNDERWATER.

Ultrasound consists of using a probe to send high-frequency sound pulses into your body.

The sound waves travel through tissue and bounce back in the form of an echo.

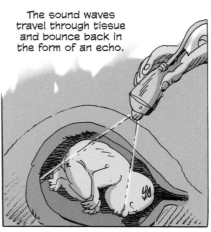

This signal is then processed by a computer that projects the image live onto a video screen.

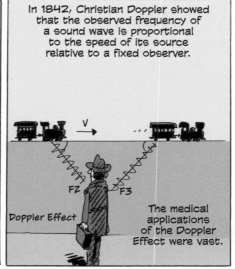

In 1842, Christian Doppler showed that the observed frequency of a sound wave is proportional to the speed of its source relative to a fixed observer.

V

F2   F3

Doppler Effect

The medical applications of the Doppler Effect were vast.

Coupled with ultrasound, the Doppler Effect helped us measure the speed of blood in blood vessels.

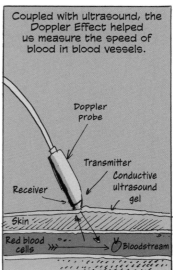

Doppler probe

Transmitter
Conductive ultrasound gel

Receiver

Skin

Red blood cells

Bloodstream

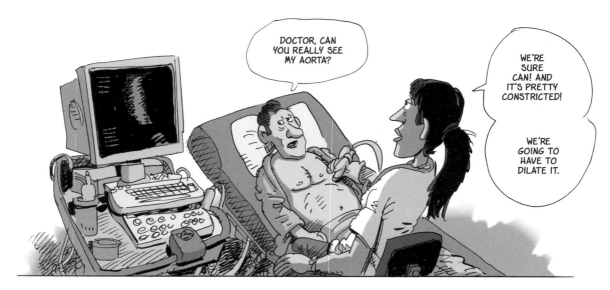

DOCTOR, CAN YOU REALLY SEE MY AORTA?

WE'RE SURE CAN! AND IT'S PRETTY CONSTRICTED!

WE'RE GOING TO HAVE TO DILATE IT.

CHAPTER 7

THE MODERN AGE DAWNS

After the Age of Enlightenment came the age of revolutions.

As always, doctors were at the mercy of global events, and were even threatened with extinction in France, only to spring back up unexpectedly at the dawn of the 19th century, achieving renown on the battlefields of the French Revolution and the Napoleonic Empire, and taking over hospitals.

For three revolutions, this time wholly medical, were to change the face of the world: the discovery of anaesthesia, the battle against infection, and experimental medicine.

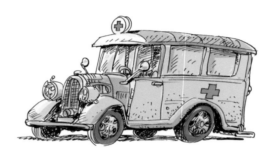

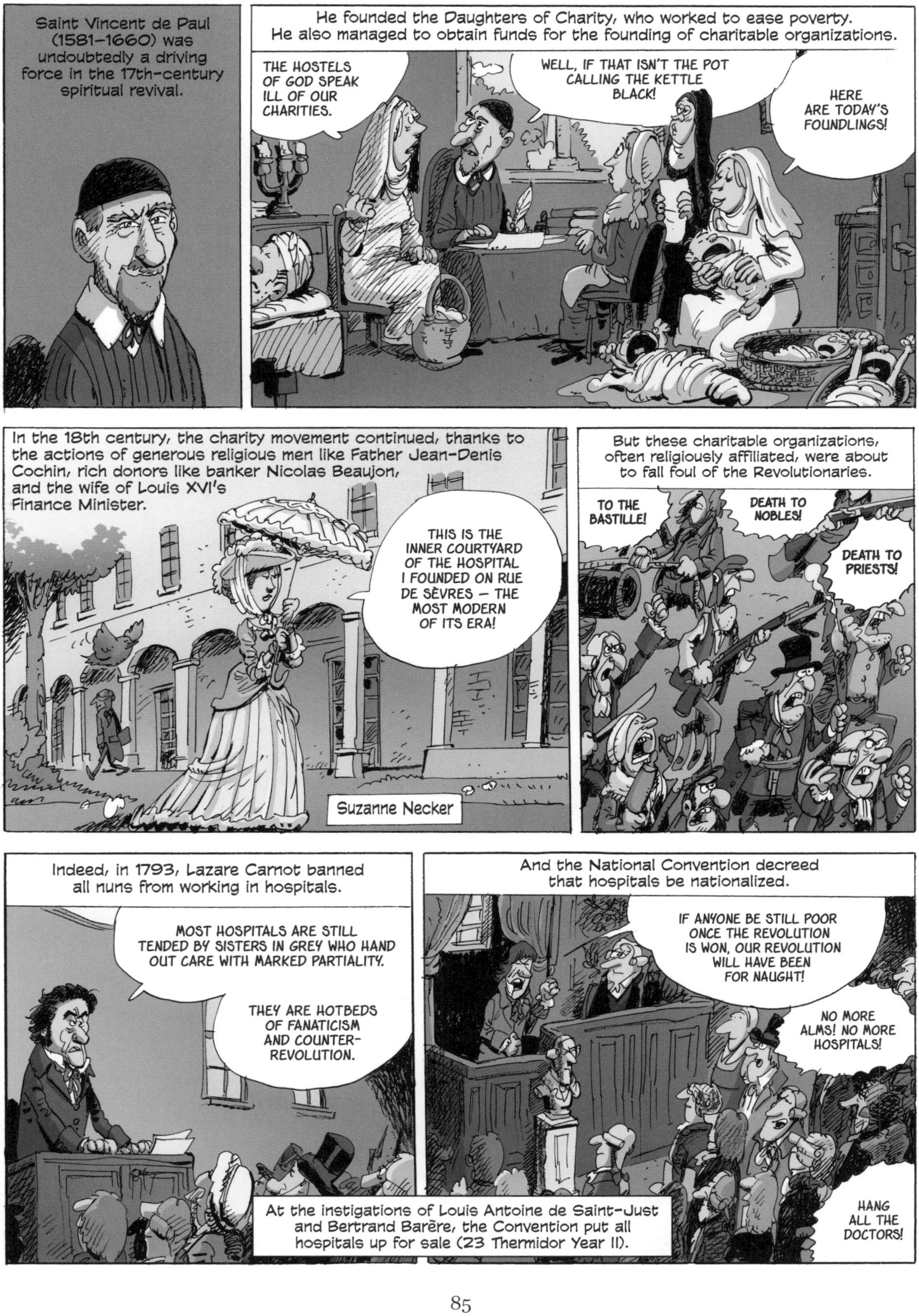
Saint Vincent de Paul (1581–1660) was undoubtedly a driving force in the 17th-century spiritual revival.
He founded the Daughters of Charity, who worked to ease poverty. He also managed to obtain funds for the founding of charitable organizations.
THE HOSTELS OF GOD SPEAK ILL OF OUR CHARITIES.
WELL, IF THAT ISN'T THE POT CALLING THE KETTLE BLACK!
HERE ARE TODAY'S FOUNDLINGS!
In the 18th century, the charity movement continued, thanks to the actions of generous religious men like Father Jean-Denis Cochin, rich donors like banker Nicolas Beaujon, and the wife of Louis XVI's Finance Minister.
THIS IS THE INNER COURTYARD OF THE HOSPITAL I FOUNDED ON RUE DE SÈVRES — THE MOST MODERN OF ITS ERA!
Suzanne Necker
But these charitable organizations, often religiously affiliated, were about to fall foul of the Revolutionaries.
TO THE BASTILLE!
DEATH TO NOBLES!
DEATH TO PRIESTS!
Indeed, in 1793, Lazare Carnot banned all nuns from working in hospitals.
MOST HOSPITALS ARE STILL TENDED BY SISTERS IN GREY WHO HAND OUT CARE WITH MARKED PARTIALITY.
THEY ARE HOTBEDS OF FANATICISM AND COUNTER-REVOLUTION.
And the National Convention decreed that hospitals be nationalized.
IF ANYONE BE STILL POOR ONCE THE REVOLUTION IS WON, OUR REVOLUTION WILL HAVE BEEN FOR NAUGHT!
NO MORE ALMS! NO MORE HOSPITALS!
At the instigations of Louis Antoine de Saint-Just and Bertrand Barère, the Convention put all hospitals up for sale (23 Thermidor Year II).
HANG ALL THE DOCTORS!

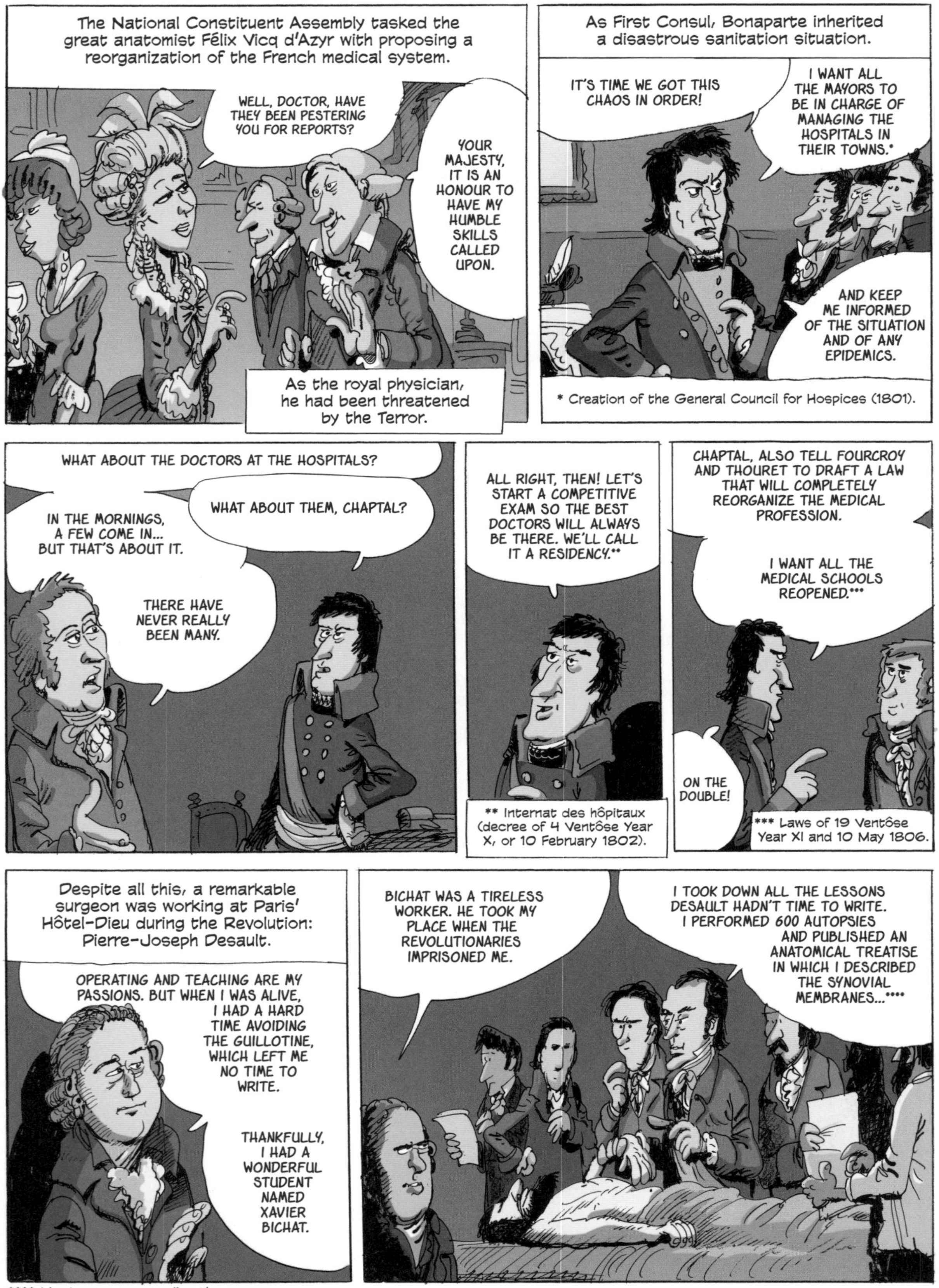

The National Constituent Assembly tasked the great anatomist Félix Vicq d'Azyr with proposing a reorganization of the French medical system.
WELL, DOCTOR, HAVE THEY BEEN PESTERING YOU FOR REPORTS?
YOUR MAJESTY, IT IS AN HONOUR TO HAVE MY HUMBLE SKILLS CALLED UPON.
As the royal physician, he had been threatened by the Terror.
As First Consul, Bonaparte inherited a disastrous sanitation situation.
IT'S TIME WE GOT THIS CHAOS IN ORDER!
I WANT ALL THE MAYORS TO BE IN CHARGE OF MANAGING THE HOSPITALS IN THEIR TOWNS.*
AND KEEP ME INFORMED OF THE SITUATION AND OF ANY EPIDEMICS.
* Creation of the General Council for Hospices (1801).
WHAT ABOUT THE DOCTORS AT THE HOSPITALS?
WHAT ABOUT THEM, CHAPTAL?
IN THE MORNINGS, A FEW COME IN... BUT THAT'S ABOUT IT.
THERE HAVE NEVER REALLY BEEN MANY.
ALL RIGHT, THEN! LET'S START A COMPETITIVE EXAM SO THE BEST DOCTORS WILL ALWAYS BE THERE. WE'LL CALL IT A RESIDENCY.**
** Internat des hôpitaux (decree of 4 Ventôse Year X, or 10 February 1802).
CHAPTAL, ALSO TELL FOURCROY AND THOURET TO DRAFT A LAW THAT WILL COMPLETELY REORGANIZE THE MEDICAL PROFESSION.
I WANT ALL THE MEDICAL SCHOOLS REOPENED.***
ON THE DOUBLE!
*** Laws of 19 Ventôse Year XI and 10 May 1806.
Despite all this, a remarkable surgeon was working at Paris' Hôtel-Dieu during the Revolution: Pierre-Joseph Desault.
OPERATING AND TEACHING ARE MY PASSIONS. BUT WHEN I WAS ALIVE, I HAD A HARD TIME AVOIDING THE GUILLOTINE, WHICH LEFT ME NO TIME TO WRITE.
THANKFULLY, I HAD A WONDERFUL STUDENT NAMED XAVIER BICHAT.
BICHAT WAS A TIRELESS WORKER. HE TOOK MY PLACE WHEN THE REVOLUTIONARIES IMPRISONED ME.
I TOOK DOWN ALL THE LESSONS DESAULT HADN'T TIME TO WRITE. I PERFORMED 600 AUTOPSIES AND PUBLISHED AN ANATOMICAL TREATISE IN WHICH I DESCRIBED THE SYNOVIAL MEMBRANES...****

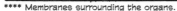

**** Membranes surrounding the organs.

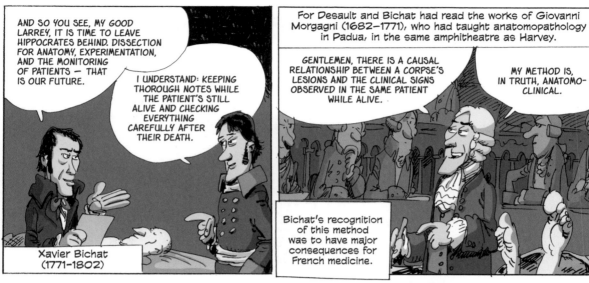

AND SO YOU SEE, MY GOOD LARREY, IT IS TIME TO LEAVE HIPPOCRATES BEHIND. DISSECTION FOR ANATOMY, EXPERIMENTATION, AND THE MONITORING OF PATIENTS — THAT IS OUR FUTURE.

I UNDERSTAND: KEEPING THOROUGH NOTES WHILE THE PATIENT'S STILL ALIVE AND CHECKING EVERYTHING CAREFULLY AFTER THEIR DEATH.

Xavier Bichat
(1771-1802)

For Desault and Bichat had read the works of Giovanni Morgagni (1682–1771), who had taught anatomopathology in Padua, in the same amphitheatre as Harvey.

GENTLEMEN, THERE IS A CAUSAL RELATIONSHIP BETWEEN A CORPSE'S LESIONS AND THE CLINICAL SIGNS OBSERVED IN THE SAME PATIENT WHILE ALIVE.

MY METHOD IS, IN TRUTH, ANATOMO-CLINICAL.

Bichat's recognition of this method was to have major consequences for French medicine.

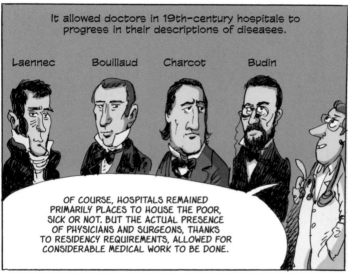

It allowed doctors in 19th-century hospitals to progress in their descriptions of diseases.

Laennec   Bouillaud   Charcot   Budin

OF COURSE, HOSPITALS REMAINED PRIMARILY PLACES TO HOUSE THE POOR, SICK OR NOT. BUT THE ACTUAL PRESENCE OF PHYSICIANS AND SURGEONS, THANKS TO RESIDENCY REQUIREMENTS, ALLOWED FOR CONSIDERABLE MEDICAL WORK TO BE DONE.

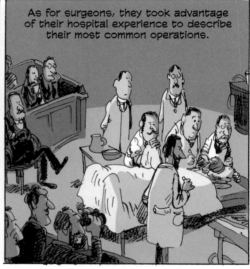

As for surgeons, they took advantage of their hospital experience to describe their most common operations.

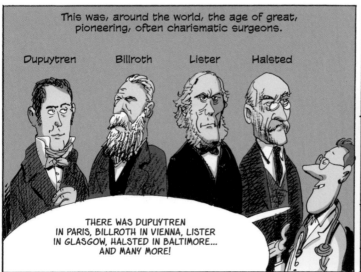

This was, around the world, the age of great, pioneering, often charismatic surgeons.

Dupuytren   Billroth   Lister   Halsted

THERE WAS DUPUYTREN IN PARIS, BILLROTH IN VIENNA, LISTER IN GLASGOW, HALSTED IN BALTIMORE... AND MANY MORE!

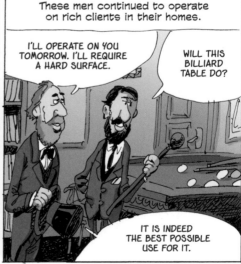

These men continued to operate on rich clients in their homes.

I'LL OPERATE ON YOU TOMORROW. I'LL REQUIRE A HARD SURFACE.

WILL THIS BILLIARD TABLE DO?

IT IS INDEED THE BEST POSSIBLE USE FOR IT.

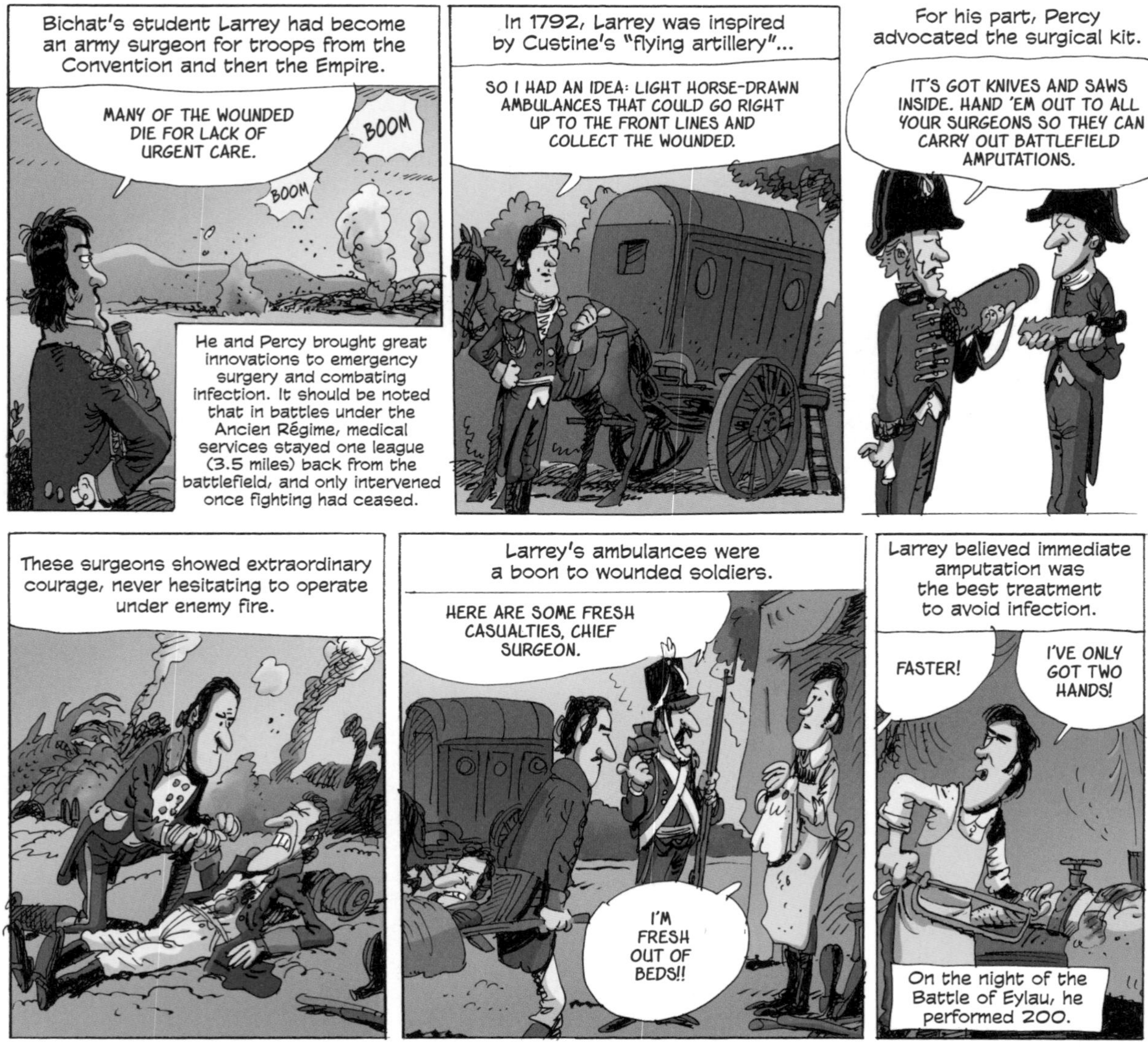
Bichat's student Larrey had become an army surgeon for troops from the Convention and then the Empire.
MANY OF THE WOUNDED DIE FOR LACK OF URGENT CARE.
BOOM
BOOM
He and Percy brought great innovations to emergency surgery and combating infection. It should be noted that in battles under the Ancien Régime, medical services stayed one league (3.5 miles) back from the battlefield, and only intervened once fighting had ceased.
In 1792, Larrey was inspired by Custine's "flying artillery"...
SO I HAD AN IDEA: LIGHT HORSE-DRAWN AMBULANCES THAT COULD GO RIGHT UP TO THE FRONT LINES AND COLLECT THE WOUNDED.
For his part, Percy advocated the surgical kit.
IT'S GOT KNIVES AND SAWS INSIDE. HAND 'EM OUT TO ALL YOUR SURGEONS SO THEY CAN CARRY OUT BATTLEFIELD AMPUTATIONS.
These surgeons showed extraordinary courage, never hesitating to operate under enemy fire.
Larrey's ambulances were a boon to wounded soldiers.
HERE ARE SOME FRESH CASUALTIES, CHIEF SURGEON.
I'M FRESH OUT OF BEDS!!
Larrey believed immediate amputation was the best treatment to avoid infection.
FASTER!
I'VE ONLY GOT TWO HANDS!
On the night of the Battle of Eylau, he performed 200.
During the Egyptian campaign, he had to adapt and find an equivalent to his "flying ambulances".
WHAT'S THAT CAMEL FOR?
IT'S THE FLYING AMBULANCE OF THE PYRAMIDS!
Larrey's reputation became world-renowned. At Waterloo, Wellington asked the Duke of Cambridge:
WHO'S THAT BRAVE SORT RUNNING AROUND UNDER OUR FIRE?
WHY, LARREY, MY LORD.
TELL THEM NOT TO FIRE AT HIM. ALLOW THE GOOD MAN TIME TO COLLECT THE WOUNDED. I SALUTE THE HONOUR AND LOYALTY ON DISPLAY!
But the 19th century would bring four fundamental discoveries that revolutionized medicine and heralded the true modern era:
• microbiology and sterilization by Koch and Pasteur,
• anaesthesia by Wells and Simpson,
• X-rays by Röntgen,
• and experimental medicine by Claude Bernard.

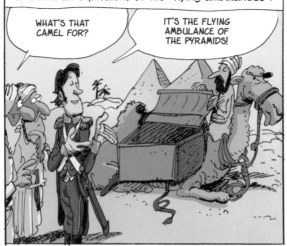

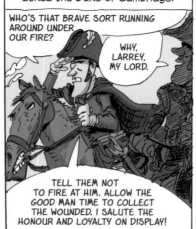

CHAPTER 8

ANAESTHESIA AT LAST!

If there is one discovery that has eased human suffering, it is without a doubt anaesthesia.

But on the battlefields of Empire, amputations were still performed without such benefits. "Bite down hard on this pipe, I'm about to start cutting," Larrey would tell soldiers. When the pipe fell and broke, it meant the patient hadn't survived the shock and atrocious pain. The expression "Casser sa pipe" has survived in French, meaning "bite the dust".

As often in the history of medicine, pure chance led to a discovery—in this case, of anaesthesia, when a dentist was out for a Sunday stroll at the fairgrounds.

As for Queen Victoria, she played a considerable part in this incredible advance without even knowing it.

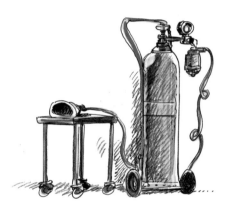

ANAESTHESIA

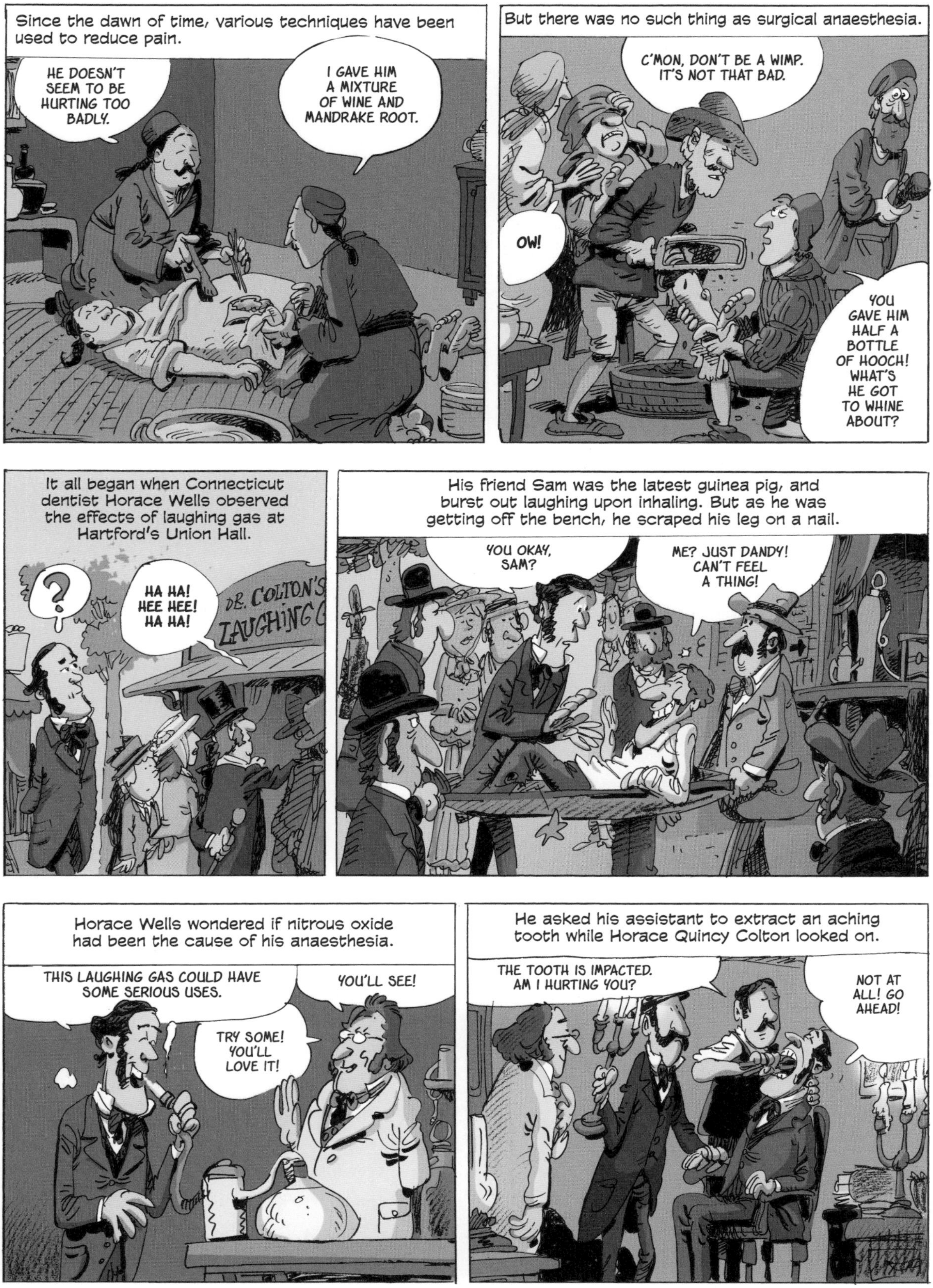
Since the dawn of time, various techniques have been used to reduce pain.
HE DOESN'T SEEM TO BE HURTING TOO BADLY.
I GAVE HIM A MIXTURE OF WINE AND MANDRAKE ROOT.
But there was no such thing as surgical anaesthesia.
C'MON, DON'T BE A WIMP. IT'S NOT THAT BAD.
OW!
YOU GAVE HIM HALF A BOTTLE OF HOOCH! WHAT'S HE GOT TO WHINE ABOUT?
It all began when Connecticut dentist Horace Wells observed the effects of laughing gas at Hartford's Union Hall.
?
HA HA! HEE HEE! HA HA!
DR. COLTON'S
LAUGHING
His friend Sam was the latest guinea pig, and burst out laughing upon inhaling. But as he was getting off the bench, he scraped his leg on a nail.
YOU OKAY, SAM?
ME? JUST DANDY! CAN'T FEEL A THING!
Horace Wells wondered if nitrous oxide had been the cause of his anaesthesia.
THIS LAUGHING GAS COULD HAVE SOME SERIOUS USES.
YOU'LL SEE!
TRY SOME! YOU'LL LOVE IT!
He asked his assistant to extract an aching tooth while Horace Quincy Colton looked on.
THE TOOTH IS IMPACTED. AM I HURTING YOU?
NOT AT ALL! GO AHEAD!

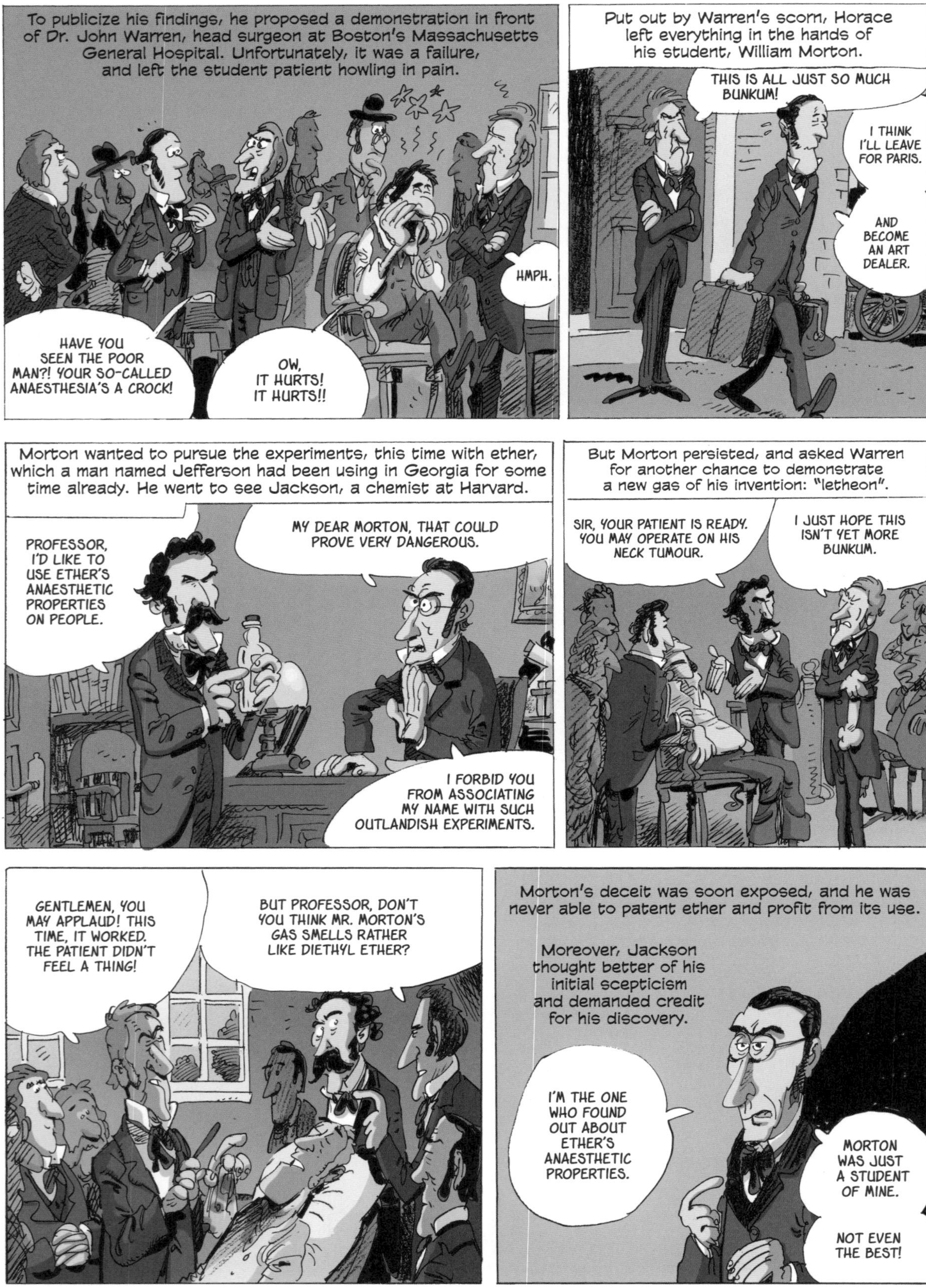
To publicize his findings, he proposed a demonstration in front of Dr. John Warren, head surgeon at Boston's Massachusetts General Hospital. Unfortunately, it was a failure, and left the student patient howling in pain.
HAVE YOU SEEN THE POOR MAN?! YOUR SO-CALLED ANAESTHESIA'S A CROCK!
OW, IT HURTS! IT HURTS!!
HMPH.
Put out by Warren's scorn, Horace left everything in the hands of his student, William Morton.
THIS IS ALL JUST SO MUCH BUNKUM!
I THINK I'LL LEAVE FOR PARIS.
AND BECOME AN ART DEALER.
Morton wanted to pursue the experiments, this time with ether, which a man named Jefferson had been using in Georgia for some time already. He went to see Jackson, a chemist at Harvard.
PROFESSOR, I'D LIKE TO USE ETHER'S ANAESTHETIC PROPERTIES ON PEOPLE.
MY DEAR MORTON, THAT COULD PROVE VERY DANGEROUS.
I FORBID YOU FROM ASSOCIATING MY NAME WITH SUCH OUTLANDISH EXPERIMENTS.
But Morton persisted, and asked Warren for another chance to demonstrate a new gas of his invention: "letheon".
SIR, YOUR PATIENT IS READY. YOU MAY OPERATE ON HIS NECK TUMOUR.
I JUST HOPE THIS ISN'T YET MORE BUNKUM.
GENTLEMEN, YOU MAY APPLAUD! THIS TIME, IT WORKED. THE PATIENT DIDN'T FEEL A THING!
BUT PROFESSOR, DON'T YOU THINK MR. MORTON'S GAS SMELLS RATHER LIKE DIETHYL ETHER?
Morton's deceit was soon exposed, and he was never able to patent ether and profit from its use.
Moreover, Jackson thought better of his initial scepticism and demanded credit for his discovery.
I'M THE ONE WHO FOUND OUT ABOUT ETHER'S ANAESTHETIC PROPERTIES.
MORTON WAS JUST A STUDENT OF MINE.
NOT EVEN THE BEST!

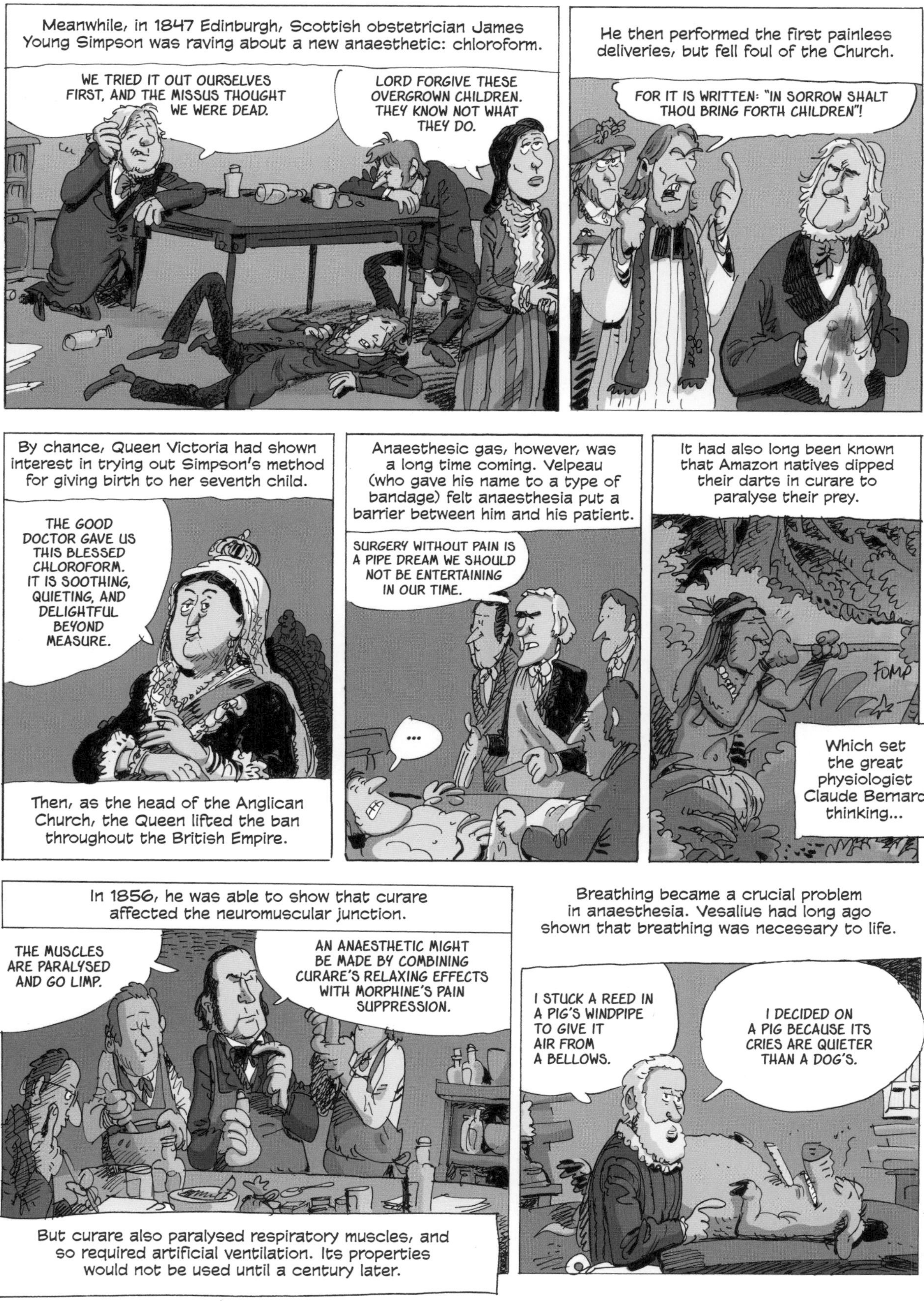
Meanwhile, in 1847 Edinburgh, Scottish obstetrician James Young Simpson was raving about a new anaesthetic: chloroform.
WE TRIED IT OUT OURSELVES FIRST, AND THE MISSUS THOUGHT WE WERE DEAD.
LORD FORGIVE THESE OVERGROWN CHILDREN. THEY KNOW NOT WHAT THEY DO.
He then performed the first painless deliveries, but fell foul of the Church.
FOR IT IS WRITTEN: "IN SORROW SHALT THOU BRING FORTH CHILDREN"!
By chance, Queen Victoria had shown interest in trying out Simpson's method for giving birth to her seventh child.
THE GOOD DOCTOR GAVE US THIS BLESSED CHLOROFORM. IT IS SOOTHING, QUIETING, AND DELIGHTFUL BEYOND MEASURE.
Then, as the head of the Anglican Church, the Queen lifted the ban throughout the British Empire.
Anaesthesic gas, however, was a long time coming. Velpeau (who gave his name to a type of bandage) felt anaesthesia put a barrier between him and his patient.
SURGERY WITHOUT PAIN IS A PIPE DREAM WE SHOULD NOT BE ENTERTAINING IN OUR TIME.
...
It had also long been known that Amazon natives dipped their darts in curare to paralyse their prey.
FOMP
Which set the great physiologist Claude Bernard thinking...
In 1856, he was able to show that curare affected the neuromuscular junction.
THE MUSCLES ARE PARALYSED AND GO LIMP.
AN ANAESTHETIC MIGHT BE MADE BY COMBINING CURARE'S RELAXING EFFECTS WITH MORPHINE'S PAIN SUPPRESSION.
But curare also paralysed respiratory muscles, and so required artificial ventilation. Its properties would not be used until a century later.
Breathing became a crucial problem in anaesthesia. Vesalius had long ago shown that breathing was necessary to life.
I STUCK A REED IN A PIG'S WINDPIPE TO GIVE IT AIR FROM A BELLOWS.
I DECIDED ON A PIG BECAUSE ITS CRIES ARE QUIETER THAN A DOG'S.

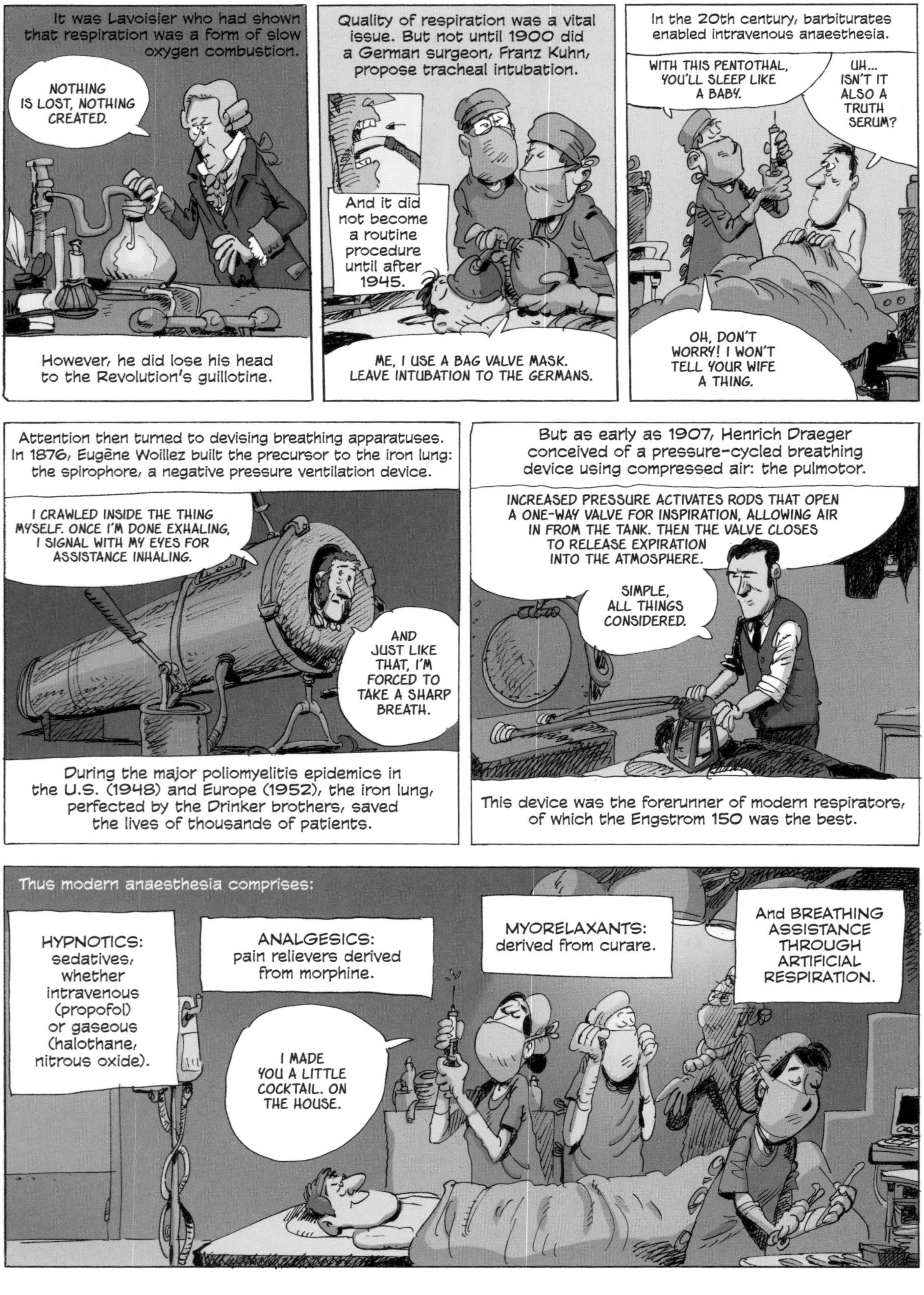
It was Lavoisier who had shown that respiration was a form of slow oxygen combustion.
NOTHING IS LOST, NOTHING CREATED.
However, he did lose his head to the Revolution's guillotine.
Quality of respiration was a vital issue. But not until 1900 did a German surgeon, Franz Kuhn, propose tracheal intubation.
And it did not become a routine procedure until after 1945.
ME, I USE A BAG VALVE MASK. LEAVE INTUBATION TO THE GERMANS.
In the 20th century, barbiturates enabled intravenous anaesthesia.
WITH THIS PENTOTHAL, YOU'LL SLEEP LIKE A BABY.
UH... ISN'T IT ALSO A TRUTH SERUM?
OH, DON'T WORRY! I WON'T TELL YOUR WIFE A THING.
Attention then turned to devising breathing apparatuses. In 1876, Eugène Woillez built the precursor to the iron lung: the spirophore, a negative pressure ventilation device.
I CRAWLED INSIDE THE THING MYSELF. ONCE I'M DONE EXHALING, I SIGNAL WITH MY EYES FOR ASSISTANCE INHALING.
AND JUST LIKE THAT, I'M FORCED TO TAKE A SHARP BREATH.
During the major poliomyelitis epidemics in the U.S. (1948) and Europe (1952), the iron lung, perfected by the Drinker brothers, saved the lives of thousands of patients.
But as early as 1907, Henrich Draeger conceived of a pressure-cycled breathing device using compressed air: the pulmotor.
INCREASED PRESSURE ACTIVATES RODS THAT OPEN A ONE-WAY VALVE FOR INSPIRATION, ALLOWING AIR IN FROM THE TANK. THEN THE VALVE CLOSES TO RELEASE EXPIRATION INTO THE ATMOSPHERE.
SIMPLE, ALL THINGS CONSIDERED.
This device was the forerunner of modern respirators, of which the Engstrom 150 was the best.
Thus modern anaesthesia comprises:
HYPNOTICS: sedatives, whether intravenous (propofol) or gaseous (halothane, nitrous oxide).
ANALGESICS: pain relievers derived from morphine.
MYORELAXANTS: derived from curare.
And BREATHING ASSISTANCE THROUGH ARTIFICIAL RESPIRATION.
I MADE YOU A LITTLE COCKTAIL. ON THE HOUSE.

CHAPTER 9

THE FIGHT AGAINST INFECTION

Robert Koch's discovery of bacteria in Germany, followed by Pasteur's invention of vaccines in France, were incontestably the greatest medical advances of the 19th century, perhaps even landmarks in the history of medicine.

These discoveries were made by exceptional figures animated by unshakeable faith in their mission and willing to make any sacrifice. So it was that Dr. Roux and his colleagues kept a loaded gun in the room during their research on rabies. Should one of them be bitten by a rabid dog, the others had vowed to kill him rather than allow him to suffer its terrible agonies.

It is a pleasure to recount such valiant deeds.

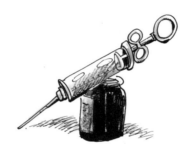

IGNAZ SEMMELWEIS

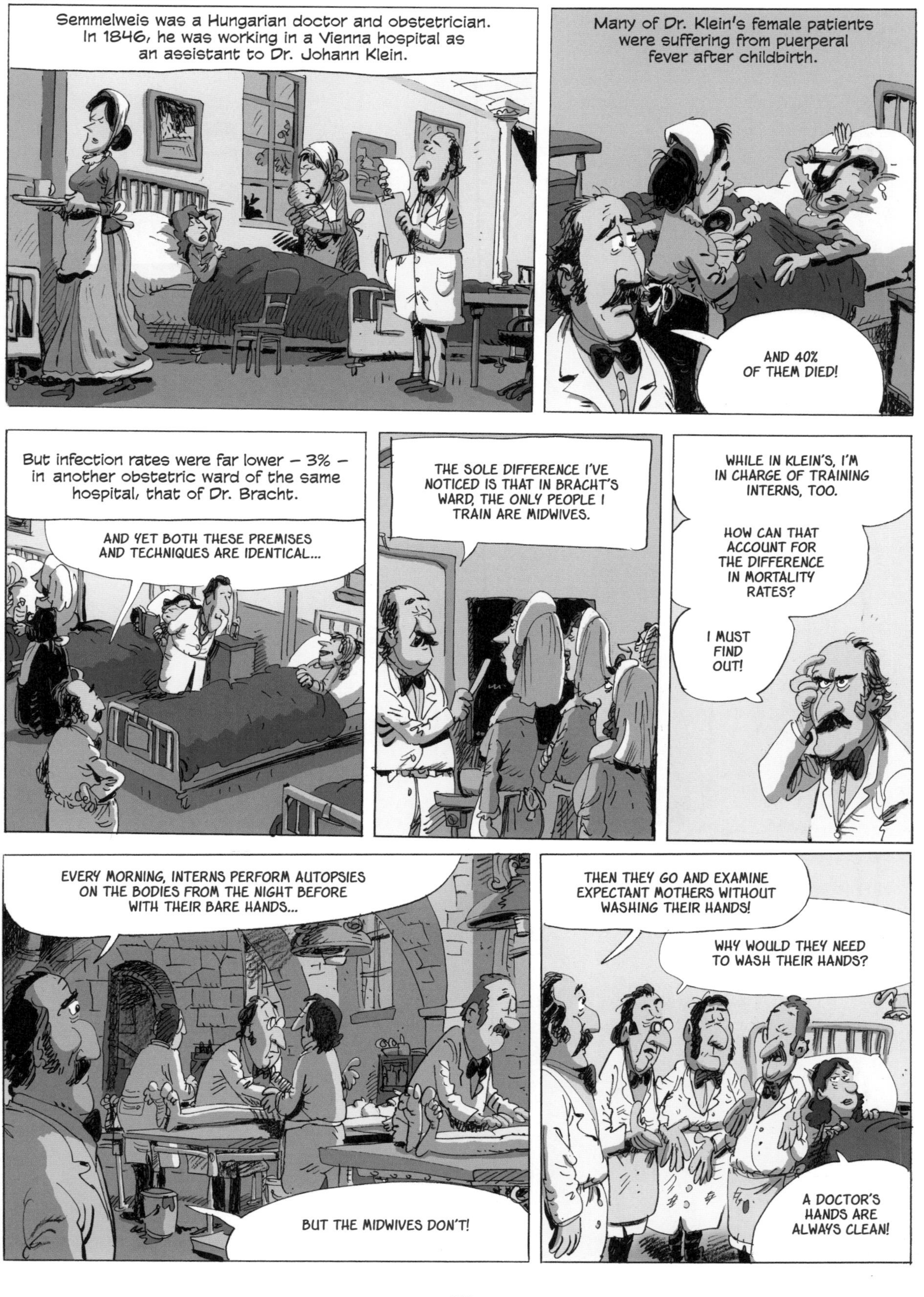
Semmelweis was a Hungarian doctor and obstetrician. In 1846, he was working in a Vienna hospital as an assistant to Dr. Johann Klein.
Many of Dr. Klein's female patients were suffering from puerperal fever after childbirth.
AND 40% OF THEM DIED!
But infection rates were far lower – 3% – in another obstetric ward of the same hospital, that of Dr. Bracht.
AND YET BOTH THESE PREMISES AND TECHNIQUES ARE IDENTICAL...
THE SOLE DIFFERENCE I'VE NOTICED IS THAT IN BRACHT'S WARD, THE ONLY PEOPLE I TRAIN ARE MIDWIVES.
WHILE IN KLEIN'S, I'M IN CHARGE OF TRAINING INTERNS, TOO.
HOW CAN THAT ACCOUNT FOR THE DIFFERENCE IN MORTALITY RATES?
I MUST FIND OUT!
EVERY MORNING, INTERNS PERFORM AUTOPSIES ON THE BODIES FROM THE NIGHT BEFORE WITH THEIR BARE HANDS...
BUT THE MIDWIVES DON'T!
THEN THEY GO AND EXAMINE EXPECTANT MOTHERS WITHOUT WASHING THEIR HANDS!
WHY WOULD THEY NEED TO WASH THEIR HANDS?
A DOCTOR'S HANDS ARE ALWAYS CLEAN!

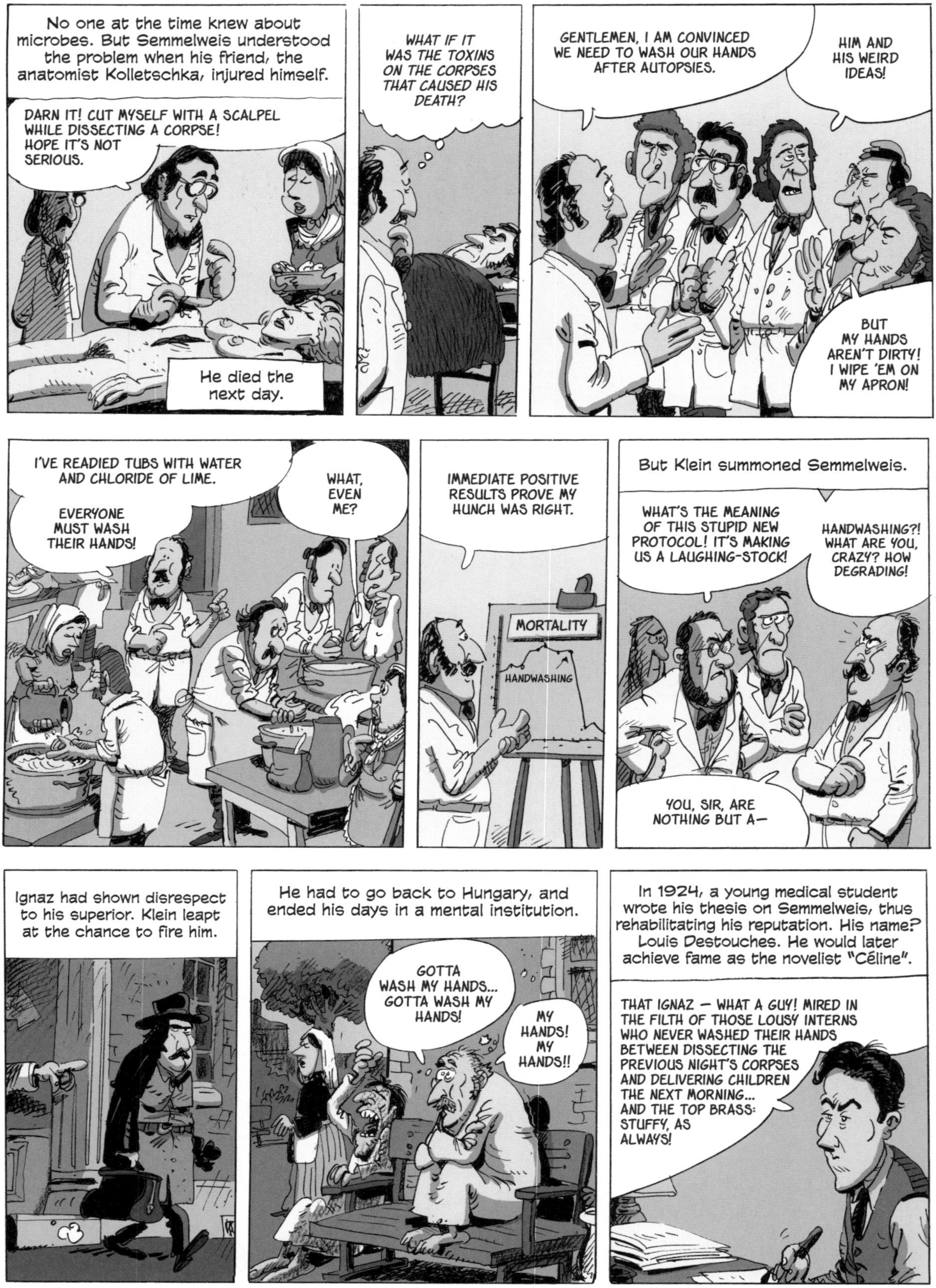
No one at the time knew about microbes. But Semmelweis understood the problem when his friend, the anatomist Kolletschka, injured himself.
DARN IT! CUT MYSELF WITH A SCALPEL WHILE DISSECTING A CORPSE! HOPE IT'S NOT SERIOUS.
He died the next day.
WHAT IF IT WAS THE TOXINS ON THE CORPSES THAT CAUSED HIS DEATH?
GENTLEMEN, I AM CONVINCED WE NEED TO WASH OUR HANDS AFTER AUTOPSIES.
HIM AND HIS WEIRD IDEAS!
BUT MY HANDS AREN'T DIRTY! I WIPE 'EM ON MY APRON!
I'VE READIED TUBS WITH WATER AND CHLORIDE OF LIME.
EVERYONE MUST WASH THEIR HANDS!
WHAT, EVEN ME?
IMMEDIATE POSITIVE RESULTS PROVE MY HUNCH WAS RIGHT.
MORTALITY
HANDWASHING
But Klein summoned Semmelweis.
WHAT'S THE MEANING OF THIS STUPID NEW PROTOCOL! IT'S MAKING US A LAUGHING-STOCK!
HANDWASHING?! WHAT ARE YOU, CRAZY? HOW DEGRADING!
YOU, SIR, ARE NOTHING BUT A—
Ignaz had shown disrespect to his superior. Klein leapt at the chance to fire him.
He had to go back to Hungary, and ended his days in a mental institution.
GOTTA WASH MY HANDS... GOTTA WASH MY HANDS!
MY HANDS! MY HANDS!!
In 1924, a young medical student wrote his thesis on Semmelweis, thus rehabilitating his reputation. His name? Louis Destouches. He would later achieve fame as the novelist "Céline".
THAT IGNAZ — WHAT A GUY! MIRED IN THE FILTH OF THOSE LOUSY INTERNS WHO NEVER WASHED THEIR HANDS BETWEEN DISSECTING THE PREVIOUS NIGHT'S CORPSES AND DELIVERING CHILDREN THE NEXT MORNING... AND THE TOP BRASS: STUFFY, AS ALWAYS!

PASTEUR AND KOCH: THE MICROBIOLOGY REVOLUTION

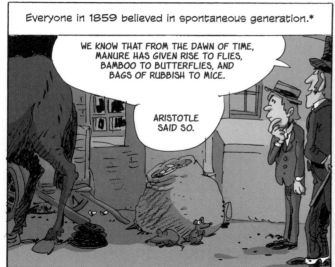

Everyone in 1859 believed in spontaneous generation.*

WE KNOW THAT FROM THE DAWN OF TIME, MANURE HAS GIVEN RISE TO FLIES, BAMBOO TO BUTTERFLIES, AND BAGS OF RUBBISH TO MICE.

ARISTOTLE SAID SO.

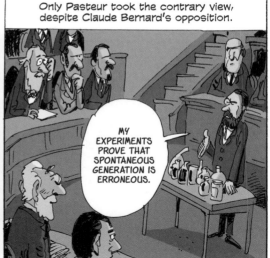

Only Pasteur took the contrary view, despite Claude Bernard's opposition.

MY EXPERIMENTS PROVE THAT SPONTANEOUS GENERATION IS ERRONEOUS.

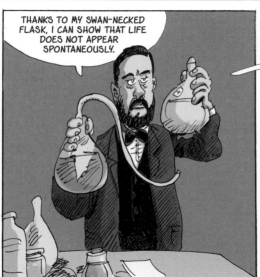

THANKS TO MY SWAN-NECKED FLASK, I CAN SHOW THAT LIFE DOES NOT APPEAR SPONTANEOUSLY.

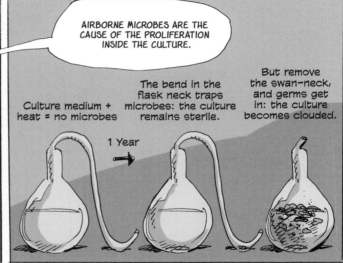

AIRBORNE MICROBES ARE THE CAUSE OF THE PROLIFERATION INSIDE THE CULTURE.

Culture medium + heat = no microbes

The bend in the flask neck traps microbes: the culture remains sterile.

But remove the swan-neck, and germs get in: the culture becomes clouded.

1 Year

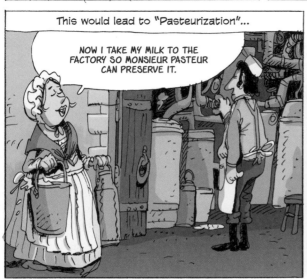

This would lead to "Pasteurization"...

NOW I TAKE MY MILK TO THE FACTORY SO MONSIEUR PASTEUR CAN PRESERVE IT.

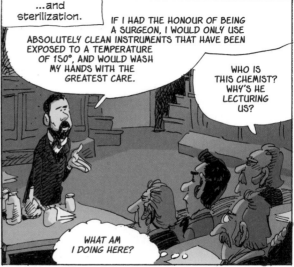

...and sterilization.

IF I HAD THE HONOUR OF BEING A SURGEON, I WOULD ONLY USE ABSOLUTELY CLEAN INSTRUMENTS THAT HAVE BEEN EXPOSED TO A TEMPERATURE OF 150°, AND WOULD WASH MY HANDS WITH THE GREATEST CARE.

WHO IS THIS CHEMIST? WHY'S HE LECTURING US?

WHAT AM I DOING HERE?

* The theory stating that all small organisms spontaneously come into being under specific conditions.

In France, Pasteur's words fell on deaf ears. But in Glasgow, in 1865, Joseph Lister started pondering...

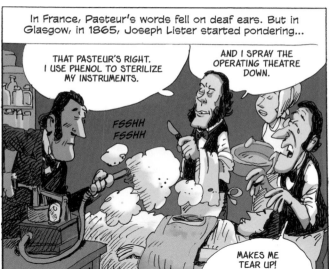

THAT PASTEUR'S RIGHT. I USE PHENOL TO STERILIZE MY INSTRUMENTS.

AND I SPRAY THE OPERATING THEATRE DOWN.

FSSHH FSSHH

MAKES ME TEAR UP!

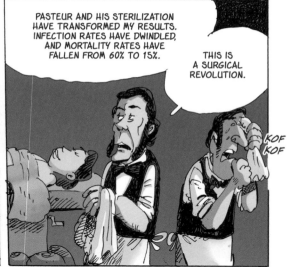

PASTEUR AND HIS STERILIZATION HAVE TRANSFORMED MY RESULTS. INFECTION RATES HAVE DWINDLED, AND MORTALITY RATES HAVE FALLEN FROM 60% TO 15%.

THIS IS A SURGICAL REVOLUTION.

KOF KOF

Meanwhile, in Berlin, Robert Koch was busy growing bacteria. He isolated them, coloured them, observed them, manipulated them, and injected them into healthy hosts. He was inventing microbiology.

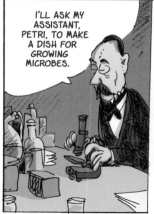

I'LL ASK MY ASSISTANT, PETRI, TO MAKE A DISH FOR GROWING MICROBES.

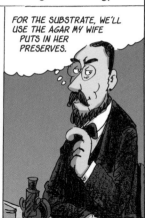

FOR THE SUBSTRATE, WE'LL USE THE AGAR MY WIFE PUTS IN HER PRESERVES.

Koch also formulated theories intended to establish a causal relationship between germs and disease.

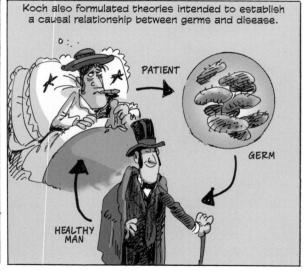

PATIENT

GERM

HEALTHY MAN

Thanks to his techniques, he discovered the main strains of bacteria.

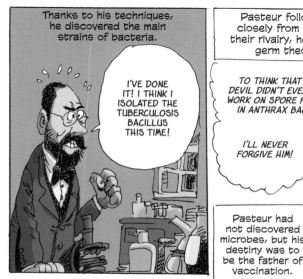

I'VE DONE IT! I THINK I ISOLATED THE TUBERCULOSIS BACILLUS THIS TIME!

Pasteur followed Koch's work closely from Paris, and despite their rivalry, he believed in Koch's germ theory of disease.

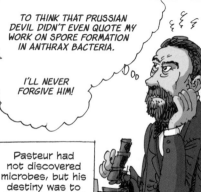

TO THINK THAT PRUSSIAN DEVIL DIDN'T EVEN QUOTE MY WORK ON SPORE FORMATION IN ANTHRAX BACTERIA.

I'LL NEVER FORGIVE HIM!

Pasteur had not discovered microbes, but his destiny was to be the father of vaccination.

It all began one day in 1880, with an outbreak of fowl cholera. Pasteur's assistant Charles Chamberland was coming back from vacation...

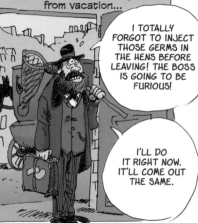

I TOTALLY FORGOT TO INJECT THOSE GERMS IN THE HENS BEFORE LEAVING! THE BOSS IS GOING TO BE FURIOUS!

I'LL DO IT RIGHT NOW. IT'LL COME OUT THE SAME.

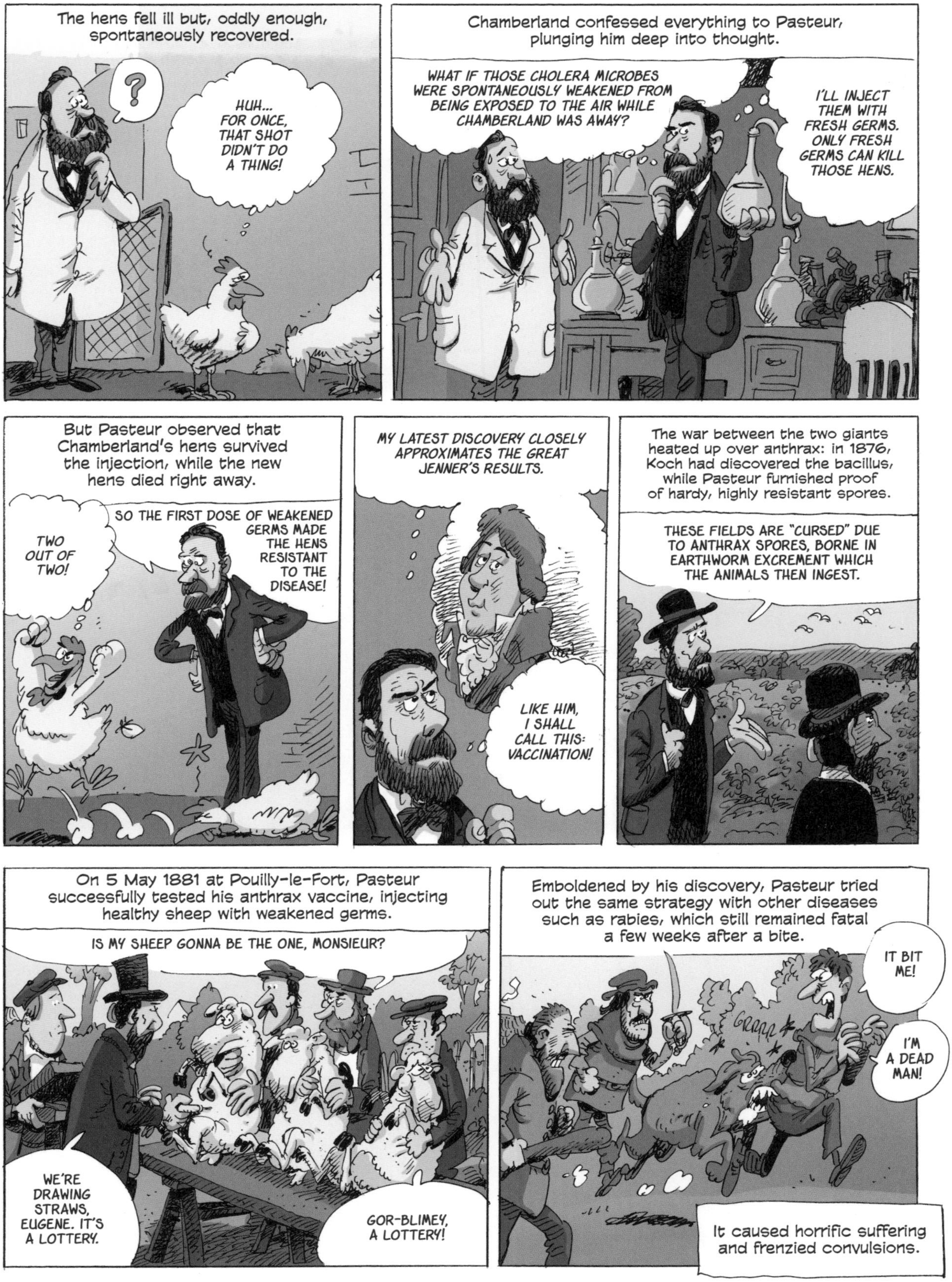
The hens fell ill but, oddly enough, spontaneously recovered.
?
HUH... FOR ONCE, THAT SHOT DIDN'T DO A THING!
Chamberland confessed everything to Pasteur, plunging him deep into thought.
WHAT IF THOSE CHOLERA MICROBES WERE SPONTANEOUSLY WEAKENED FROM BEING EXPOSED TO THE AIR WHILE CHAMBERLAND WAS AWAY?
I'LL INJECT THEM WITH FRESH GERMS. ONLY FRESH GERMS CAN KILL THOSE HENS.
But Pasteur observed that Chamberland's hens survived the injection, while the new hens died right away.
TWO OUT OF TWO!
SO THE FIRST DOSE OF WEAKENED GERMS MADE THE HENS RESISTANT TO THE DISEASE!
MY LATEST DISCOVERY CLOSELY APPROXIMATES THE GREAT JENNER'S RESULTS.
LIKE HIM, I SHALL CALL THIS: VACCINATION!
The war between the two giants heated up over anthrax: in 1876, Koch had discovered the bacillus, while Pasteur furnished proof of hardy, highly resistant spores.
THESE FIELDS ARE "CURSED" DUE TO ANTHRAX SPORES, BORNE IN EARTHWORM EXCREMENT WHICH THE ANIMALS THEN INGEST.
On 5 May 1881 at Pouilly-le-Fort, Pasteur successfully tested his anthrax vaccine, injecting healthy sheep with weakened germs.
IS MY SHEEP GONNA BE THE ONE, MONSIEUR?
WE'RE DRAWING STRAWS, EUGENE. IT'S A LOTTERY.
GOR-BLIMEY, A LOTTERY!
Emboldened by his discovery, Pasteur tried out the same strategy with other diseases such as rabies, which still remained fatal a few weeks after a bite.
IT BIT ME!
I'M A DEAD MAN!
GRRRR
It caused horrific suffering and frenzied convulsions.

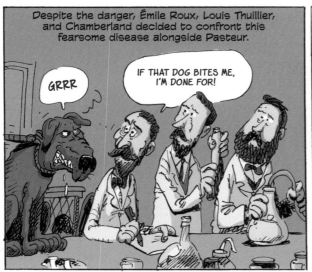

Despite the danger, Émile Roux, Louis Thuillier, and Chamberland decided to confront this fearsome disease alongside Pasteur.

GRRR

IF THAT DOG BITES ME, I'M DONE FOR!

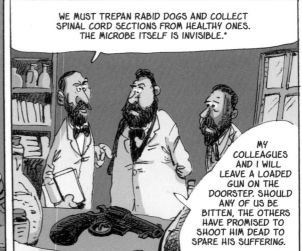

WE MUST TREPAN RABID DOGS AND COLLECT SPINAL CORD SECTIONS FROM HEALTHY ONES. THE MICROBE ITSELF IS INVISIBLE.*

MY COLLEAGUES AND I WILL LEAVE A LOADED GUN ON THE DOORSTEP. SHOULD ANY OF US BE BITTEN, THE OTHERS HAVE PROMISED TO SHOOT HIM DEAD TO SPARE HIS SUFFERING.

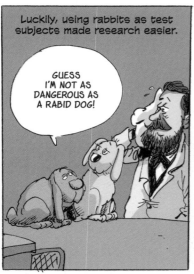

Luckily, using rabbits as test subjects made research easier.

GUESS I'M NOT AS DANGEROUS AS A RABID DOG!

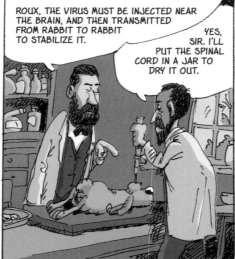

ROUX, THE VIRUS MUST BE INJECTED NEAR THE BRAIN, AND THEN TRANSMITTED FROM RABBIT TO RABBIT TO STABILIZE IT.

YES, SIR. I'LL PUT THE SPINAL CORD IN A JAR TO DRY IT OUT.

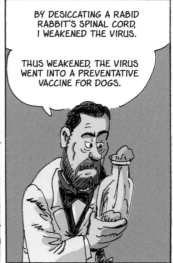

BY DESICCATING A RABID RABBIT'S SPINAL CORD, I WEAKENED THE VIRUS.

THUS WEAKENED, THE VIRUS WENT INTO A PREVENTATIVE VACCINE FOR DOGS.

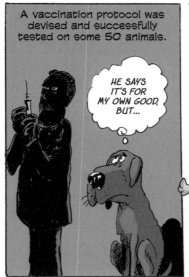

A vaccination protocol was devised and successfully tested on some 50 animals.

HE SAYS IT'S FOR MY OWN GOOD, BUT...

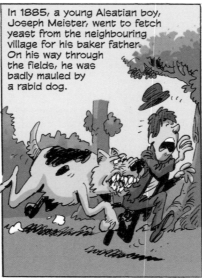

In 1885, a young Alsatian boy, Joseph Meister, went to fetch yeast from the neighbouring village for his baker father. On his way through the fields, he was badly mauled by a rabid dog.

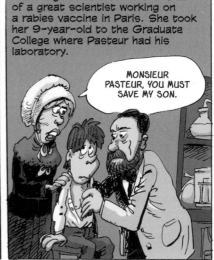

The village doctor told his mother of a great scientist working on a rabies vaccine in Paris. She took her 9-year-old to the Graduate College where Pasteur had his laboratory.

MONSIEUR PASTEUR, YOU MUST SAVE MY SON.

* In fact, it is a virus, which can only be seen with an electron microscope.

At the time, Pasteur was not yet the scientific giant he would later become.

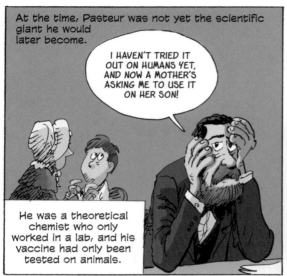

I HAVEN'T TRIED IT OUT ON HUMANS YET, AND NOW A MOTHER'S ASKING ME TO USE IT ON HER SON!

He was a theoretical chemist who only worked in a lab, and his vaccine had only been tested on animals.

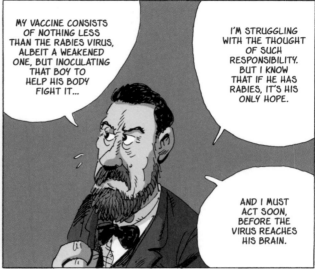

MY VACCINE CONSISTS OF NOTHING LESS THAN THE RABIES VIRUS, ALBEIT A WEAKENED ONE, BUT INOCULATING THAT BOY TO HELP HIS BODY FIGHT IT...

I'M STRUGGLING WITH THE THOUGHT OF SUCH RESPONSIBILITY. BUT I KNOW THAT IF HE HAS RABIES, IT'S HIS ONLY HOPE.

AND I MUST ACT SOON, BEFORE THE VIRUS REACHES HIS BRAIN.

Pasteur hesitated, but two eminent physicians, Professor Alfred Vulpian and Dr. Jacques-Joseph Grancher, administered the 13 injections, each with a more virulent strain.

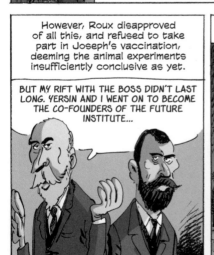

6 July 1885.

To put the matter beyond doubt, Pasteur took the risk of inoculating Joseph secondarily with a particularly aggressive form of rabies... and he continued to do just fine. The vaccine had been effective.

OKAY, SO I EXPERIMENTED ON A HUMAN BEING...

BUT SO DID JENNER!

However, Roux disapproved of all this, and refused to take part in Joseph's vaccination, deeming the animal experiments insufficiently conclusive as yet.

BUT MY RIFT WITH THE BOSS DIDN'T LAST LONG. YERSIN AND I WENT ON TO BECOME THE CO-FOUNDERS OF THE FUTURE INSTITUTE...

...which opened on 14 November 1888.

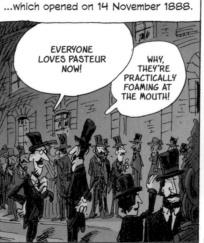

EVERYONE LOVES PASTEUR NOW!

WHY, THEY'RE PRACTICALLY FOAMING AT THE MOUTH!

As for young Joseph Meister, he became the Pasteur Institute's caretaker.

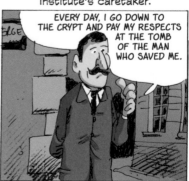

EVERY DAY, I GO DOWN TO THE CRYPT AND PAY MY RESPECTS AT THE TOMB OF THE MAN WHO SAVED ME.

Meister committed suicide in 1940, unable to bear – it is said – the prospect of Nazi stormtroopers marching through the doors of the crypt.

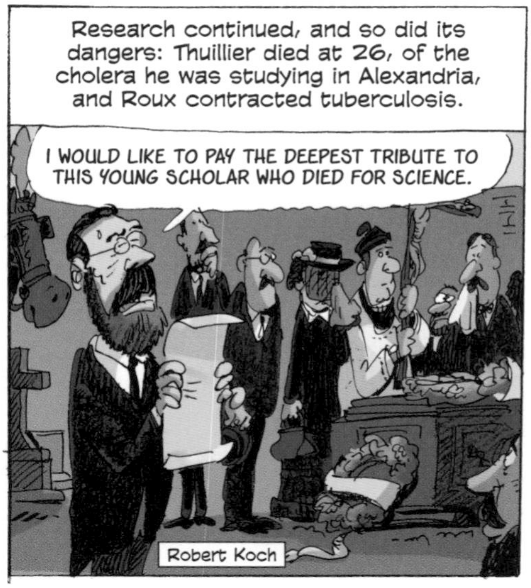
Research continued, and so did its dangers: Thuillier died at 26, of the cholera he was studying in Alexandria, and Roux contracted tuberculosis.
I WOULD LIKE TO PAY THE DEEPEST TRIBUTE TO THIS YOUNG SCHOLAR WHO DIED FOR SCIENCE.
Robert Koch

But it was still unclear how our bodies naturally fought off germs, and how vaccines worked. The task of finding out fell to the students of Koch and Pasteur.

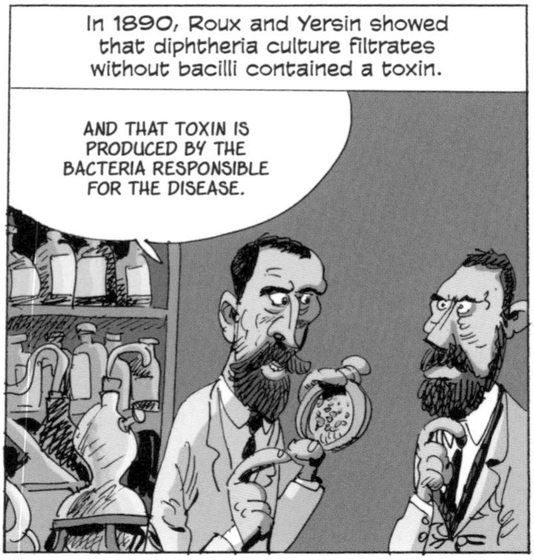
In 1890, Roux and Yersin showed that diphtheria culture filtrates without bacilli contained a toxin.
AND THAT TOXIN IS PRODUCED BY THE BACTERIA RESPONSIBLE FOR THE DISEASE.

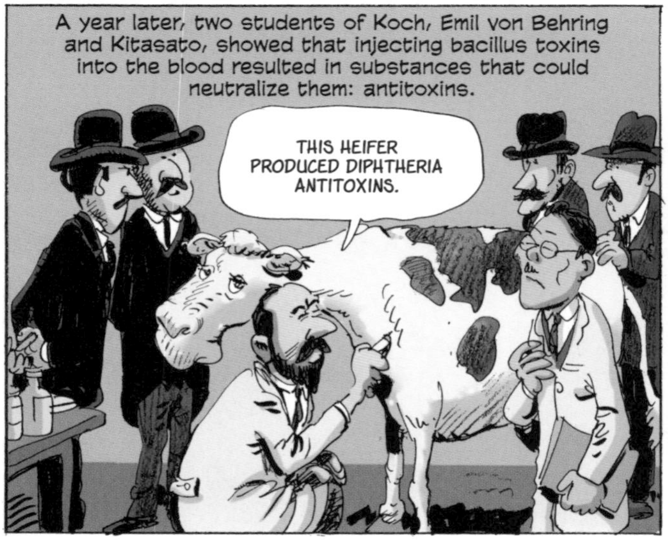
A year later, two students of Koch, Emil von Behring and Kitasato, showed that injecting bacillus toxins into the blood resulted in substances that could neutralize them: antitoxins.
THIS HEIFER PRODUCED DIPHTHERIA ANTITOXINS.

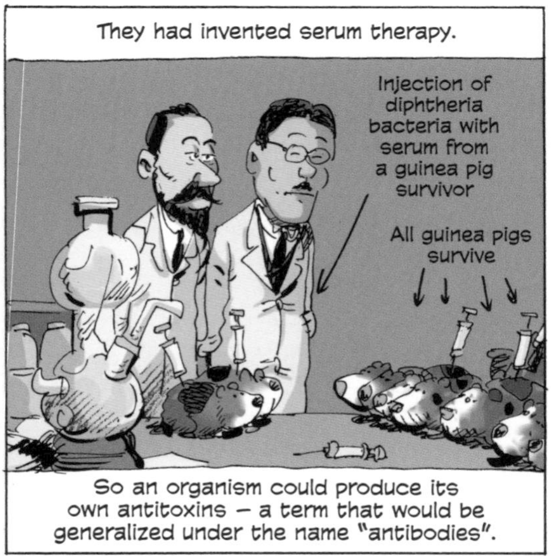
They had invented serum therapy.
Injection of diphtheria bacteria with serum from a guinea pig survivor
All guinea pigs survive
So an organism could produce its own antitoxins — a term that would be generalized under the name "antibodies".

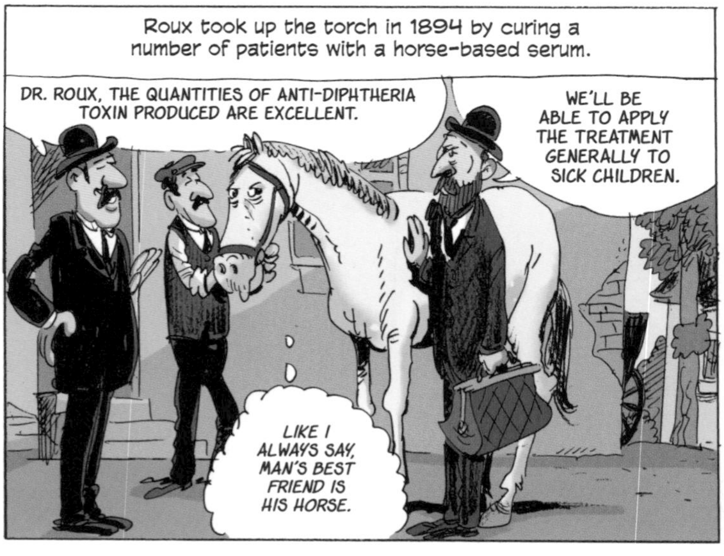
Roux took up the torch in 1894 by curing a number of patients with a horse-based serum.
DR. ROUX, THE QUANTITIES OF ANTI-DIPHTHERIA TOXIN PRODUCED ARE EXCELLENT.
WE'LL BE ABLE TO APPLY THE TREATMENT GENERALLY TO SICK CHILDREN.
LIKE I ALWAYS SAY, MAN'S BEST FRIEND IS HIS HORSE.

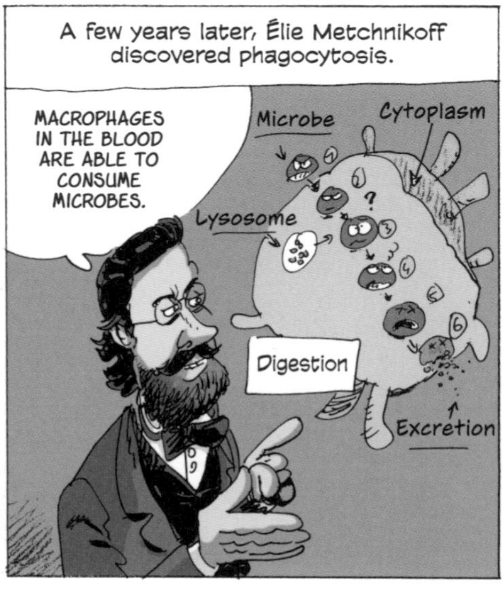
A few years later, Élie Metchnikoff discovered phagocytosis.
MACROPHAGES IN THE BLOOD ARE ABLE TO CONSUME MICROBES.
Microbe
Cytoplasm
Lysosome
Digestion
Excretion

The body defended itself against microbes, either by making antibodies, or by mobilizing white blood cells.

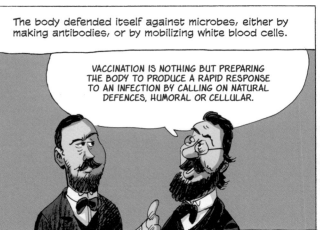

VACCINATION IS NOTHING BUT PREPARING THE BODY TO PRODUCE A RAPID RESPONSE TO AN INFECTION BY CALLING ON NATURAL DEFENCES, HUMORAL OR CELLULAR.

Behring and Metchnikoff had just invented a new science: immunology.

Koch had discovered the tuberculosis bacillus (B.K.), but he needed a vaccine. Two of Pasteur's men set to it.

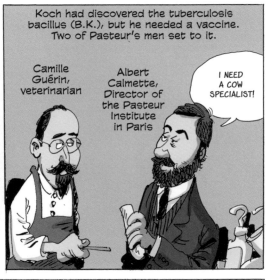

Camille Guérin, veterinarian

Albert Calmette, Director of the Pasteur Institute in Paris

I NEED A COW SPECIALIST!

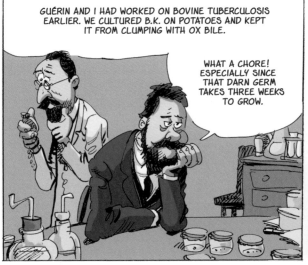

GUÉRIN AND I HAD WORKED ON BOVINE TUBERCULOSIS EARLIER. WE CULTURED B.K. ON POTATOES AND KEPT IT FROM CLUMPING WITH OX BILE.

WHAT A CHORE! ESPECIALLY SINCE THAT DARN GERM TAKES THREE WEEKS TO GROW.

WE HAD TO KEEP SUBCULTURING OUR STRAIN TO MULTIPLY IT. WE NOTED THAT THIS LOWERED ITS VIRULENCE.

I HAD TO SUBCULTURE IT 230 TIMES OVER 13 YEARS!

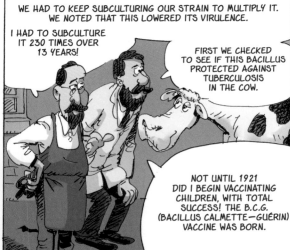

FIRST WE CHECKED TO SEE IF THIS BACILLUS PROTECTED AGAINST TUBERCULOSIS IN THE COW.

NOT UNTIL 1921 DID I BEGIN VACCINATING CHILDREN, WITH TOTAL SUCCESS! THE B.C.G. (BACILLUS CALMETTE—GUÉRIN) VACCINE WAS BORN.

At the time, using the optical microscope, students of Koch and Pasteur were able to clearly see bacteria they had coloured.

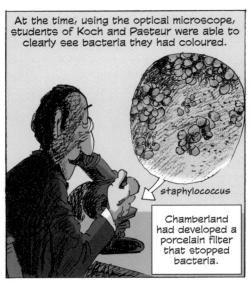

staphylococcus

Chamberland had developed a porcelain filter that stopped bacteria.

But in Delft in 1898, Martinus Beijerinck, working on tobacco mosaic disease, ground up infected leaves...

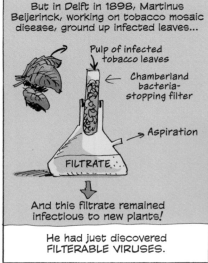

Pulp of infected tobacco leaves

← Chamberland bacteria-stopping filter

→ Aspiration

FILTRATE

And this filtrate remained infectious to new plants!

He had just discovered FILTERABLE VIRUSES.

But these viruses would remain unseen till the electron microscope.

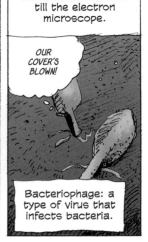

OUR COVER'S BLOWN!

Bacteriophage: a type of virus that infects bacteria.

HALSTED AND THE GLOVES OF LOVE

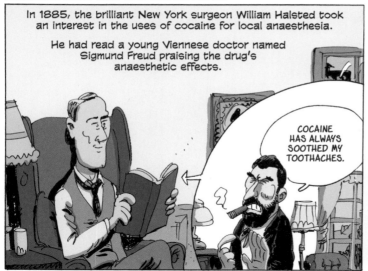

In 1885, the brilliant New York surgeon William Halsted took an interest in the uses of cocaine for local anaesthesia.

He had read a young Viennese doctor named Sigmund Freud praising the drug's anaesthetic effects.

COCAINE HAS ALWAYS SOOTHED MY TOOTHACHES.

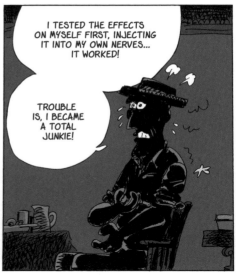

I TESTED THE EFFECTS ON MYSELF FIRST, INJECTING IT INTO MY OWN NERVES... IT WORKED!

TROUBLE IS, I BECAME A TOTAL JUNKIE!

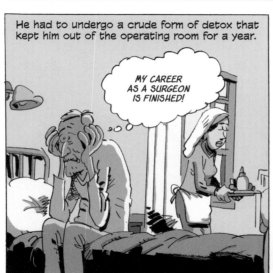

He had to undergo a crude form of detox that kept him out of the operating room for a year.

MY CAREER AS A SURGEON IS FINISHED!

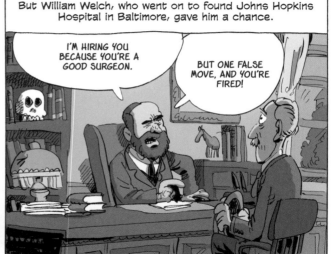

But William Welch, who went on to found Johns Hopkins Hospital in Baltimore, gave him a chance.

I'M HIRING YOU BECAUSE YOU'RE A GOOD SURGEON.

BUT ONE FALSE MOVE, AND YOU'RE FIRED!

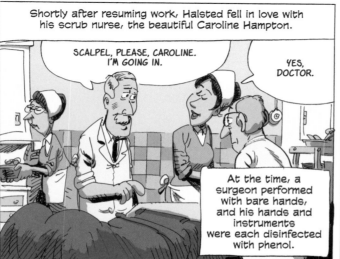

Shortly after resuming work, Halsted fell in love with his scrub nurse, the beautiful Caroline Hampton.

SCALPEL, PLEASE, CAROLINE. I'M GOING IN.

YES, DOCTOR.

At the time, a surgeon performed with bare hands, and his hands and instruments were each disinfected with phenol.

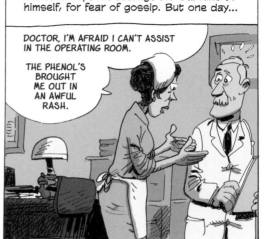

Halsted kept his feelings for Caroline to himself, for fear of gossip. But one day...

DOCTOR, I'M AFRAID I CAN'T ASSIST IN THE OPERATING ROOM.

THE PHENOL'S BROUGHT ME OUT IN AN AWFUL RASH.

Halsted, who could not bear the thought of losing Caroline, paid a visit to Charles Goodyear, who had just invented a new substance: rubber.

WOULD YOU BE ABLE TO MAKE A PAIR OF GLOVES THAT WOULD FIT MISS HAMPTON LIKE A SECOND SKIN AND PROTECT HER FROM ANTISEPTICS?

HMM... COULD DO!

Caroline was able to stay with her surgeon.

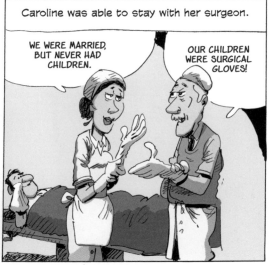

WE WERE MARRIED, BUT NEVER HAD CHILDREN.

OUR CHILDREN WERE SURGICAL GLOVES!

And so it was that surgical gloves came to be invented... out of love!

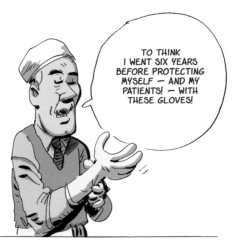

TO THINK I WENT SIX YEARS BEFORE PROTECTING MYSELF — AND MY PATIENTS! — WITH THESE GLOVES!

Halsted indeed went on to perform great acts of surgery, as Welch had predicted.

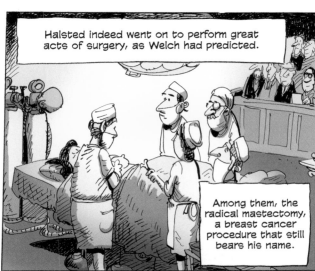

Among them, the radical mastectomy, a breast cancer procedure that still bears his name.

He became a professor, and along with William Welch, William Osler, and Horace Kelly, founded Johns Hopkins Hospital.

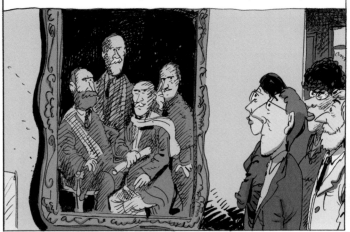

And his drug habit?

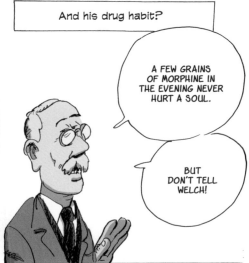

A FEW GRAINS OF MORPHINE IN THE EVENING NEVER HURT A SOUL.

BUT DON'T TELL WELCH!

THE DISCOVERY OF VITAMINS

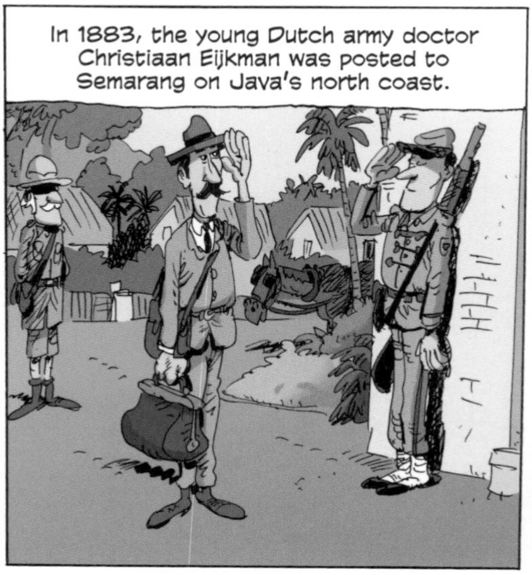
In 1883, the young Dutch army doctor Christiaan Eijkman was posted to Semarang on Java's north coast.

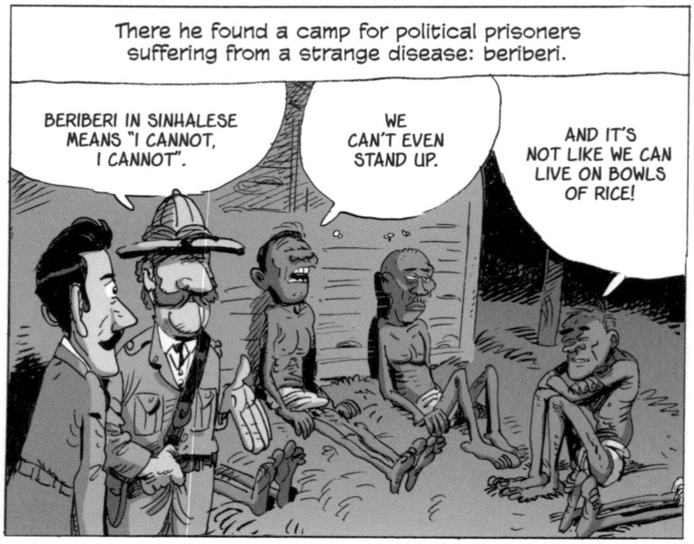
There he found a camp for political prisoners suffering from a strange disease: beriberi.
BERIBERI IN SINHALESE MEANS "I CANNOT, I CANNOT".
WE CAN'T EVEN STAND UP.
AND IT'S NOT LIKE WE CAN LIVE ON BOWLS OF RICE!

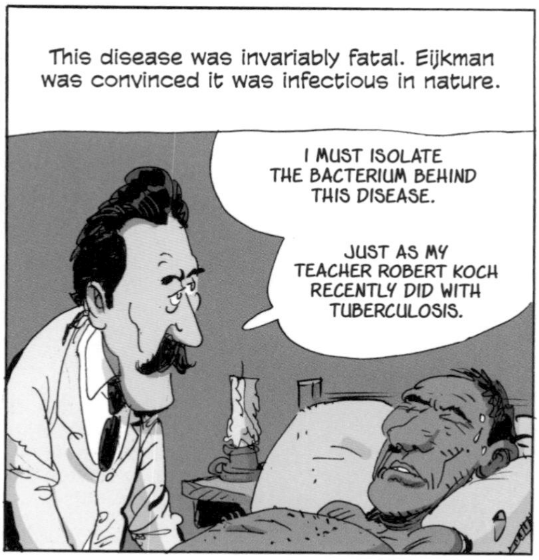
This disease was invariably fatal. Eijkman was convinced it was infectious in nature.
I MUST ISOLATE THE BACTERIUM BEHIND THIS DISEASE.
JUST AS MY TEACHER ROBERT KOCH RECENTLY DID WITH TUBERCULOSIS.

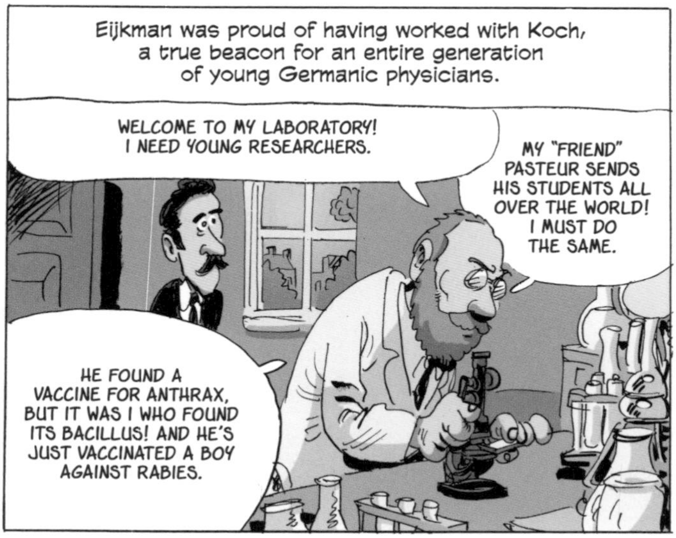
Eijkman was proud of having worked with Koch, a true beacon for an entire generation of young Germanic physicians.
WELCOME TO MY LABORATORY! I NEED YOUNG RESEARCHERS.
MY "FRIEND" PASTEUR SENDS HIS STUDENTS ALL OVER THE WORLD! I MUST DO THE SAME.
HE FOUND A VACCINE FOR ANTHRAX, BUT IT WAS I WHO FOUND ITS BACILLUS! AND HE'S JUST VACCINATED A BOY AGAINST RABIES.

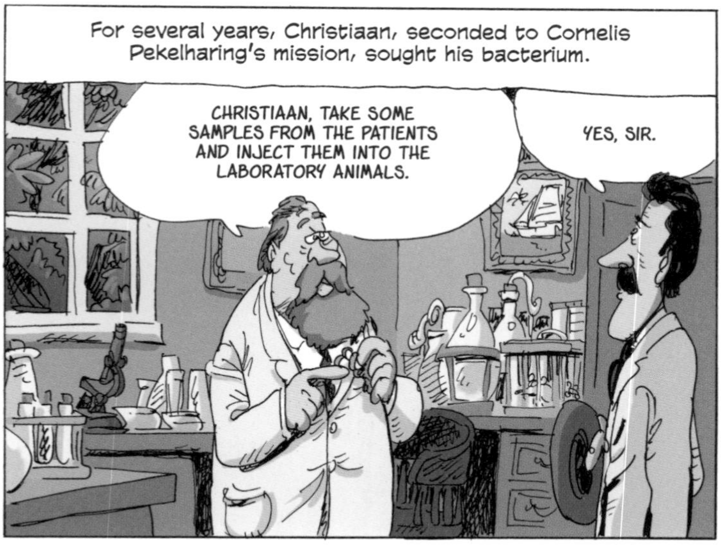
For several years, Christiaan, seconded to Cornelis Pekelharing's mission, sought his bacterium.
CHRISTIAAN, TAKE SOME SAMPLES FROM THE PATIENTS AND INJECT THEM INTO THE LABORATORY ANIMALS.
YES, SIR.

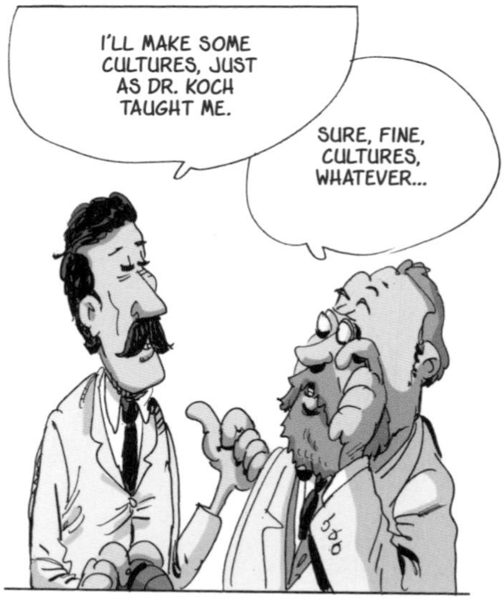
I'LL MAKE SOME CULTURES, JUST AS DR. KOCH TAUGHT ME.
SURE, FINE, CULTURES, WHATEVER...

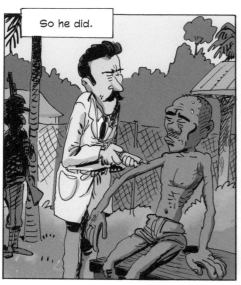

So he did.

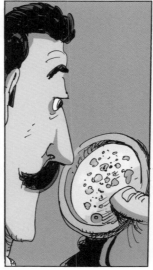

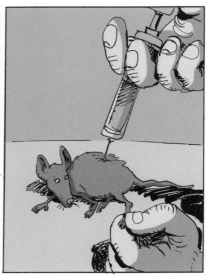

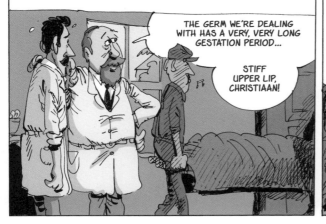

But his results were disappointing, and the inoculations didn't work. The prisoners kept dying. Not that the soldiers really cared.

THE GERM WE'RE DEALING WITH HAS A VERY, VERY LONG GESTATION PERIOD...

STIFF UPPER LIP, CHRISTIAAN!

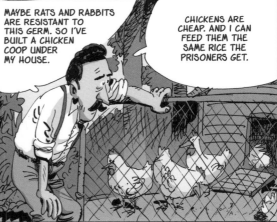

Eijkman decided to switch species and picked hens as his new test subjects.

MAYBE RATS AND RABBITS ARE RESISTANT TO THIS GERM. SO I'VE BUILT A CHICKEN COOP UNDER MY HOUSE.

CHICKENS ARE CHEAP. AND I CAN FEED THEM THE SAME RICE THE PRISONERS GET.

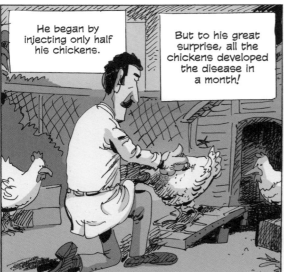

He began by injecting only half his chickens.

But to his great surprise, all the chickens developed the disease in a month!

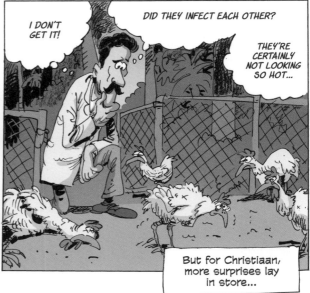

I DON'T GET IT!

DID THEY INFECT EACH OTHER?

THEY'RE CERTAINLY NOT LOOKING SO HOT...

But for Christiaan, more surprises lay in store...

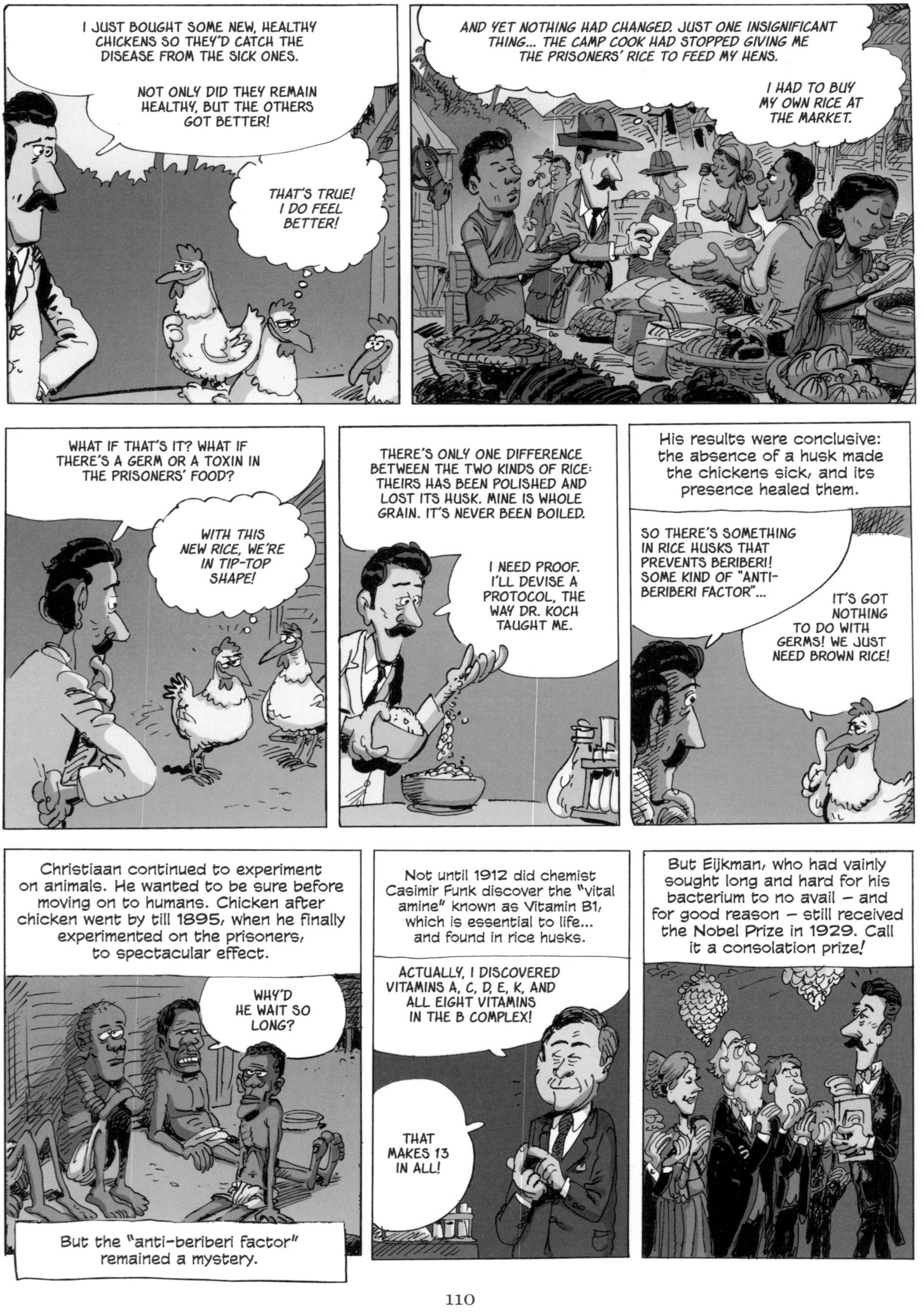
I JUST BOUGHT SOME NEW, HEALTHY CHICKENS SO THEY'D CATCH THE DISEASE FROM THE SICK ONES.
NOT ONLY DID THEY REMAIN HEALTHY, BUT THE OTHERS GOT BETTER!
THAT'S TRUE! I DO FEEL BETTER!
AND YET NOTHING HAD CHANGED. JUST ONE INSIGNIFICANT THING... THE CAMP COOK HAD STOPPED GIVING ME THE PRISONERS' RICE TO FEED MY HENS.
I HAD TO BUY MY OWN RICE AT THE MARKET.
WHAT IF THAT'S IT? WHAT IF THERE'S A GERM OR A TOXIN IN THE PRISONERS' FOOD?
WITH THIS NEW RICE, WE'RE IN TIP-TOP SHAPE!
THERE'S ONLY ONE DIFFERENCE BETWEEN THE TWO KINDS OF RICE: THEIRS HAS BEEN POLISHED AND LOST ITS HUSK. MINE IS WHOLE GRAIN. IT'S NEVER BEEN BOILED.
I NEED PROOF. I'LL DEVISE A PROTOCOL, THE WAY DR. KOCH TAUGHT ME.
His results were conclusive: the absence of a husk made the chickens sick, and its presence healed them.
SO THERE'S SOMETHING IN RICE HUSKS THAT PREVENTS BERIBERI! SOME KIND OF "ANTI-BERIBERI FACTOR"...
IT'S GOT NOTHING TO DO WITH GERMS! WE JUST NEED BROWN RICE!
Christiaan continued to experiment on animals. He wanted to be sure before moving on to humans. Chicken after chicken went by till 1895, when he finally experimented on the prisoners, to spectacular effect.
WHY'D HE WAIT SO LONG?
But the "anti-beriberi factor" remained a mystery.
Not until 1912 did chemist Casimir Funk discover the "vital amine" known as Vitamin B1, which is essential to life... and found in rice husks.
ACTUALLY, I DISCOVERED VITAMINS A, C, D, E, K, AND ALL EIGHT VITAMINS IN THE B COMPLEX!
THAT MAKES 13 IN ALL!
But Eijkman, who had vainly sought long and hard for his bacterium to no avail – and for good reason – still received the Nobel Prize in 1929. Call it a consolation prize!

CHAPTER 10

EXPERIMENTAL MEDICINE

The last of the great 19th-century medical revolutions was that of Magendie, in particular his student Claude Bernard's introduction of experimental medicine. Their goal was to understand how organs worked, and analyse the composition of blood. They would not be satisfied by merely describing, as had been the practice until then, but only by performing actual experiments.

The beginning was rocky, faced with the ignorance, even the downright contempt, of many physicians of the time.

And yet experimental medicine heralded the astonishing leap of modern medicine.

This is yet another of the great turning points in the history of medicine—and history itself.

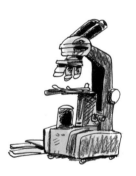

In the early 19th century, physicians were not interested in biology, and no one knew what blood was made up of.

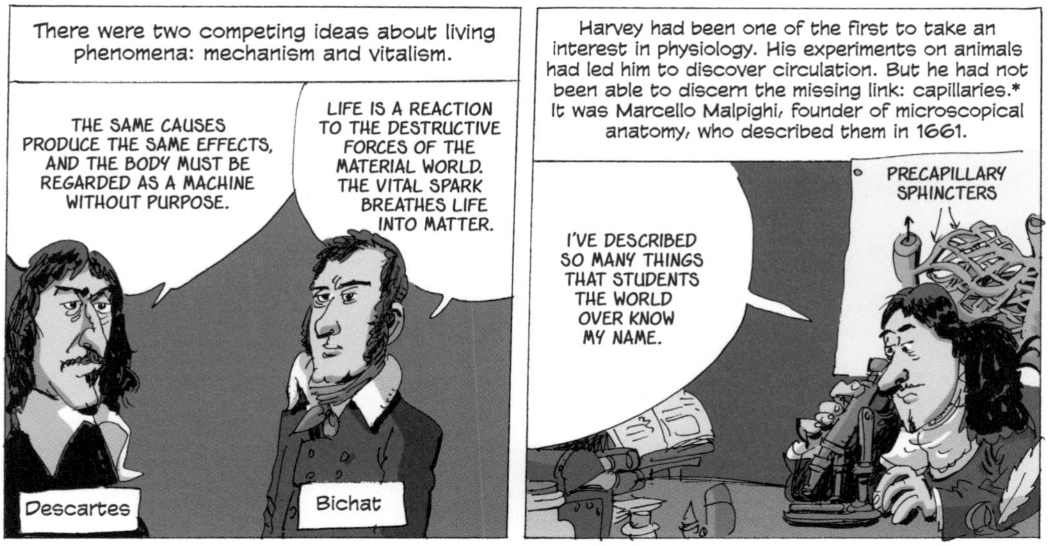
There were two competing ideas about living phenomena: mechanism and vitalism.
THE SAME CAUSES PRODUCE THE SAME EFFECTS, AND THE BODY MUST BE REGARDED AS A MACHINE WITHOUT PURPOSE.
LIFE IS A REACTION TO THE DESTRUCTIVE FORCES OF THE MATERIAL WORLD. THE VITAL SPARK BREATHES LIFE INTO MATTER.
Descartes
Bichat
Harvey had been one of the first to take an interest in physiology. His experiments on animals had led him to discover circulation. But he had not been able to discern the missing link: capillaries.* It was Marcello Malpighi, founder of microscopical anatomy, who described them in 1661.
I'VE DESCRIBED SO MANY THINGS THAT STUDENTS THE WORLD OVER KNOW MY NAME.
PRECAPILLARY SPHINCTERS

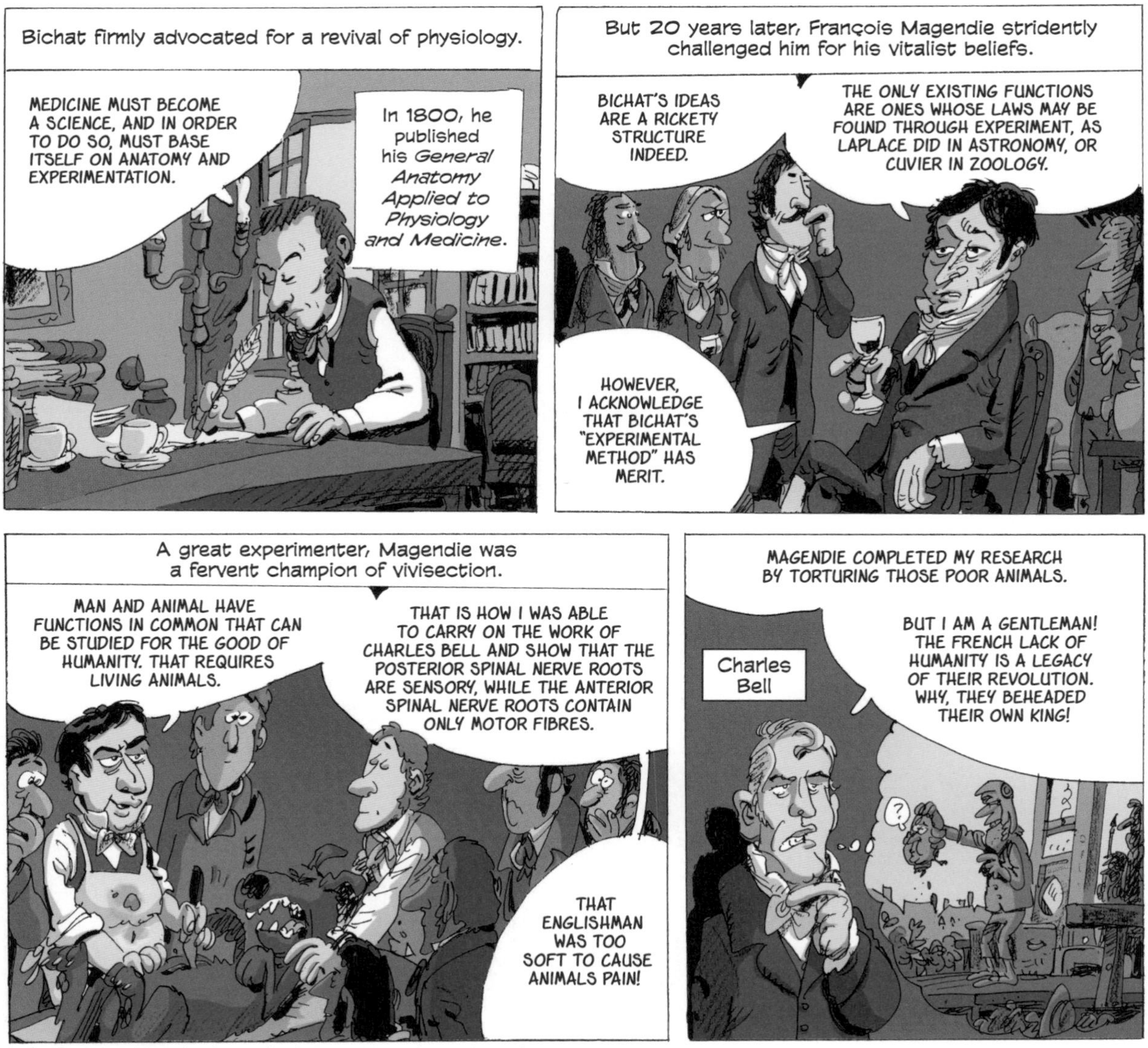
Bichat firmly advocated for a revival of physiology.
MEDICINE MUST BECOME A SCIENCE, AND IN ORDER TO DO SO, MUST BASE ITSELF ON ANATOMY AND EXPERIMENTATION.
In 1800, he published his *General Anatomy Applied to Physiology and Medicine*.
But 20 years later, François Magendie stridently challenged him for his vitalist beliefs.
BICHAT'S IDEAS ARE A RICKETY STRUCTURE INDEED.
THE ONLY EXISTING FUNCTIONS ARE ONES WHOSE LAWS MAY BE FOUND THROUGH EXPERIMENT, AS LAPLACE DID IN ASTRONOMY, OR CUVIER IN ZOOLOGY.
HOWEVER, I ACKNOWLEDGE THAT BICHAT'S "EXPERIMENTAL METHOD" HAS MERIT.
A great experimenter, Magendie was a fervent champion of vivisection.
MAN AND ANIMAL HAVE FUNCTIONS IN COMMON THAT CAN BE STUDIED FOR THE GOOD OF HUMANITY. THAT REQUIRES LIVING ANIMALS.
THAT IS HOW I WAS ABLE TO CARRY ON THE WORK OF CHARLES BELL AND SHOW THAT THE POSTERIOR SPINAL NERVE ROOTS ARE SENSORY, WHILE THE ANTERIOR SPINAL NERVE ROOTS CONTAIN ONLY MOTOR FIBRES.
THAT ENGLISHMAN WAS TOO SOFT TO CAUSE ANIMALS PAIN!
MAGENDIE COMPLETED MY RESEARCH BY TORTURING THOSE POOR ANIMALS.
Charles Bell
BUT I AM A GENTLEMAN! THE FRENCH LACK OF HUMANITY IS A LEGACY OF THEIR REVOLUTION. WHY, THEY BEHEADED THEIR OWN KING!

* The fine branching blood vessels that connect veins and arteries.

It wasn't as if Magendie's positions didn't draw their own fair share of criticism...

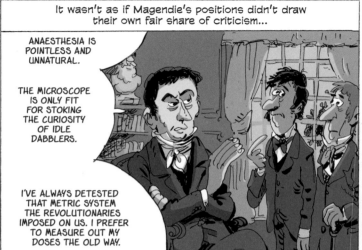

ANAESTHESIA IS POINTLESS AND UNNATURAL.

THE MICROSCOPE IS ONLY FIT FOR STOKING THE CURIOSITY OF IDLE DABBLERS.

I'VE ALWAYS DETESTED THAT METRIC SYSTEM THE REVOLUTIONARIES IMPOSED ON US. I PREFER TO MEASURE OUT MY DOSES THE OLD WAY.

But he was a brilliant physician and founded the Chair of Physiology at the Collège de France.

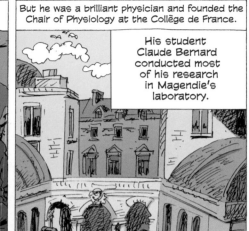

His student Claude Bernard conducted most of his research in Magendie's laboratory.

Taking up his teacher's methods, Bernard went on to invent experimental medicine and the concept of medical biology.

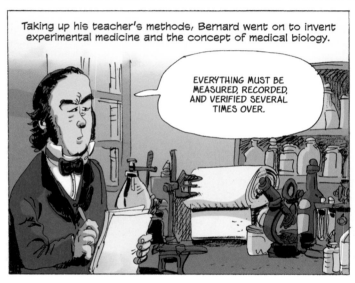

EVERYTHING MUST BE MEASURED, RECORDED, AND VERIFIED SEVERAL TIMES OVER.

So it was that he demonstrated curare's paralysing effects on a frog.

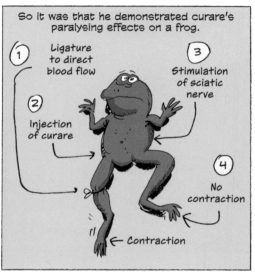

1 Ligature to direct blood flow

2 Injection of curare

3 Stimulation of sciatic nerve

4 No contraction

← Contraction

He also showed the role played by blood: an internal medium in which the body's cells dwelled and communicated.

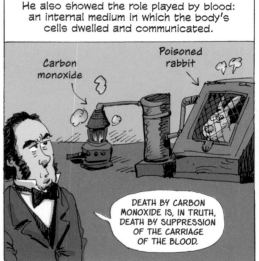

Carbon monoxide

Poisoned rabbit

DEATH BY CARBON MONOXIDE IS, IN TRUTH, DEATH BY SUPPRESSION OF THE CARRIAGE OF THE BLOOD.

And he was greatly interested in sugar.

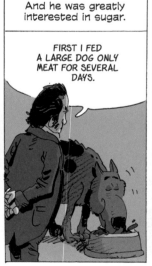

FIRST I FED A LARGE DOG ONLY MEAT FOR SEVERAL DAYS.

THEN I EXCISED THE LIVER AND SUBJECTED IT TO A COLD WATER RINSE TO REMOVE ALL THE BLOOD.

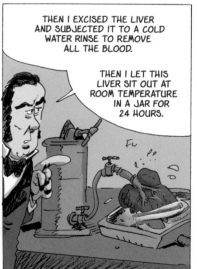

THEN I LET THIS LIVER SIT OUT AT ROOM TEMPERATURE IN A JAR FOR 24 HOURS.

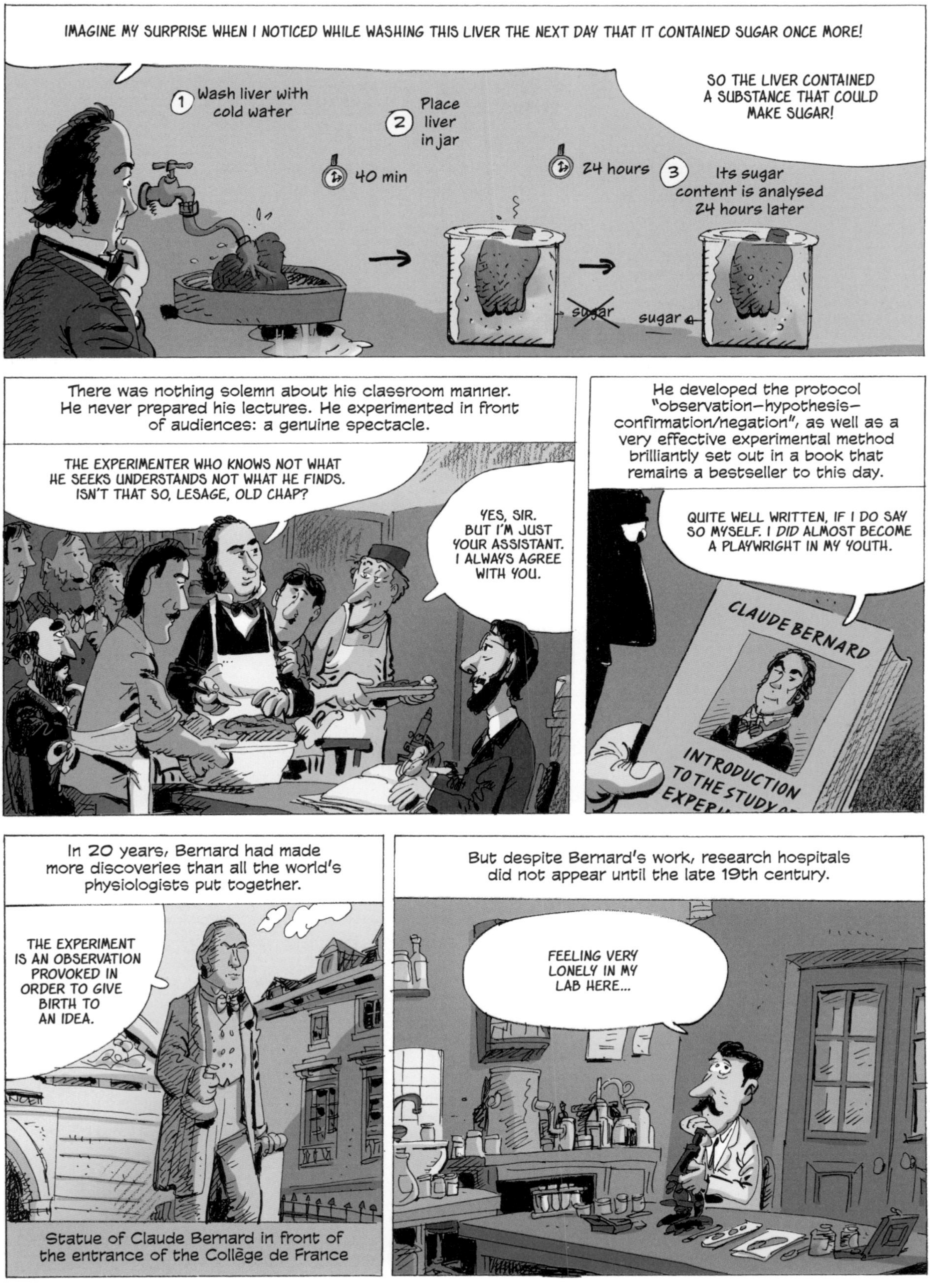
IMAGINE MY SURPRISE WHEN I NOTICED WHILE WASHING THIS LIVER THE NEXT DAY THAT IT CONTAINED SUGAR ONCE MORE!
1 Wash liver with cold water
2 Place liver in jar
40 min
24 hours
3 Its sugar content is analysed 24 hours later
SO THE LIVER CONTAINED A SUBSTANCE THAT COULD MAKE SUGAR!
sugar
sugar
There was nothing solemn about his classroom manner. He never prepared his lectures. He experimented in front of audiences: a genuine spectacle.
THE EXPERIMENTER WHO KNOWS NOT WHAT HE SEEKS UNDERSTANDS NOT WHAT HE FINDS. ISN'T THAT SO, LESAGE, OLD CHAP?
YES, SIR. BUT I'M JUST YOUR ASSISTANT. I ALWAYS AGREE WITH YOU.
He developed the protocol "observation–hypothesis–confirmation/negation", as well as a very effective experimental method brilliantly set out in a book that remains a bestseller to this day.
QUITE WELL WRITTEN, IF I DO SAY SO MYSELF. I *DID* ALMOST BECOME A PLAYWRIGHT IN MY YOUTH.
CLAUDE BERNARD
INTRODUCTION TO THE STUDY
In 20 years, Bernard had made more discoveries than all the world's physiologists put together.
THE EXPERIMENT IS AN OBSERVATION PROVOKED IN ORDER TO GIVE BIRTH TO AN IDEA.
Statue of Claude Bernard in front of the entrance of the Collège de France
But despite Bernard's work, research hospitals did not appear until the late 19th century.
FEELING VERY LONELY IN MY LAB HERE...

CHAPTER 11

CHILDREN'S MEDICINE

For a long time, doctors overlooked children. Infant mortality was an unbearably heavy burden that had to be endured, and only God could decide who would live and who would die.

The unquestionable force of destiny was such that even the great Montaigne himself admitted to having "lost two or three children at nurse, if not without regret, at least without repining".

Only in the 18th century, under the influence of Jean-Jacques Rousseau, at a time of slightly improved living conditions, was childhood considered an actual period in a person's life, a time to be devoted to learning.

Physicians began to take an interest in these little creatures...

But—significantly—according to the *Oxford English Dictionary*, the word "paediatric" did not begin to be used until 1880.

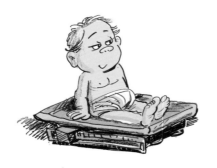

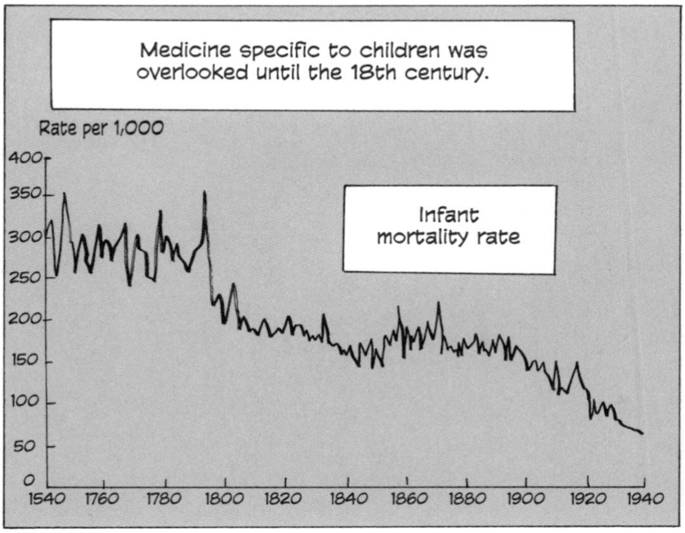
Medicine specific to children was overlooked until the 18th century.
Rate per 1,000
400
350
300
250
200
150
100
50
0
1540
1760
1780
1800
1820
1840
1860
1880
1900
1920
1940
Infant mortality rate

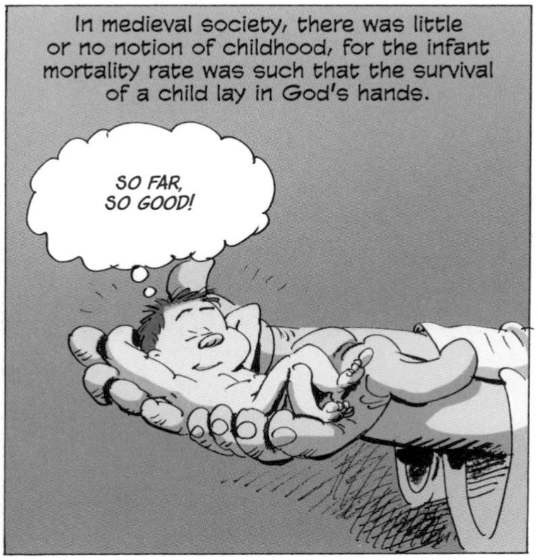
In medieval society, there was little or no notion of childhood, for the infant mortality rate was such that the survival of a child lay in God's hands.
SO FAR, SO GOOD!

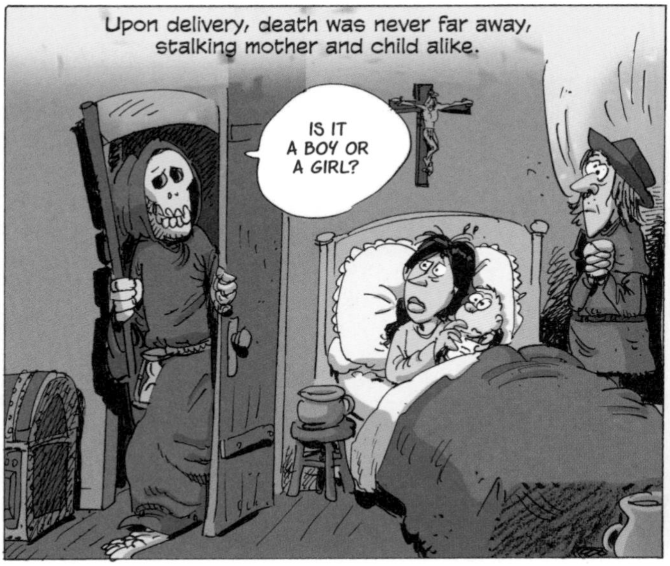
Upon delivery, death was never far away, stalking mother and child alike.
IS IT A BOY OR A GIRL?

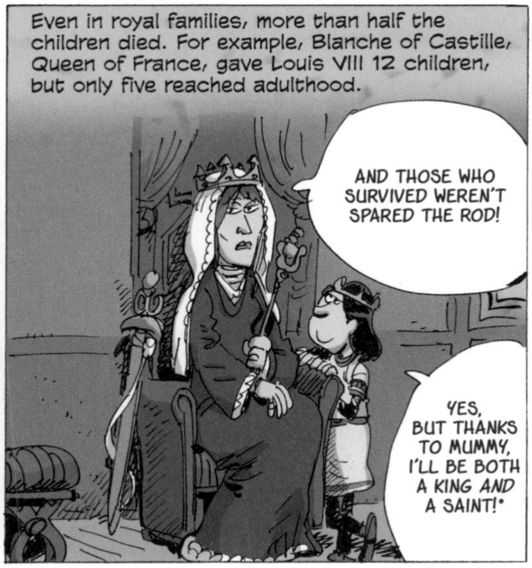
Even in royal families, more than half the children died. For example, Blanche of Castille, Queen of France, gave Louis VIII 12 children, but only five reached adulthood.
AND THOSE WHO SURVIVED WEREN'T SPARED THE ROD!
YES, BUT THANKS TO MUMMY, I'LL BE BOTH A KING *AND* A SAINT!*

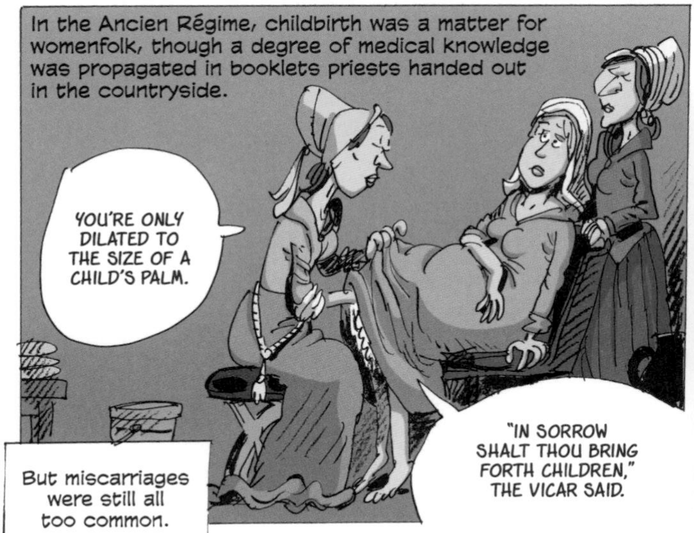
In the Ancien Régime, childbirth was a matter for womenfolk, though a degree of medical knowledge was propagated in booklets priests handed out in the countryside.
YOU'RE ONLY DILATED TO THE SIZE OF A CHILD'S PALM.
"IN SORROW SHALT THOU BRING FORTH CHILDREN," THE VICAR SAID.
But miscarriages were still all too common.

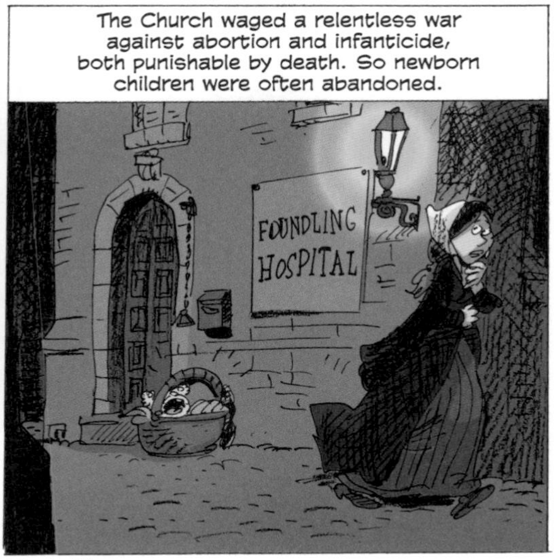
The Church waged a relentless war against abortion and infanticide, both punishable by death. So newborn children were often abandoned.
FOUNDLING HOSPITAL

* Louis IX.

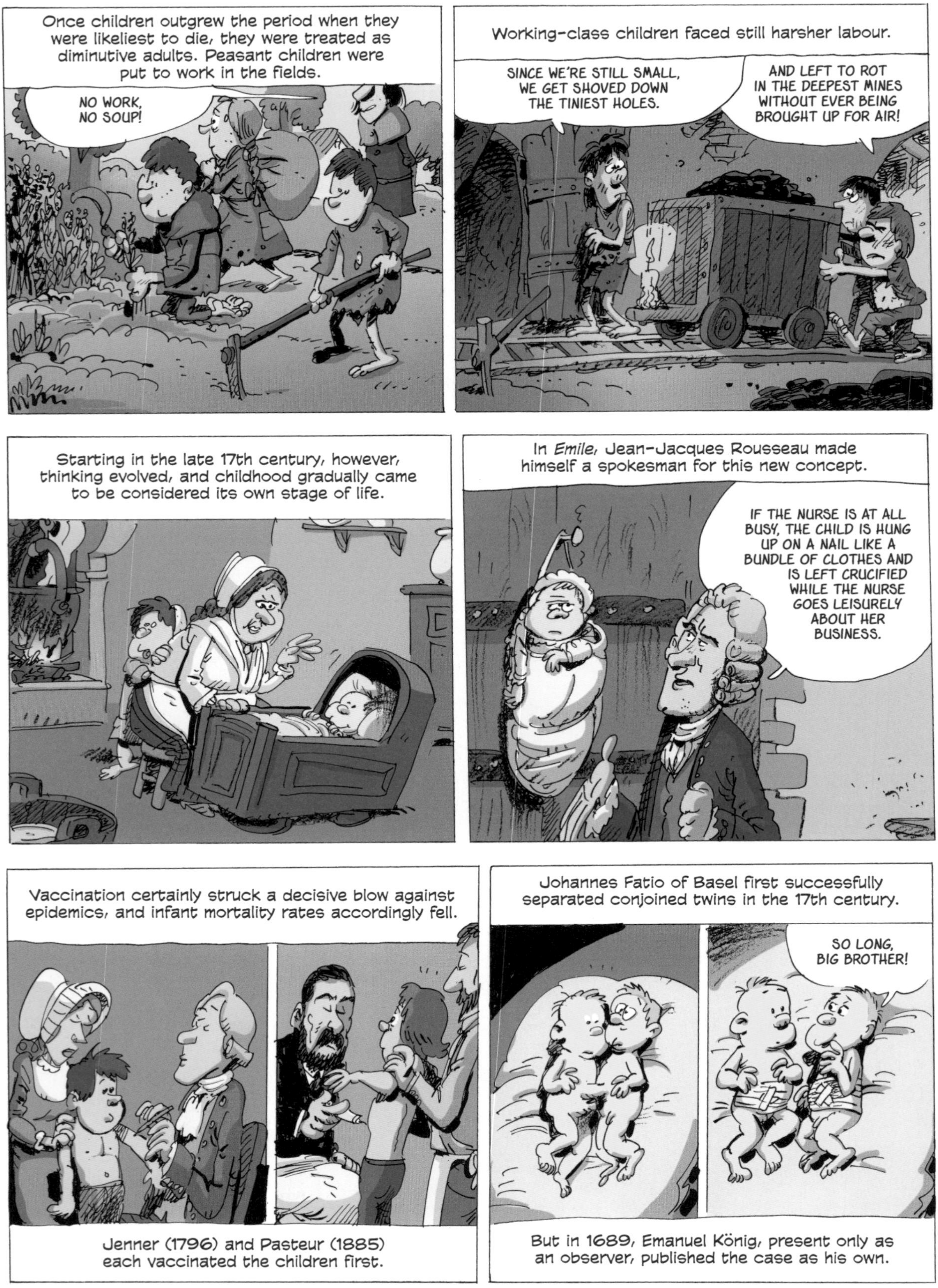
Once children outgrew the period when they were likeliest to die, they were treated as diminutive adults. Peasant children were put to work in the fields.
NO WORK, NO SOUP!
Working-class children faced still harsher labour.
SINCE WE'RE STILL SMALL, WE GET SHOVED DOWN THE TINIEST HOLES.
AND LEFT TO ROT IN THE DEEPEST MINES WITHOUT EVER BEING BROUGHT UP FOR AIR!
Starting in the late 17th century, however, thinking evolved, and childhood gradually came to be considered its own stage of life.
In *Emile*, Jean-Jacques Rousseau made himself a spokesman for this new concept.
IF THE NURSE IS AT ALL BUSY, THE CHILD IS HUNG UP ON A NAIL LIKE A BUNDLE OF CLOTHES AND IS LEFT CRUCIFIED WHILE THE NURSE GOES LEISURELY ABOUT HER BUSINESS.
Vaccination certainly struck a decisive blow against epidemics, and infant mortality rates accordingly fell.
Jenner (1796) and Pasteur (1885) each vaccinated the children first.
Johannes Fatio of Basel first successfully separated conjoined twins in the 17th century.
SO LONG, BIG BROTHER!
But in 1689, Emanuel König, present only as an observer, published the case as his own.

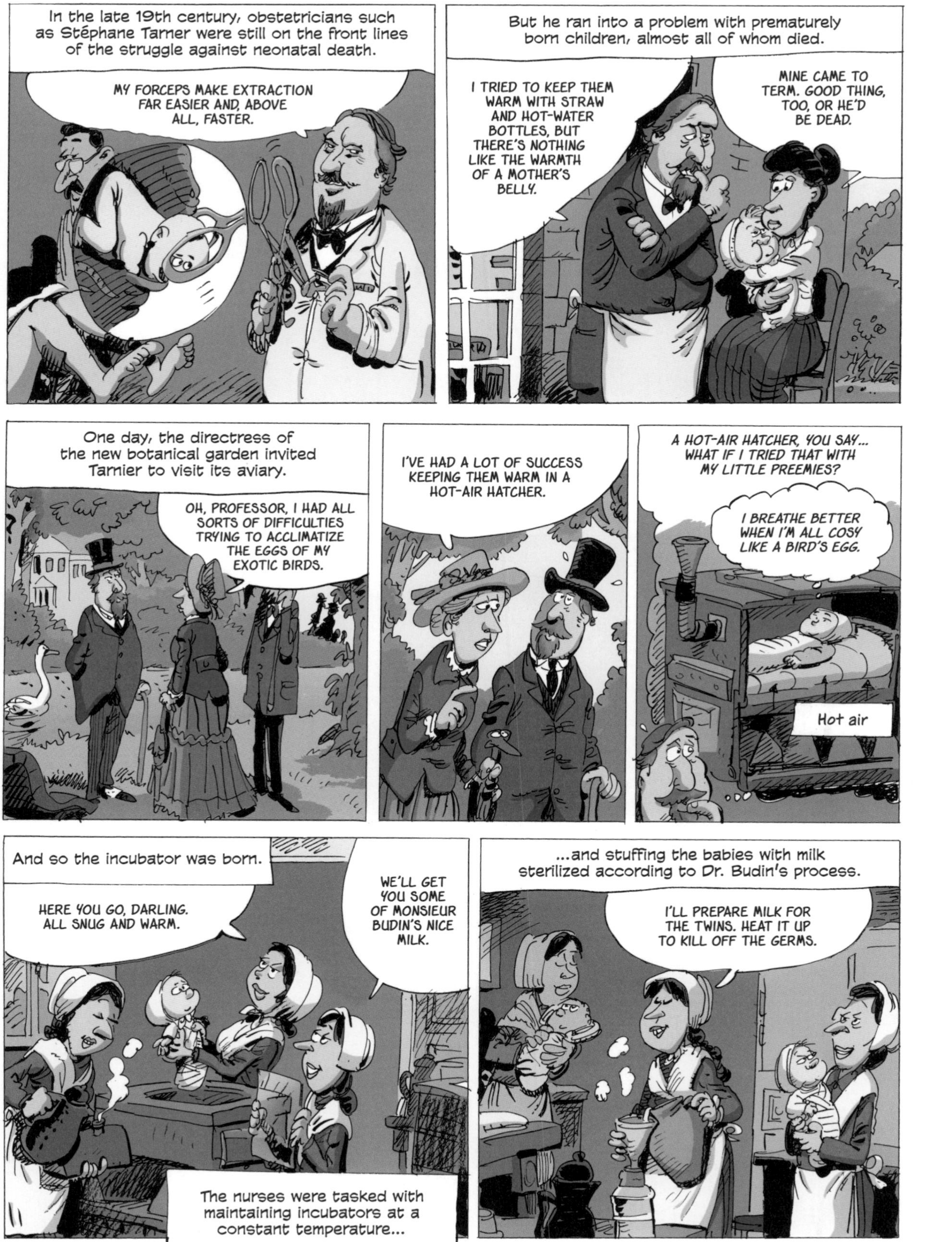
In the late 19th century, obstetricians such as Stéphane Tarner were still on the front lines of the struggle against neonatal death.
MY FORCEPS MAKE EXTRACTION FAR EASIER AND, ABOVE ALL, FASTER.
But he ran into a problem with prematurely born children, almost all of whom died.
I TRIED TO KEEP THEM WARM WITH STRAW AND HOT-WATER BOTTLES, BUT THERE'S NOTHING LIKE THE WARMTH OF A MOTHER'S BELLY.
MINE CAME TO TERM. GOOD THING, TOO, OR HE'D BE DEAD.
One day, the directress of the new botanical garden invited Tarnier to visit its aviary.
OH, PROFESSOR, I HAD ALL SORTS OF DIFFICULTIES TRYING TO ACCLIMATIZE THE EGGS OF MY EXOTIC BIRDS.
I'VE HAD A LOT OF SUCCESS KEEPING THEM WARM IN A HOT-AIR HATCHER.
A HOT-AIR HATCHER, YOU SAY... WHAT IF I TRIED THAT WITH MY LITTLE PREEMIES?
I BREATHE BETTER WHEN I'M ALL COSY LIKE A BIRD'S EGG.
Hot air
And so the incubator was born.
HERE YOU GO, DARLING. ALL SNUG AND WARM.
WE'LL GET YOU SOME OF MONSIEUR BUDIN'S NICE MILK.
The nurses were tasked with maintaining incubators at a constant temperature...
...and stuffing the babies with milk sterilized according to Dr. Budin's process.
I'LL PREPARE MILK FOR THE TWINS. HEAT IT UP TO KILL OFF THE GERMS.

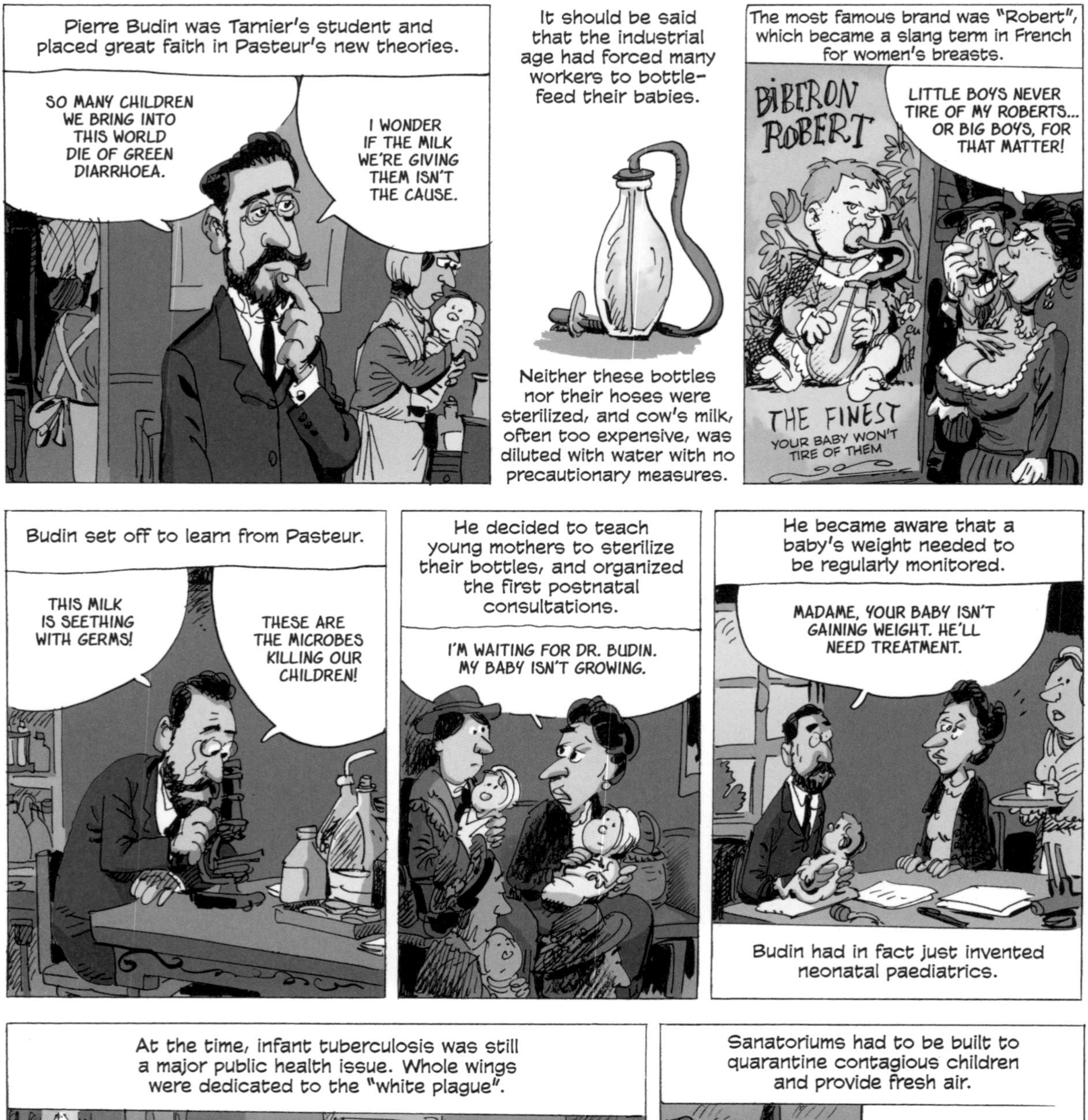
Pierre Budin was Tarnier's student and placed great faith in Pasteur's new theories.
SO MANY CHILDREN WE BRING INTO THIS WORLD DIE OF GREEN DIARRHOEA.
I WONDER IF THE MILK WE'RE GIVING THEM ISN'T THE CAUSE.
It should be said that the industrial age had forced many workers to bottle-feed their babies.
Neither these bottles nor their hoses were sterilized, and cow's milk, often too expensive, was diluted with water with no precautionary measures.
The most famous brand was "Robert", which became a slang term in French for women's breasts.
BIBERON ROBERT
THE FINEST
YOUR BABY WON'T TIRE OF THEM
LITTLE BOYS NEVER TIRE OF MY ROBERTS... OR BIG BOYS, FOR THAT MATTER!
Budin set off to learn from Pasteur.
THIS MILK IS SEETHING WITH GERMS!
THESE ARE THE MICROBES KILLING OUR CHILDREN!
He decided to teach young mothers to sterilize their bottles, and organized the first postnatal consultations.
I'M WAITING FOR DR. BUDIN. MY BABY ISN'T GROWING.
He became aware that a baby's weight needed to be regularly monitored.
MADAME, YOUR BABY ISN'T GAINING WEIGHT. HE'LL NEED TREATMENT.
Budin had in fact just invented neonatal paediatrics.
At the time, infant tuberculosis was still a major public health issue. Whole wings were dedicated to the "white plague".
KOFF
Sanatoriums had to be built to quarantine contagious children and provide fresh air.
HEY, WAIT... WHY WAS THE FIRST ONE BUILT ON THE COAST, IN BERCK?
IT'S NOT EXACTLY THE SUNNIEST PLACE IN FRANCE!

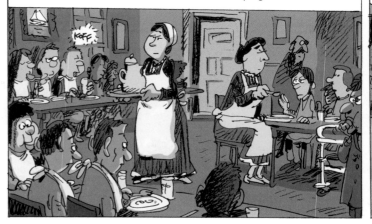

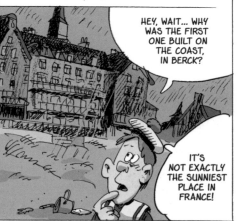

This is a good place to tell the story of "Lonely Marianne" of Berck, who took her charges out to the beach every day to take in the good salt air.

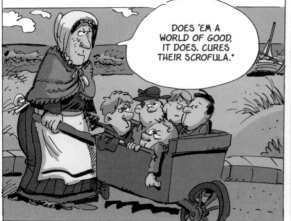

DOES 'EM A WORLD OF GOOD, IT DOES. CURES THEIR SCROFULA.*

Astonished by her good results, Dr. Perrochaud of Montreuil-sur-Mer decided to entrust her with eight consumptive children, who also quickly recovered.

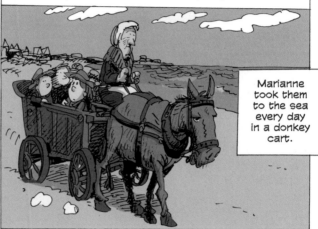

Marianne took them to the sea every day in a donkey cart.

In 1861, Perrochaud managed to convince the Director of Welfare in Paris to send him consumptive children and build a hospital of wood for them by the beach.

Then, in 1869, a hospital with 500 beds: the Hôpital Napoléon.

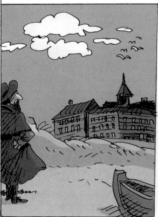

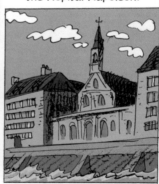

Faced with the frequency of tuberculous arthritis, the hospital specialized in treating the effects of Pott's disease.

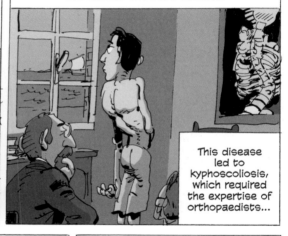

This disease led to kyphoscoliosis, which required the expertise of orthopaedists...

...and for which the treatment at the time was a plaster corset.

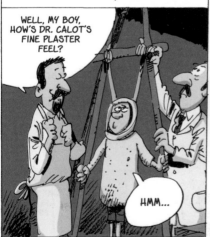

WELL, MY BOY, HOW'S DR. CALOT'S FINE PLASTER FEEL?

HMM...

But Jean-François Calot wanted to go further, and to flatten humps under anaesthesia. He was known as the "straightener of hunchbacks".

IT'S A SPINE-TINGLING TECHNIQUE!

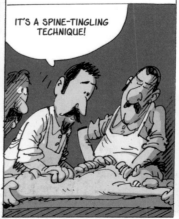

It was an international success. The whole world flocked to see Calot operate in Berck.

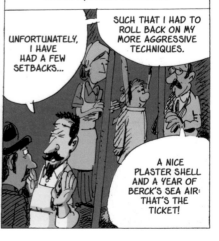

UNFORTUNATELY, I HAVE HAD A FEW SETBACKS...

SUCH THAT I HAD TO ROLL BACK ON MY MORE AGGRESSIVE TECHNIQUES.

A NICE PLASTER SHELL AND A YEAR OF BERCK'S SEA AIR: THAT'S THE TICKET!

* An old-fashioned term referring to glandular swelling.

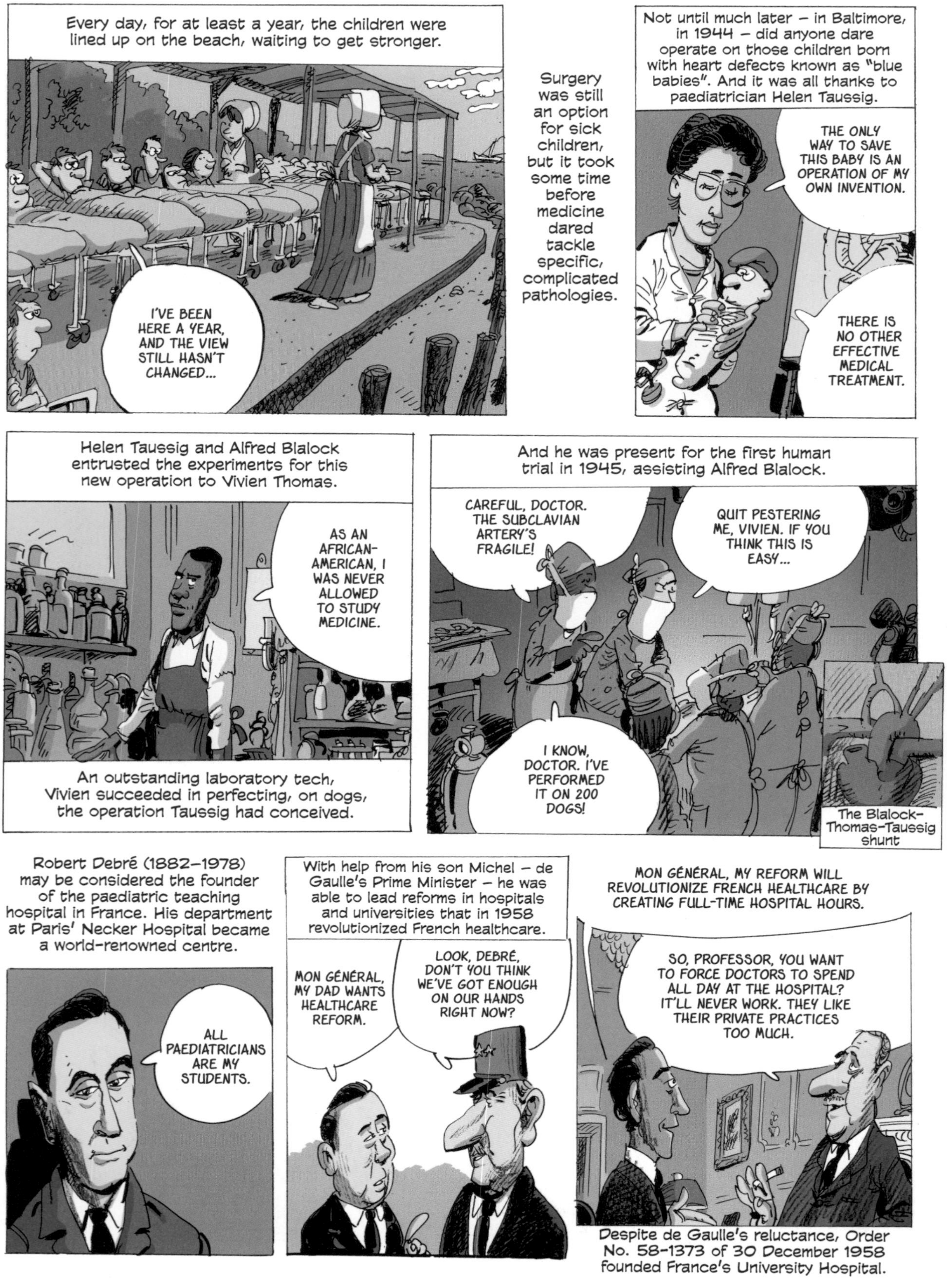
Every day, for at least a year, the children were lined up on the beach, waiting to get stronger.
I'VE BEEN HERE A YEAR, AND THE VIEW STILL HASN'T CHANGED...
Surgery was still an option for sick children, but it took some time before medicine dared tackle specific, complicated pathologies.
Not until much later – in Baltimore, in 1944 – did anyone dare operate on those children born with heart defects known as "blue babies". And it was all thanks to paediatrician Helen Taussig.
THE ONLY WAY TO SAVE THIS BABY IS AN OPERATION OF MY OWN INVENTION.
THERE IS NO OTHER EFFECTIVE MEDICAL TREATMENT.
Helen Taussig and Alfred Blalock entrusted the experiments for this new operation to Vivien Thomas.
AS AN AFRICAN-AMERICAN, I WAS NEVER ALLOWED TO STUDY MEDICINE.
An outstanding laboratory tech, Vivien succeeded in perfecting, on dogs, the operation Taussig had conceived.
And he was present for the first human trial in 1945, assisting Alfred Blalock.
CAREFUL, DOCTOR. THE SUBCLAVIAN ARTERY'S FRAGILE!
QUIT PESTERING ME, VIVIEN. IF YOU THINK THIS IS EASY...
I KNOW, DOCTOR. I'VE PERFORMED IT ON 200 DOGS!
The Blalock-Thomas-Taussig shunt
Robert Debré (1882–1978) may be considered the founder of the paediatric teaching hospital in France. His department at Paris' Necker Hospital became a world-renowned centre.
ALL PAEDIATRICIANS ARE MY STUDENTS.
With help from his son Michel – de Gaulle's Prime Minister – he was able to lead reforms in hospitals and universities that in 1958 revolutionized French healthcare.
MON GÉNÉRAL, MY DAD WANTS HEALTHCARE REFORM.
LOOK, DEBRÉ, DON'T YOU THINK WE'VE GOT ENOUGH ON OUR HANDS RIGHT NOW?
MON GÉNÉRAL, MY REFORM WILL REVOLUTIONIZE FRENCH HEALTHCARE BY CREATING FULL-TIME HOSPITAL HOURS.
SO, PROFESSOR, YOU WANT TO FORCE DOCTORS TO SPEND ALL DAY AT THE HOSPITAL? IT'LL NEVER WORK. THEY LIKE THEIR PRIVATE PRACTICES TOO MUCH.
Despite de Gaulle's reluctance, Order No. 58-1373 of 30 December 1958 founded France's University Hospital.

Meanwhile, paediatric research advanced. In 1958, Debré's student Marthe Gautier was sent to Harvard, where she specialized in cell culture.

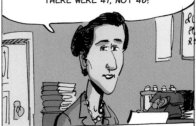

I WAS WORKING WITH DOWN'S SYNDROME FIBROBLASTS. ONE DAY, I COUNTED THE CHROMOSOMES: THERE WERE 47, NOT 46!

She'd just discovered Trisomy 21.

Advances in genetics allowed inherited diseases to be diagnosed. Apart from diseases linked to chromosomes, there were also diseases due to one or several genes (D.N.A.).

These could reveal themselves at birth, such as:

Mucoviscidosis (Cystic fibrosis)   or   Duchenne muscular dystrophy

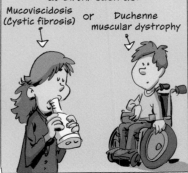

Smaller instruments, more effective optics, and especially advances in intensive care let surgeons operate on newborns, and even envisage *in utero* operations.

GOOD THING I'VE GOT MY BIG GLASSES ON!

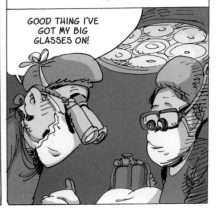

So it was that, in the great tradition of Tarnier and Budin, Gilbert Huault created neonatal intensive care.

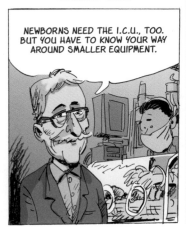

NEWBORNS NEED THE I.C.U., TOO. BUT YOU HAVE TO KNOW YOUR WAY AROUND SMALLER EQUIPMENT.

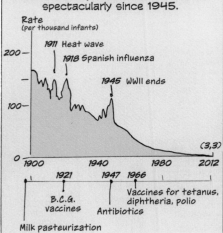

Thanks to vaccines and antibiotics, infant mortality rates have decreased spectacularly since 1945.

Rate
(per thousand infants)

200 —

1911 Heat wave

1918 Spanish influenza

1945 WWII ends

100 —

(3,3)

0
1900   1940   1980   2012

1921   1947   1966

B.C.G. vaccines

Antibiotics

Vaccines for tetanus, diphtheria, polio

Milk pasteurization

And yet some fundamental insights awaited discovery in the second half of the 20th century, till which time, for example, newborns were still thought of as digestive tracts unable to experience pain and without feeling.

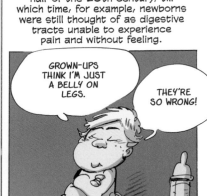

GROWN-UPS THINK I'M JUST A BELLY ON LEGS.

THEY'RE SO WRONG!

In fact, babies' nervous systems were thought to be insufficiently developed to feel anything. Medical and even surgical procedures were performed on them without analgesics.* Indian anaesthetist Dr. Kanwaljeet Anand only remedied this in 1987.

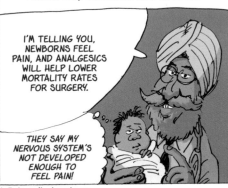

I'M TELLING YOU, NEWBORNS FEEL PAIN, AND ANALGESICS WILL HELP LOWER MORTALITY RATES FOR SURGERY.

THEY SAY MY NERVOUS SYSTEM'S NOT DEVELOPED ENOUGH TO FEEL PAIN!

Françoise Dolto – a student of Jacques Lacan – took a keen interest in child psychology.

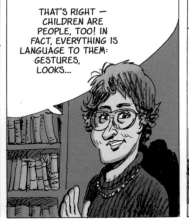

THAT'S RIGHT – CHILDREN ARE PEOPLE, TOO! IN FACT, EVERYTHING IS LANGUAGE TO THEM: GESTURES, LOOKS...

Her essential contribution was the assertion that children were just as much beings as adults, making them patients in their own right.

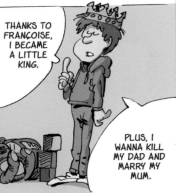

THANKS TO FRANÇOISE, I BECAME A LITTLE KING.

PLUS, I WANNA KILL MY DAD AND MARRY MY MUM.

* Pain-relieving drugs.

CHAPTER 12

IN SEARCH OF MENTAL ILLNESS

Like the ancients, René Descartes (1596–1650) believed the mind an immaterial substance distinct from the brain. Two centuries later, Ernest Renan (1823–1892) taught just the opposite: that the brain produced thoughts in the same way as the liver produced bile.

To this day, the discovery of mental illnesses remains marked by this duality between neurology (which rationally matches a problem to a physical anomaly) and psychiatry, first and foremost a metaphysics of the mind, which inevitably entails the notion of madness. However, a more modern vision of psychiatry now conceives of the possible involvement of organic dysfunction.

The ways in which our knowledge has evolved show the part that neurotransmitter anomalies play in mental illness. Perhaps, in the future, psychiatry will seem but a facet of the abnormal expression of chemistry and connections in the brain.

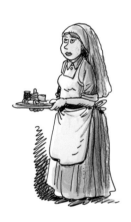

PART ONE: PSYCHIATRY, OR SPIRITUAL DISEASE

Hippocrates had begun to differentiate among mental afflictions with his theory of humours.

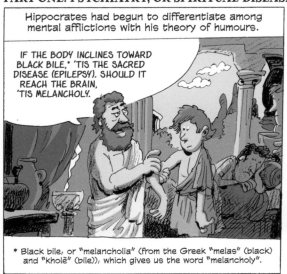

IF THE BODY INCLINES TOWARD BLACK BILE,* 'TIS THE SACRED DISEASE (EPILEPSY). SHOULD IT REACH THE BRAIN, 'TIS MELANCHOLY.

* Black bile, or "melancholia" (from the Greek "melas" (black) and "kholē" (bile)), which gives us the word "melancholy".

For hysteria, he espoused the theory of the "wandering womb".

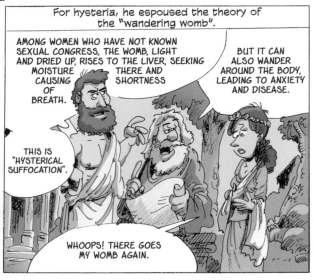

AMONG WOMEN WHO HAVE NOT KNOWN SEXUAL CONGRESS, THE WOMB, LIGHT AND DRIED UP, RISES TO THE LIVER, SEEKING MOISTURE THERE AND CAUSING SHORTNESS OF BREATH.

BUT IT CAN ALSO WANDER AROUND THE BODY, LEADING TO ANXIETY AND DISEASE.

THIS IS "HYSTERICAL SUFFOCATION".

WHOOPS! THERE GOES MY WOMB AGAIN.

In the Middle Ages, mental illness was seen as demonic possession.

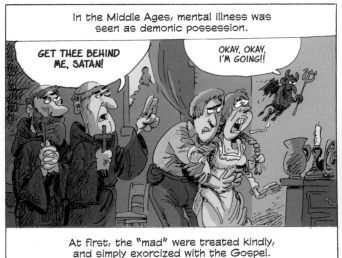

GET THEE BEHIND ME, SATAN!

OKAY, OKAY, I'M GOING!!

At first, the "mad" were treated kindly, and simply exorcized with the Gospel.

Unfortunately, they were later lumped in with heretics and witches, and burned at the stake.

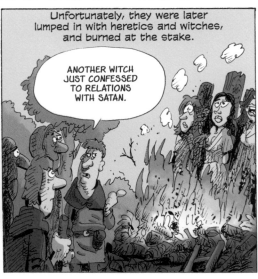

ANOTHER WITCH JUST CONFESSED TO RELATIONS WITH SATAN.

Starting in the 17th century, the insane were subjected to the "great confinement". They were imprisoned and stripped of their belongings.

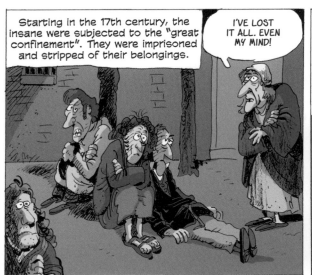

I'VE LOST IT ALL. EVEN MY MIND!

In 1777, the Scotsman William Cullen was the first to suggest a new way to approach mental illness.

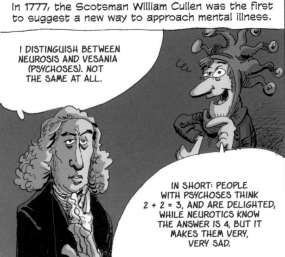

I DISTINGUISH BETWEEN NEUROSIS AND VESANIA (PSYCHOSES). NOT THE SAME AT ALL.

IN SHORT: PEOPLE WITH PSYCHOSES THINK 2 + 2 = 3, AND ARE DELIGHTED, WHILE NEUROTICS KNOW THE ANSWER IS 4, BUT IT MAKES THEM VERY, VERY SAD.

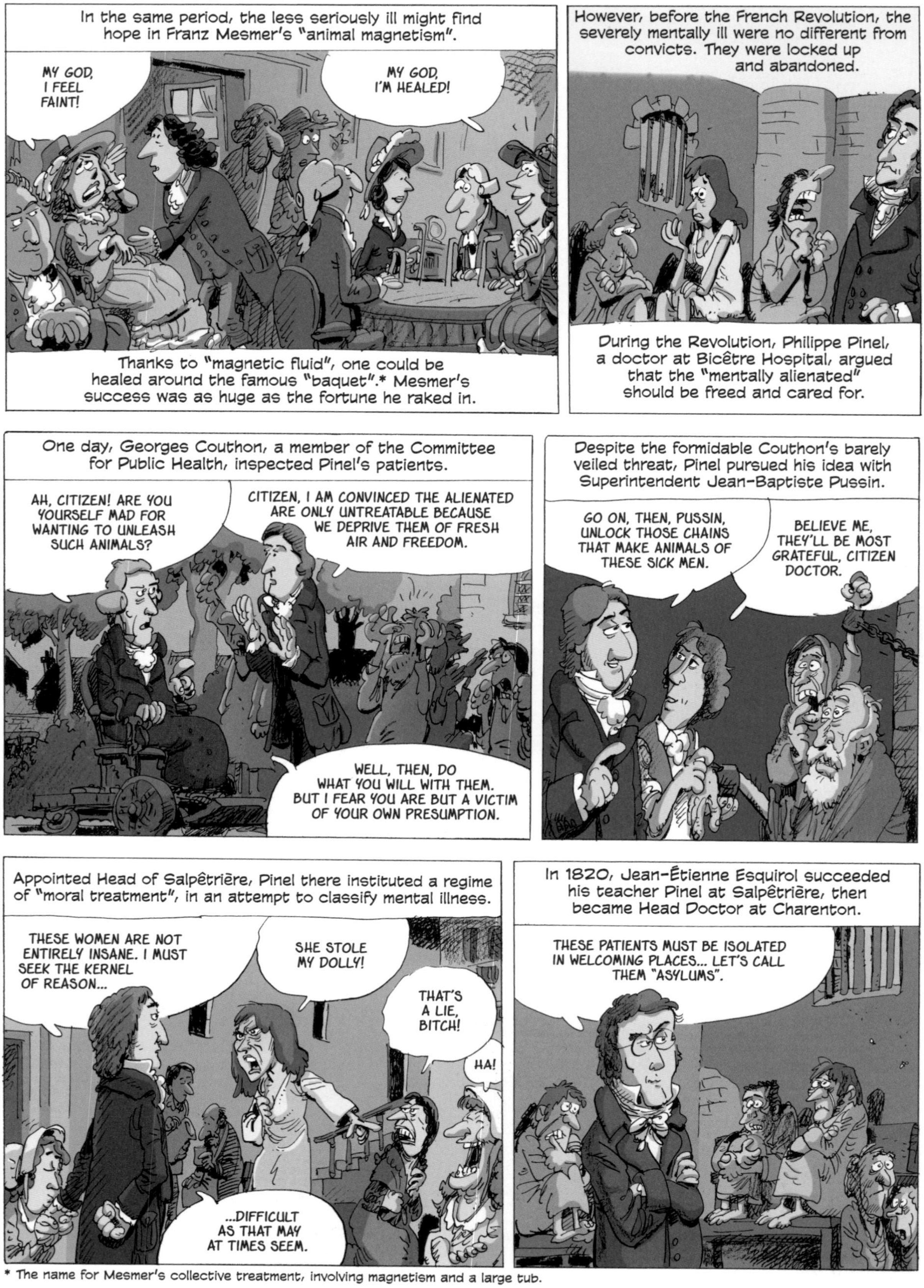
In the same period, the less seriously ill might find hope in Franz Mesmer's "animal magnetism".
MY GOD, I FEEL FAINT!
MY GOD, I'M HEALED!
Thanks to "magnetic fluid", one could be healed around the famous "baquet".* Mesmer's success was as huge as the fortune he raked in.
However, before the French Revolution, the severely mentally ill were no different from convicts. They were locked up and abandoned.
During the Revolution, Philippe Pinel, a doctor at Bicêtre Hospital, argued that the "mentally alienated" should be freed and cared for.
One day, Georges Couthon, a member of the Committee for Public Health, inspected Pinel's patients.
AH, CITIZEN! ARE YOU YOURSELF MAD FOR WANTING TO UNLEASH SUCH ANIMALS?
CITIZEN, I AM CONVINCED THE ALIENATED ARE ONLY UNTREATABLE BECAUSE WE DEPRIVE THEM OF FRESH AIR AND FREEDOM.
WELL, THEN, DO WHAT YOU WILL WITH THEM. BUT I FEAR YOU ARE BUT A VICTIM OF YOUR OWN PRESUMPTION.
Despite the formidable Couthon's barely veiled threat, Pinel pursued his idea with Superintendent Jean-Baptiste Pussin.
GO ON, THEN, PUSSIN, UNLOCK THOSE CHAINS THAT MAKE ANIMALS OF THESE SICK MEN.
BELIEVE ME, THEY'LL BE MOST GRATEFUL, CITIZEN DOCTOR.
Appointed Head of Salpêtrière, Pinel there instituted a regime of "moral treatment", in an attempt to classify mental illness.
THESE WOMEN ARE NOT ENTIRELY INSANE. I MUST SEEK THE KERNEL OF REASON...
SHE STOLE MY DOLLY!
THAT'S A LIE, BITCH!
HA!
...DIFFICULT AS THAT MAY AT TIMES SEEM.
In 1820, Jean-Étienne Esquirol succeeded his teacher Pinel at Salpêtrière, then became Head Doctor at Charenton.
THESE PATIENTS MUST BE ISOLATED IN WELCOMING PLACES... LET'S CALL THEM "ASYLUMS".

* The name for Mesmer's collective treatment, involving magnetism and a large tub.

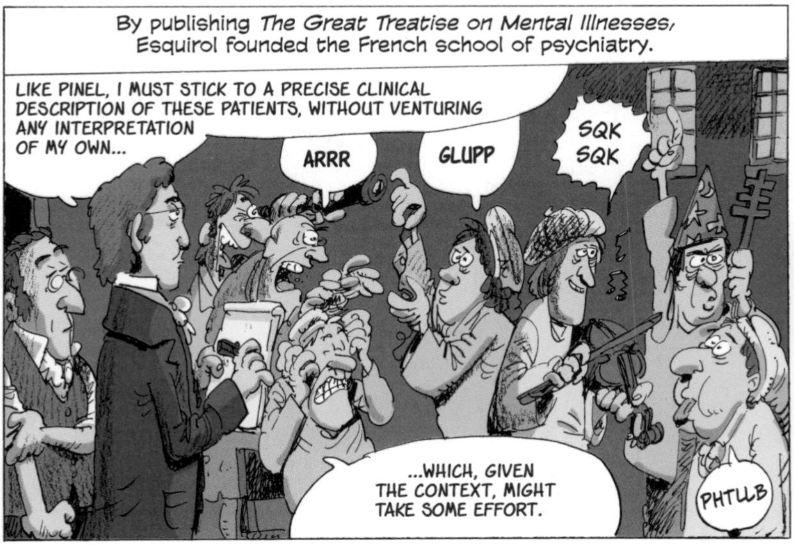
By publishing The Great Treatise on Mental Illnesses, Esquirol founded the French school of psychiatry.
LIKE PINEL, I MUST STICK TO A PRECISE CLINICAL DESCRIPTION OF THESE PATIENTS, WITHOUT VENTURING ANY INTERPRETATION OF MY OWN...
ARRR
GLUPP
SQK SQK
...WHICH, GIVEN THE CONTEXT, MIGHT TAKE SOME EFFORT.
PHTLLB

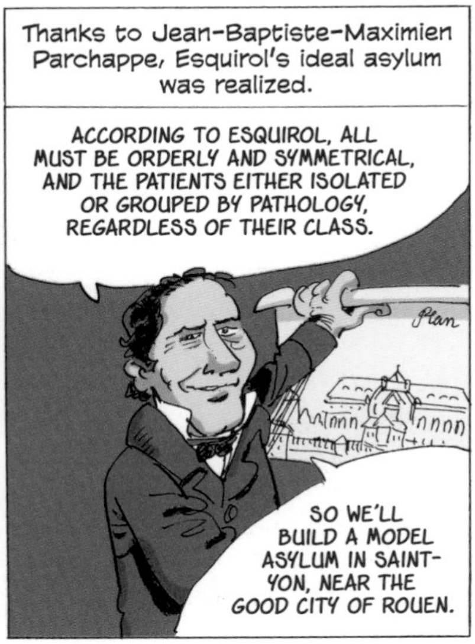
Thanks to Jean-Baptiste-Maximien Parchappe, Esquirol's ideal asylum was realized.
ACCORDING TO ESQUIROL, ALL MUST BE ORDERLY AND SYMMETRICAL, AND THE PATIENTS EITHER ISOLATED OR GROUPED BY PATHOLOGY, REGARDLESS OF THEIR CLASS.
Plan
SO WE'LL BUILD A MODEL ASYLUM IN SAINT-YON, NEAR THE GOOD CITY OF ROUEN.

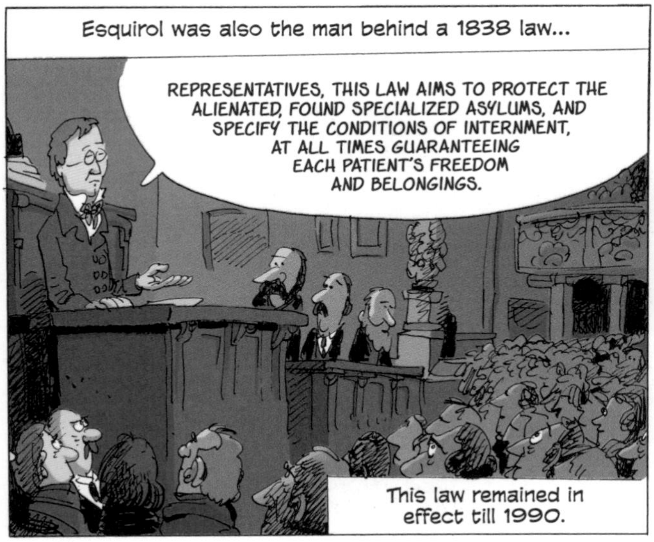
Esquirol was also the man behind a 1838 law...
REPRESENTATIVES, THIS LAW AIMS TO PROTECT THE ALIENATED, FOUND SPECIALIZED ASYLUMS, AND SPECIFY THE CONDITIONS OF INTERNMENT, AT ALL TIMES GUARANTEEING EACH PATIENT'S FREEDOM AND BELONGINGS.
This law remained in effect till 1990.

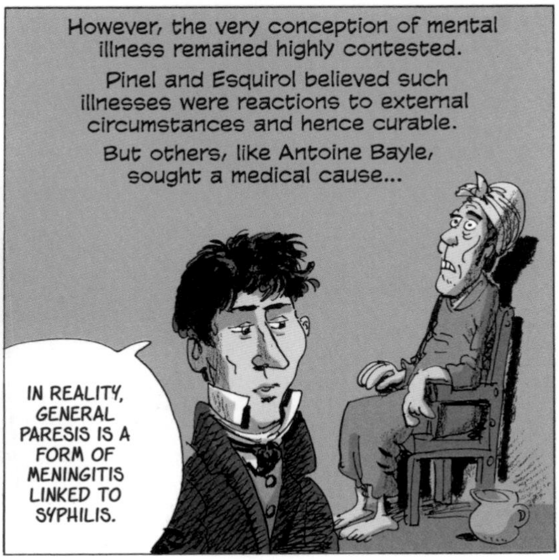
However, the very conception of mental illness remained highly contested.
Pinel and Esquirol believed such illnesses were reactions to external circumstances and hence curable.
But others, like Antoine Bayle, sought a medical cause...
IN REALITY, GENERAL PARESIS IS A FORM OF MENINGITIS LINKED TO SYPHILIS.

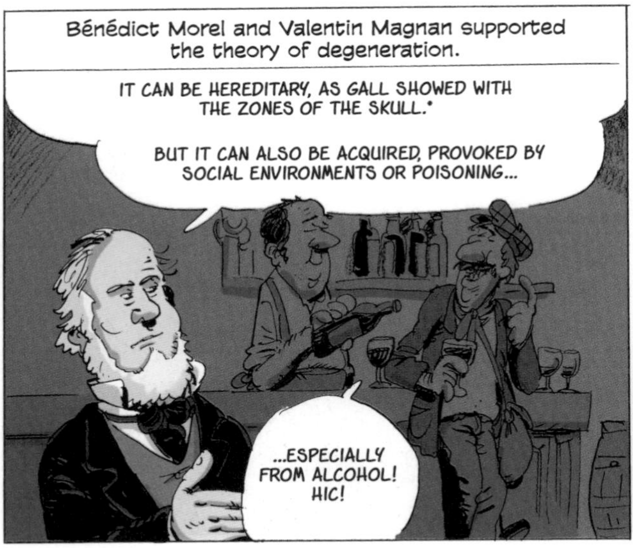
Bénédict Morel and Valentin Magnan supported the theory of degeneration.
IT CAN BE HEREDITARY, AS GALL SHOWED WITH THE ZONES OF THE SKULL.*
BUT IT CAN ALSO BE ACQUIRED, PROVOKED BY SOCIAL ENVIRONMENTS OR POISONING...
...ESPECIALLY FROM ALCOHOL! HIC!

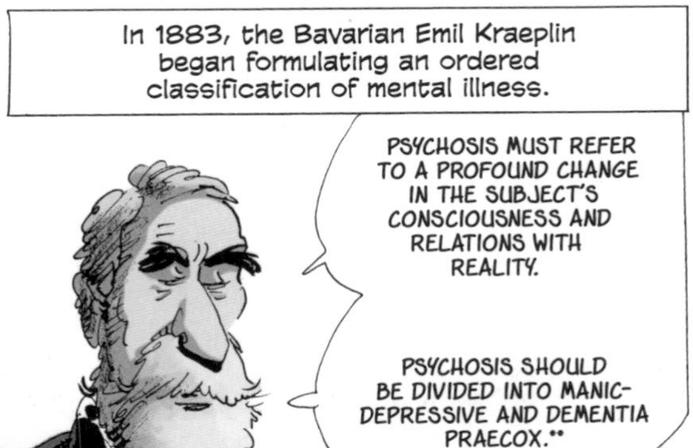
In 1883, the Bavarian Emil Kraeplin began formulating an ordered classification of mental illness.
PSYCHOSIS MUST REFER TO A PROFOUND CHANGE IN THE SUBJECT'S CONSCIOUSNESS AND RELATIONS WITH REALITY.
PSYCHOSIS SHOULD BE DIVIDED INTO MANIC-DEPRESSIVE AND DEMENTIA PRAECOX.**
** Eugen Bleuler would later name this "schizophrenia".

* See page 139.

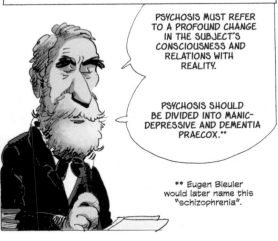

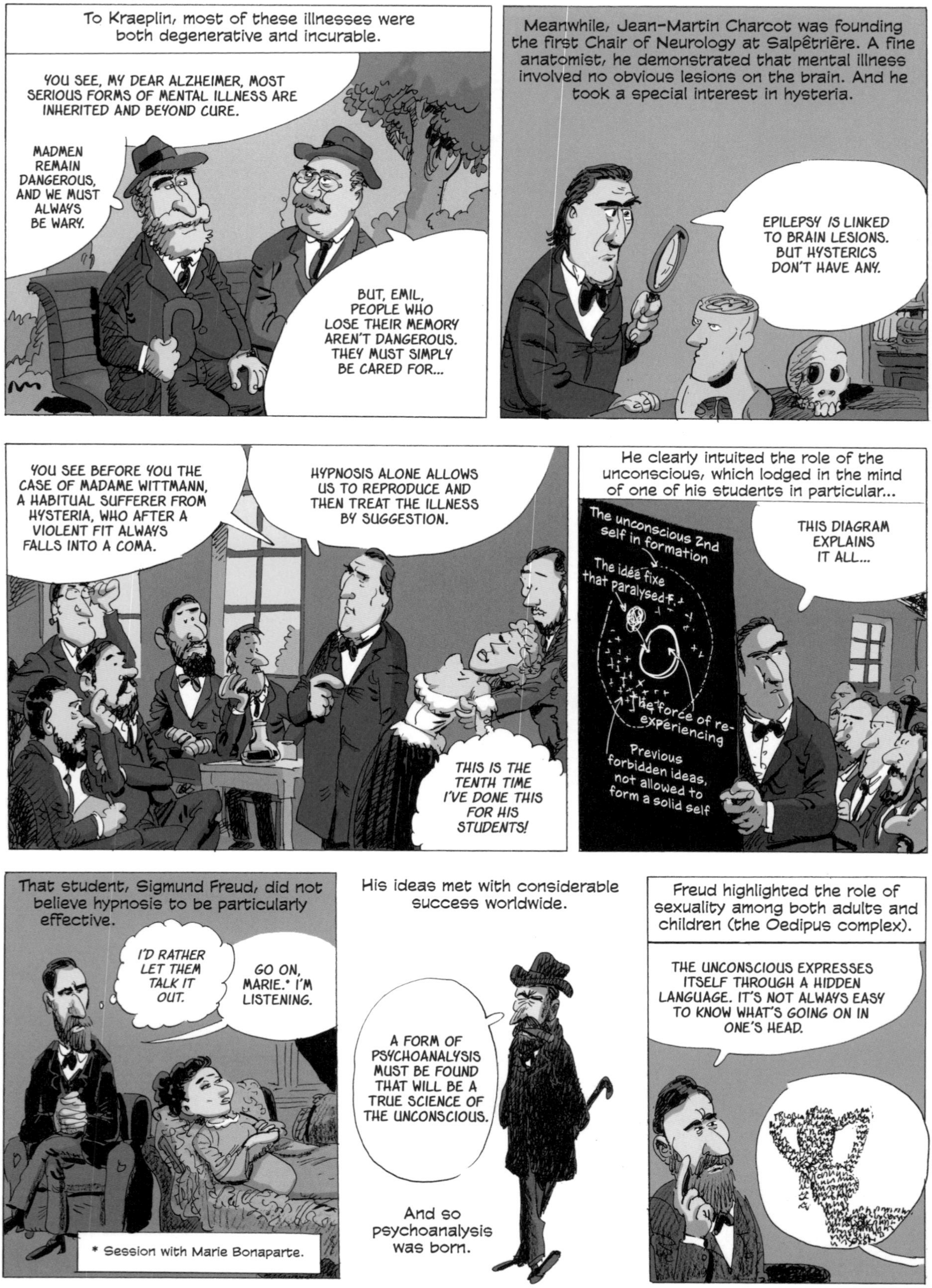
To Kraeplin, most of these illnesses were both degenerative and incurable.
YOU SEE, MY DEAR ALZHEIMER, MOST SERIOUS FORMS OF MENTAL ILLNESS ARE INHERITED AND BEYOND CURE.
MADMEN REMAIN DANGEROUS, AND WE MUST ALWAYS BE WARY.
BUT, EMIL, PEOPLE WHO LOSE THEIR MEMORY AREN'T DANGEROUS. THEY MUST SIMPLY BE CARED FOR...
Meanwhile, Jean-Martin Charcot was founding the first Chair of Neurology at Salpêtrière. A fine anatomist, he demonstrated that mental illness involved no obvious lesions on the brain. And he took a special interest in hysteria.
EPILEPSY IS LINKED TO BRAIN LESIONS. BUT HYSTERICS DON'T HAVE ANY.
YOU SEE BEFORE YOU THE CASE OF MADAME WITTMANN, A HABITUAL SUFFERER FROM HYSTERIA, WHO AFTER A VIOLENT FIT ALWAYS FALLS INTO A COMA.
HYPNOSIS ALONE ALLOWS US TO REPRODUCE AND THEN TREAT THE ILLNESS BY SUGGESTION.
THIS IS THE TENTH TIME I'VE DONE THIS FOR HIS STUDENTS!
He clearly intuited the role of the unconscious, which lodged in the mind of one of his students in particular...
The unconscious 2nd self in formation
The idée fixe that paralysed
The force of re-experiencing
Previous forbidden ideas, not allowed to form a solid self
THIS DIAGRAM EXPLAINS IT ALL...
That student, Sigmund Freud, did not believe hypnosis to be particularly effective.
I'D RATHER LET THEM TALK IT OUT.
GO ON, MARIE.* I'M LISTENING.
* Session with Marie Bonaparte.
His ideas met with considerable success worldwide.
A FORM OF PSYCHOANALYSIS MUST BE FOUND THAT WILL BE A TRUE SCIENCE OF THE UNCONSCIOUS.
And so psychoanalysis was born.
Freud highlighted the role of sexuality among both adults and children (the Oedipus complex).
THE UNCONSCIOUS EXPRESSES ITSELF THROUGH A HIDDEN LANGUAGE. IT'S NOT ALWAYS EASY TO KNOW WHAT'S GOING ON IN ONE'S HEAD.

But Freud's heirs were clear about their divergent views...

For Adler, the origin of neurosis was not sexuality...

...BUT THE FEELING OF INFERIORITY.

And for Carl Jung, it was all about the archetypes of the collective unconscious.

SO TO SUM UP, DOCTOR, MY NEUROSIS IS ALL ABOUT THE SERPENT TEMPTER, THE VIRGIN BIRTH, THE CREATION OF THE WORLD, ACHILLES' HEEL, AND THE VASTNESS OF THE OCEAN?

ER... WELL, LET'S TRY TO REFINE THAT A BIT...

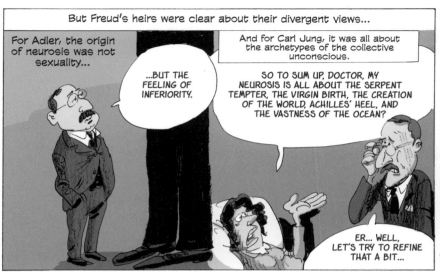

In 1953, Jacques Lacan, who had introduced linguistics into psychoanalysis, added a fourth stage, the "mirror", to the three Freud had proposed (the oral, anal, and phallic).

THAT IDIOT AGAIN. I'LL TEACH HIM TO STEAL MY MUMMY FROM ME!

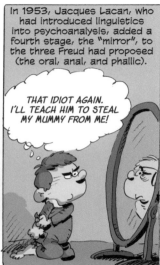

Pierre Janet was committed to making the study of psychology truly scientific.

IT'S TIME TO FREE PSYCHOLOGY FROM ITS OLD PHILOSOPHICAL CLASSIFICATION.

WE MUST APPLY EXPERIMENTAL METHODS IN LABORATORY SETTINGS, AS MY TEACHER THÉODULE-ARMAND RIBOT SUGGESTED.

Among his successors, Jean Piaget was interested in the child's psychological development.

PUFF

Meanwhile, the ideal asylums Esquirol had dreamed of had become veritable "straitjackets of stone". All transgressions were severely punished there, while treatments were few and far between, and often barbaric.

WE'VE BEEN BAD BOYS AND GIRLS!

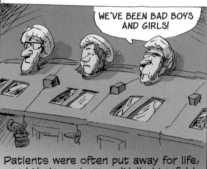

Patients were often put away for life, and their numbers multiplied tenfold in just one century.

The response to wild agitation or aggressive behaviour was invariably incarceration with inhumane treatment, including freezing showers...

TAKE THAT, YOU BIG BOYS. THAT'LL SET YOU STRAIGHT.

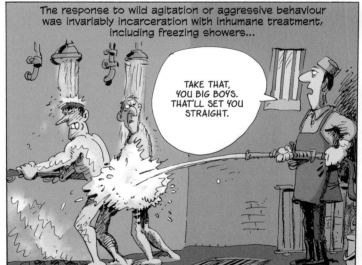

Electroshock...

ZAP! A SHOCK TO THE SYSTEM.

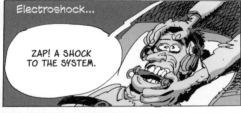

Or the straitjacket.

THESE THINGS'LL DRIVE YOU CRAZY!

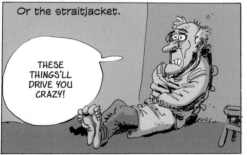

Worst of all was lobotomy (surgery on white matter of the frontal lobe).
MY TECHNIQUE INVOLVES AN ICE-PICK I STICK THROUGH THE EYE SOCKET INTO THE FRONTAL LOBE. I'M ON MY 4,000TH PATIENT!
From the 1950s on, serious doubts put an end to this practice, but its creator, the Portuguese Egas Moniz, had won the Nobel Prize in 1949.
Biological therapies began to address psychoses in 1917.
Malariotherapy consisted of intentionally infecting patients with malaria to induce a fever.
IT'S GREAT FOR HEADACHES!
Whereas insulin shock therapy sought to induce a coma.
UPON EMERGING FROM THE COMA, I EMERGE FROM MY BODY.
After World War Two, there was a great awakening.
The Nazis had exterminated the mentally ill.
In France, they had starved to death in asylums.
Psychiatrists who had been in concentration camps realized their patients had undergone the same ordeal that they had just gone through.
Starting in 1960, psychiatry in France would be divided into sectors. It privileged treatments outside asylums, which were now seen as prison camps.
Support shelters
Private or public clinics
Liaison psychiatry
Psychiatric hospital
Outpatient services
But the real revolution was the discovery of psychotropic drugs.
In 1952, the great medical visionary Henri Laborit suggested using chlorpromazine to treat shock.
AS A NAVY MEDIC, I'D NOTICED THAT LARGACTIL PLUNGED PATIENTS INTO A STATE OF APATHY AND INDIFFERENCE.
At St. Anne's Hospital, Jean Delay and Pierre Deniker prescribed chlorpromazine for their schizophrenic patients.
LARGACTIL IS ACTUALLY AN ANTIPSYCHOTIC, BUT IT CAN ALSO BE USED TO TREAT SYMPTOMS OF CONFUSION.

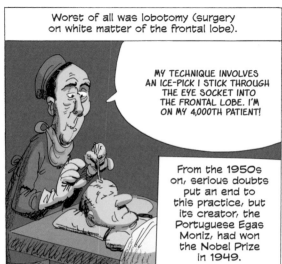

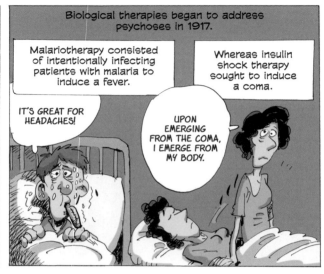

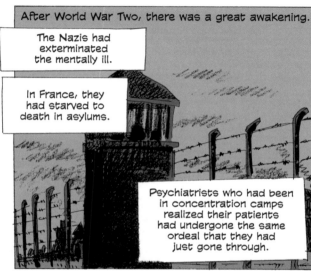

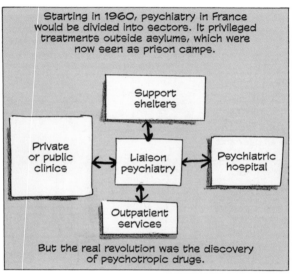

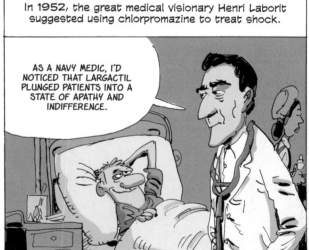

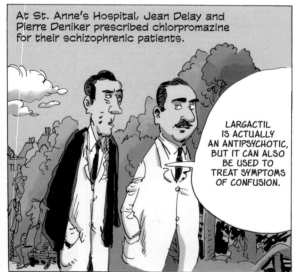

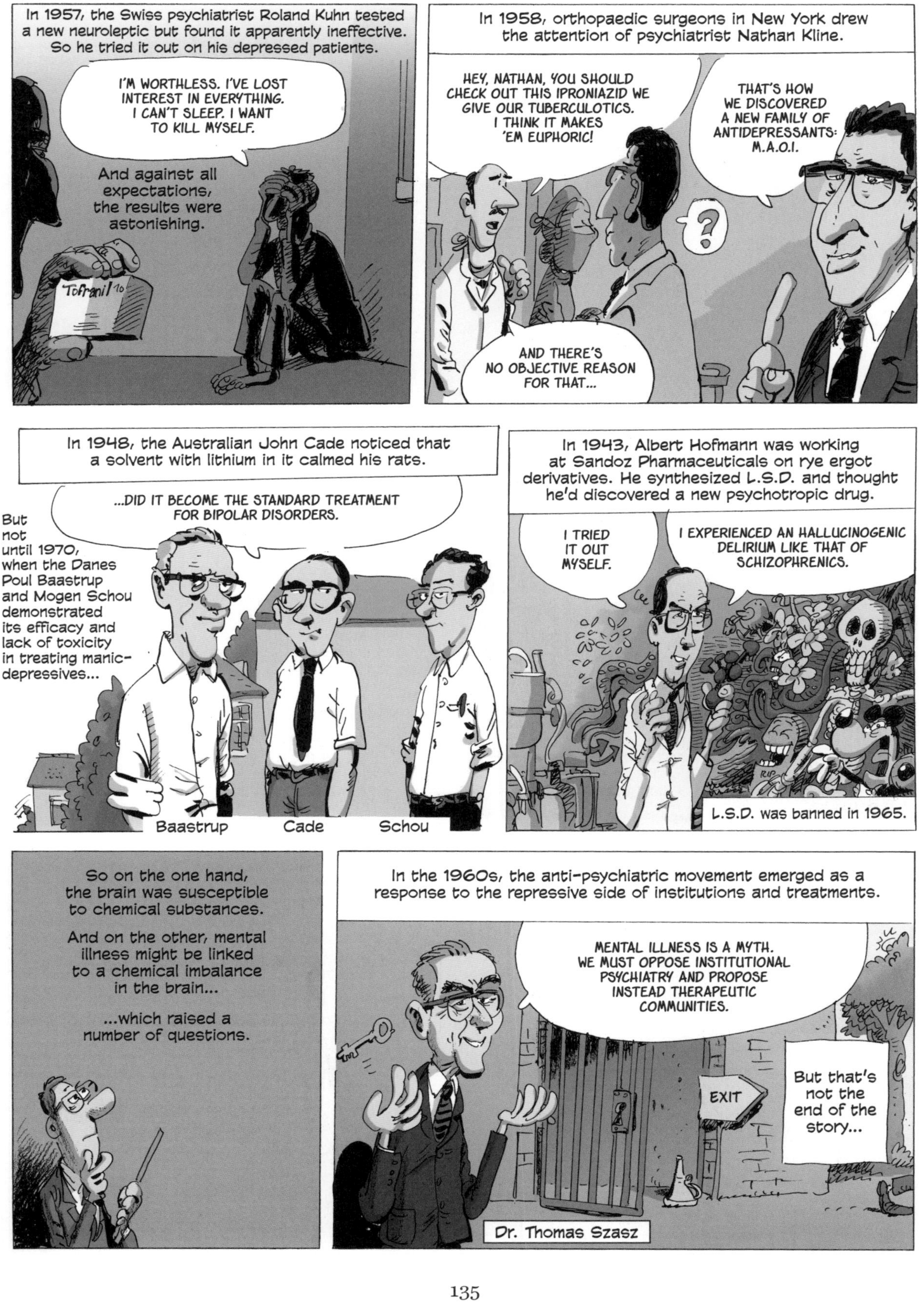

In 1957, the Swiss psychiatrist Roland Kuhn tested a new neuroleptic but found it apparently ineffective. So he tried it out on his depressed patients.
I'M WORTHLESS. I'VE LOST INTEREST IN EVERYTHING. I CAN'T SLEEP. I WANT TO KILL MYSELF.
And against all expectations, the results were astonishing.
Tofranil
In 1958, orthopaedic surgeons in New York drew the attention of psychiatrist Nathan Kline.
HEY, NATHAN, YOU SHOULD CHECK OUT THIS IPRONIAZID WE GIVE OUR TUBERCULOTICS. I THINK IT MAKES 'EM EUPHORIC!
AND THERE'S NO OBJECTIVE REASON FOR THAT...
?
THAT'S HOW WE DISCOVERED A NEW FAMILY OF ANTIDEPRESSANTS: M.A.O.I.
In 1948, the Australian John Cade noticed that a solvent with lithium in it calmed his rats.
But not until 1970, when the Danes Poul Baastrup and Mogen Schou demonstrated its efficacy and lack of toxicity in treating manic-depressives...
...DID IT BECOME THE STANDARD TREATMENT FOR BIPOLAR DISORDERS.
Baastrup
Cade
Schou
In 1943, Albert Hofmann was working at Sandoz Pharmaceuticals on rye ergot derivatives. He synthesized L.S.D. and thought he'd discovered a new psychotropic drug.
I TRIED IT OUT MYSELF.
I EXPERIENCED AN HALLUCINOGENIC DELIRIUM LIKE THAT OF SCHIZOPHRENICS.
L.S.D. was banned in 1965.
So on the one hand, the brain was susceptible to chemical substances.
And on the other, mental illness might be linked to a chemical imbalance in the brain...
...which raised a number of questions.
In the 1960s, the anti-psychiatric movement emerged as a response to the repressive side of institutions and treatments.
MENTAL ILLNESS IS A MYTH. WE MUST OPPOSE INSTITUTIONAL PSYCHIATRY AND PROPOSE INSTEAD THERAPEUTIC COMMUNITIES.
EXIT
But that's not the end of the story...
Dr. Thomas Szasz

PART TWO: THE DISCOVERY OF THE MYSTERIOUS BRAIN

The brain's role was hotly debated in Antiquity. The Egyptians gave more importance to the heart.

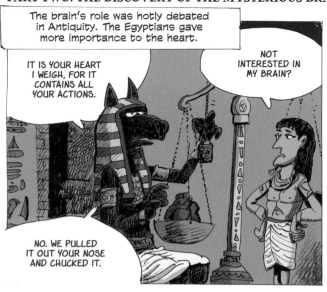

IT IS YOUR HEART I WEIGH, FOR IT CONTAINS ALL YOUR ACTIONS.

NOT INTERESTED IN MY BRAIN?

NO. WE PULLED IT OUT YOUR NOSE AND CHUCKED IT.

The seat of thought also divided Greek physicians.

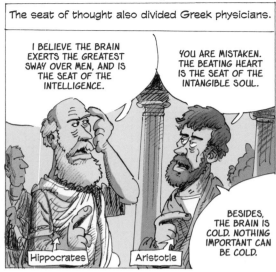

I BELIEVE THE BRAIN EXERTS THE GREATEST SWAY OVER MEN, AND IS THE SEAT OF THE INTELLIGENCE.

YOU ARE MISTAKEN. THE BEATING HEART IS THE SEAT OF THE INTANGIBLE SOUL.

BESIDES, THE BRAIN IS COLD. NOTHING IMPORTANT CAN BE COLD.

Hippocrates · Aristotle

Herophilos described the cerebral ventricles...

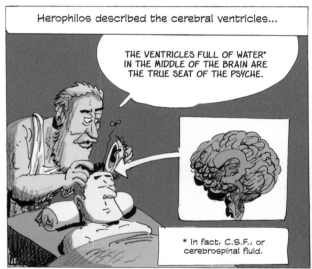

THE VENTRICLES FULL OF WATER* IN THE MIDDLE OF THE BRAIN ARE THE TRUE SEAT OF THE PSYCHE.

* In fact, C.S.F., or cerebrospinal fluid.

...while his accomplice Erasistratus compared the brains of animals.

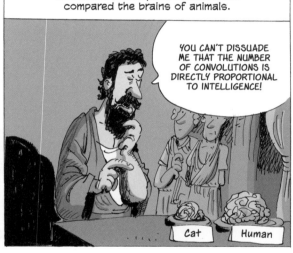

YOU CAN'T DISSUADE ME THAT THE NUMBER OF CONVOLUTIONS IS DIRECTLY PROPORTIONAL TO INTELLIGENCE!

Cat · Human

Galen believed the seat of the soul and thought was indeed the cerebral ventricles.

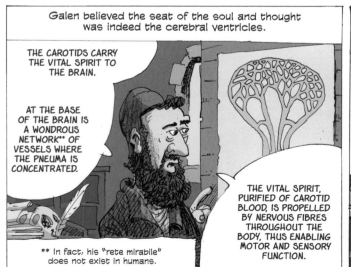

THE CAROTIDS CARRY THE VITAL SPIRIT TO THE BRAIN.

AT THE BASE OF THE BRAIN IS A WONDROUS NETWORK** OF VESSELS WHERE THE PNEUMA IS CONCENTRATED.

THE VITAL SPIRIT, PURIFIED OF CAROTID BLOOD, IS PROPELLED BY NERVOUS FIBRES THROUGHOUT THE BODY, THUS ENABLING MOTOR AND SENSORY FUNCTION.

** In fact, his "rete mirabile" does not exist in humans.

Backed by the Church, Galen's opinions prevailed until the 17th century. Saint Augustine said:

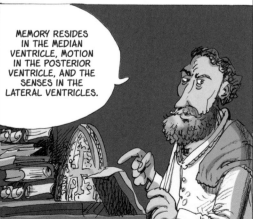

MEMORY RESIDES IN THE MEDIAN VENTRICLE, MOTION IN THE POSTERIOR VENTRICLE, AND THE SENSES IN THE LATERAL VENTRICLES.

And Avicenna, a devoted Galenist, believed the same.

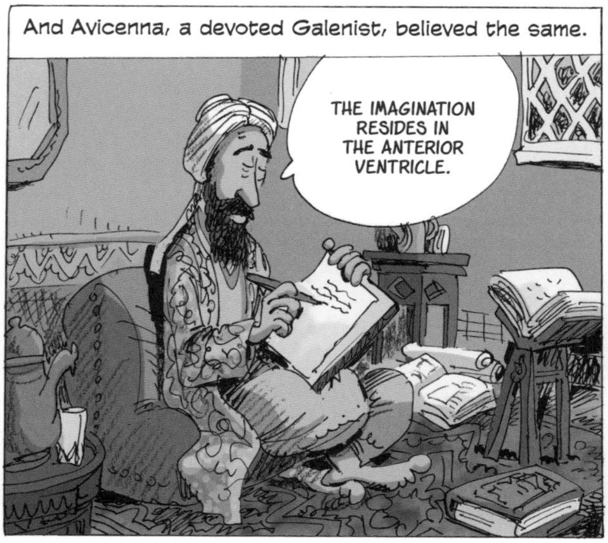
THE IMAGINATION RESIDES IN THE ANTERIOR VENTRICLE.

Vesalius still mentions the "rete mirabile" in the first edition of his *Fabrica*.

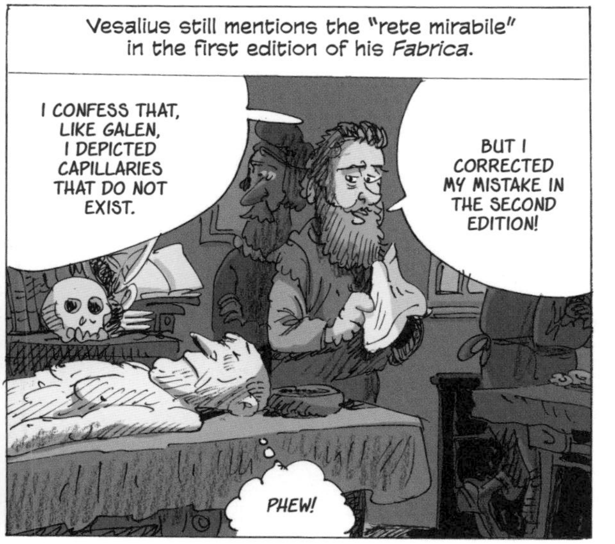
I CONFESS THAT, LIKE GALEN, I DEPICTED CAPILLARIES THAT DO NOT EXIST.
BUT I CORRECTED MY MISTAKE IN THE SECOND EDITION!
PHEW!

Descartes' conception of the brain remained quite Galenic as well.

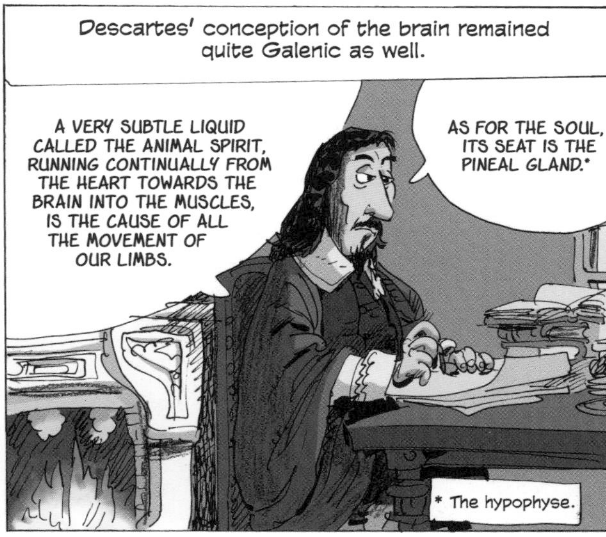
A VERY SUBTLE LIQUID CALLED THE ANIMAL SPIRIT, RUNNING CONTINUALLY FROM THE HEART TOWARDS THE BRAIN INTO THE MUSCLES, IS THE CAUSE OF ALL THE MOVEMENT OF OUR LIMBS.
AS FOR THE SOUL, ITS SEAT IS THE PINEAL GLAND.*

* The hypophyse.

But in 1664, the *Cerebri Anatome* of English doctor Thomas Willis proved a decisive advance.

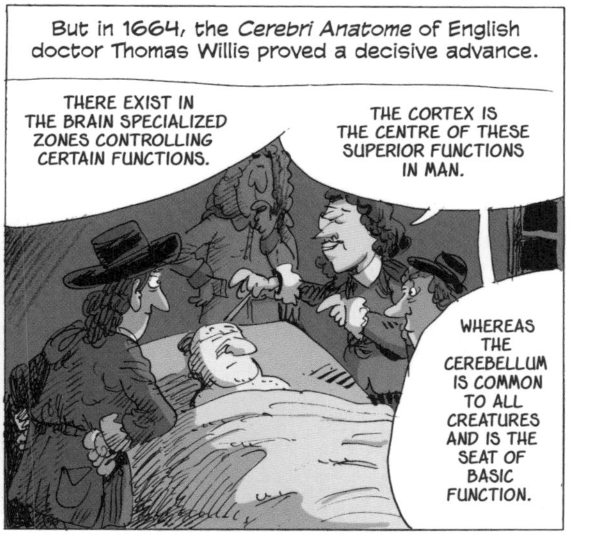
THERE EXIST IN THE BRAIN SPECIALIZED ZONES CONTROLLING CERTAIN FUNCTIONS.
THE CORTEX IS THE CENTRE OF THESE SUPERIOR FUNCTIONS IN MAN.
WHEREAS THE CEREBELLUM IS COMMON TO ALL CREATURES AND IS THE SEAT OF BASIC FUNCTION.

The king of neologisms, he invented the terms "neurology" and "psychology", which met with some success...

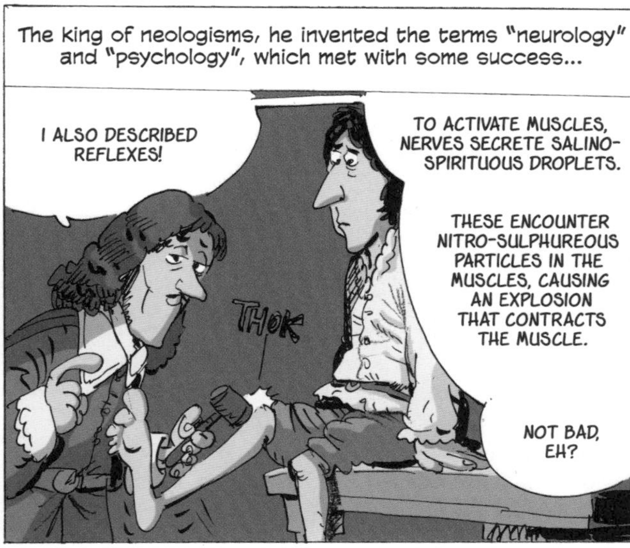
I ALSO DESCRIBED REFLEXES!
TO ACTIVATE MUSCLES, NERVES SECRETE SALINO-SPIRITUOUS DROPLETS.
THESE ENCOUNTER NITRO-SULPHUREOUS PARTICLES IN THE MUSCLES, CAUSING AN EXPLOSION THAT CONTRACTS THE MUSCLE.
THOK
NOT BAD, EH?

ANIMAL ELECTRICITY

Luigi Galvani was an anatomy professor in Bologna. In 1791, he showed that lightning striking a frog's leg via a lightning rod would make the leg twitch.

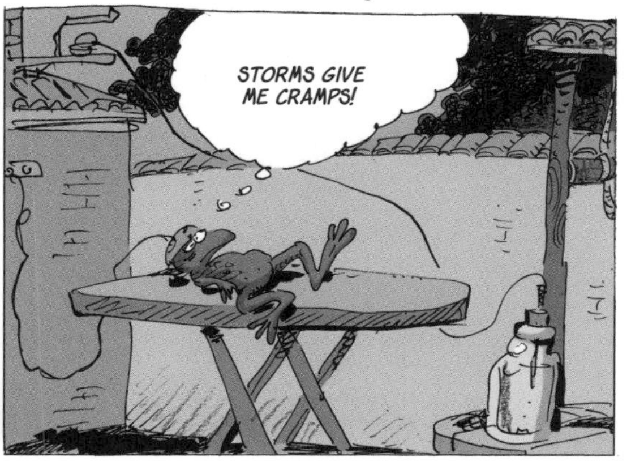
STORMS GIVE ME CRAMPS!

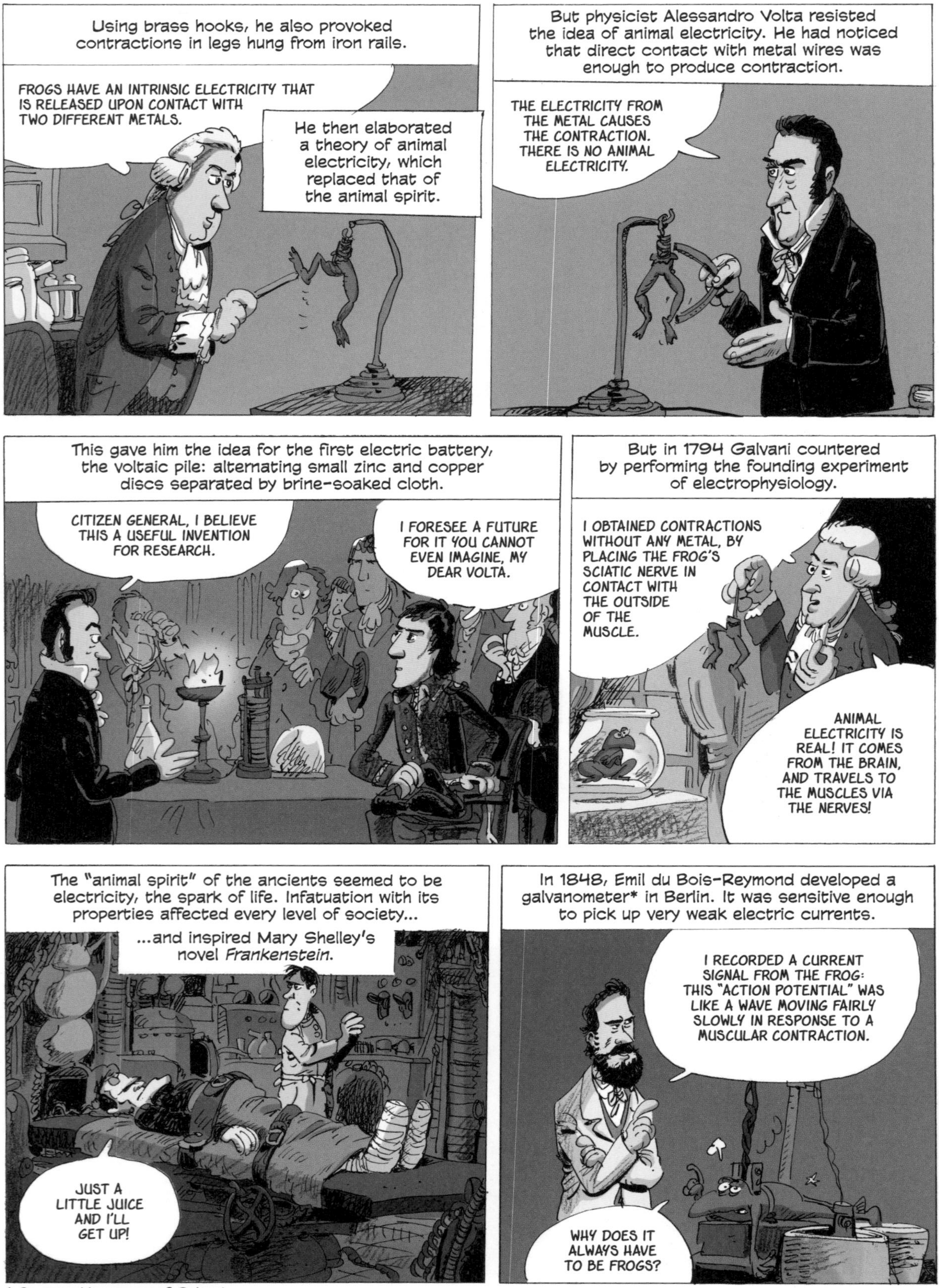
Using brass hooks, he also provoked contractions in legs hung from iron rails.
FROGS HAVE AN INTRINSIC ELECTRICITY THAT IS RELEASED UPON CONTACT WITH TWO DIFFERENT METALS.
He then elaborated a theory of animal electricity, which replaced that of the animal spirit.
But physicist Alessandro Volta resisted the idea of animal electricity. He had noticed that direct contact with metal wires was enough to produce contraction.
THE ELECTRICITY FROM THE METAL CAUSES THE CONTRACTION. THERE IS NO ANIMAL ELECTRICITY.
This gave him the idea for the first electric battery, the voltaic pile: alternating small zinc and copper discs separated by brine-soaked cloth.
CITIZEN GENERAL, I BELIEVE THIS A USEFUL INVENTION FOR RESEARCH.
I FORESEE A FUTURE FOR IT YOU CANNOT EVEN IMAGINE, MY DEAR VOLTA.
But in 1794 Galvani countered by performing the founding experiment of electrophysiology.
I OBTAINED CONTRACTIONS WITHOUT ANY METAL, BY PLACING THE FROG'S SCIATIC NERVE IN CONTACT WITH THE OUTSIDE OF THE MUSCLE.
ANIMAL ELECTRICITY IS REAL! IT COMES FROM THE BRAIN, AND TRAVELS TO THE MUSCLES VIA THE NERVES!
The "animal spirit" of the ancients seemed to be electricity, the spark of life. Infatuation with its properties affected every level of society...
...and inspired Mary Shelley's novel *Frankenstein*.
JUST A LITTLE JUICE AND I'LL GET UP!
In 1848, Emil du Bois-Reymond developed a galvanometer* in Berlin. It was sensitive enough to pick up very weak electric currents.
I RECORDED A CURRENT SIGNAL FROM THE FROG: THIS "ACTION POTENTIAL" WAS LIKE A WAVE MOVING FAIRLY SLOWLY IN RESPONSE TO A MUSCULAR CONTRACTION.
WHY DOES IT ALWAYS HAVE TO BE FROGS?

* So named in memory of Galvani.

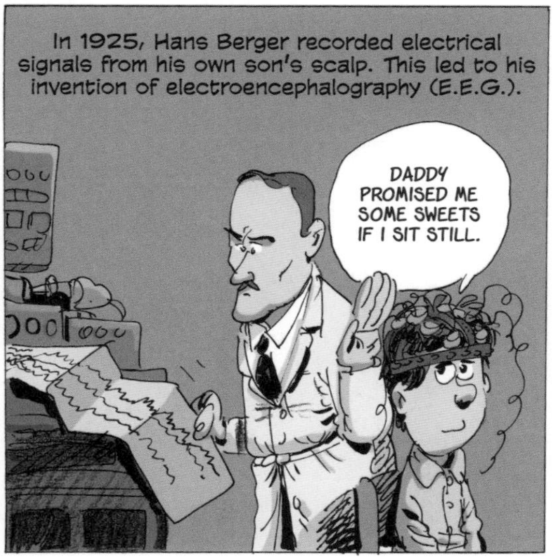
In 1925, Hans Berger recorded electrical signals from his own son's scalp. This led to his invention of electroencephalography (E.E.G.).
DADDY PROMISED ME SOME SWEETS IF I SIT STILL.

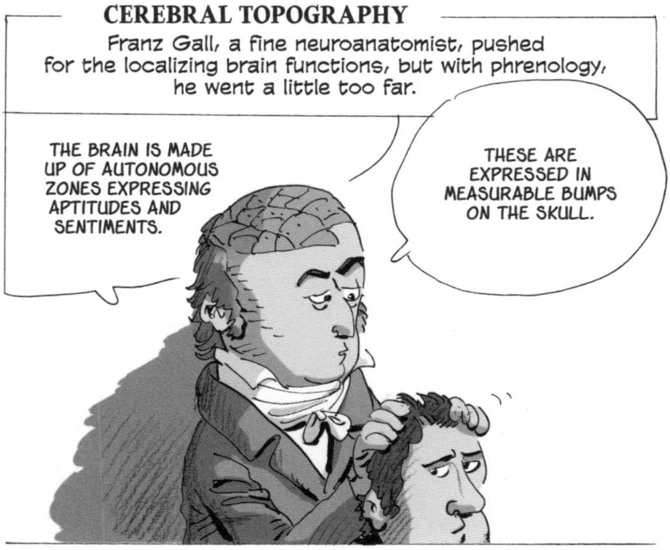
CEREBRAL TOPOGRAPHY
Franz Gall, a fine neuroanatomist, pushed for the localizing brain functions, but with phrenology, he went a little too far.
THE BRAIN IS MADE UP OF AUTONOMOUS ZONES EXPRESSING APTITUDES AND SENTIMENTS.
THESE ARE EXPRESSED IN MEASURABLE BUMPS ON THE SKULL.

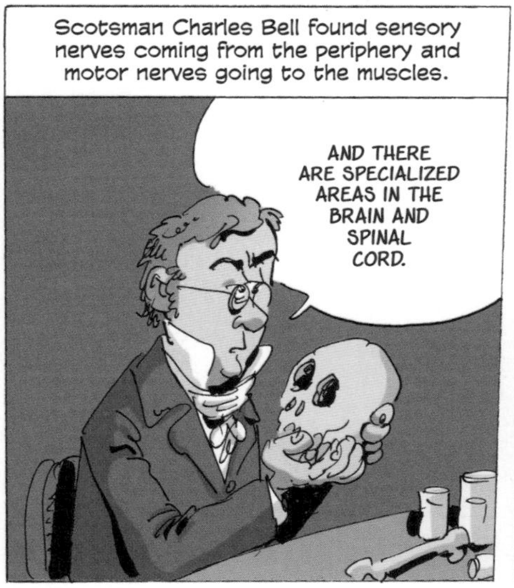
Scotsman Charles Bell found sensory nerves coming from the periphery and motor nerves going to the muscles.
AND THERE ARE SPECIALIZED AREAS IN THE BRAIN AND SPINAL CORD.

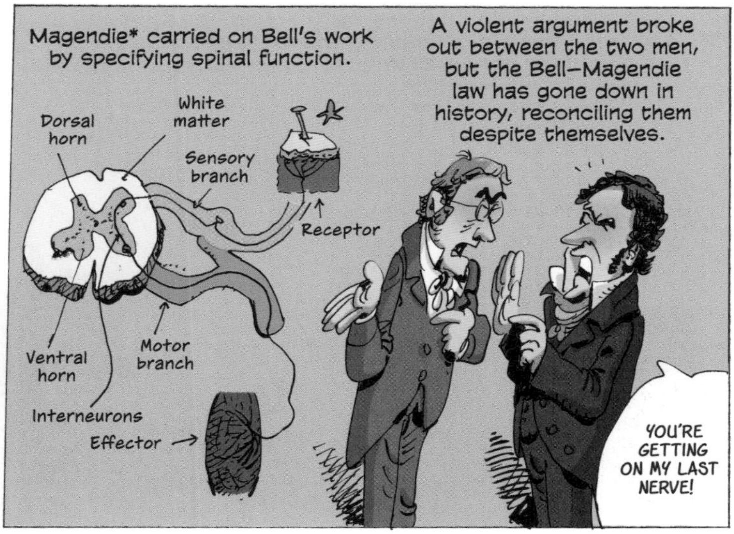
Magendie* carried on Bell's work by specifying spinal function.
Dorsal horn
White matter
Sensory branch
Receptor
Ventral horn
Motor branch
Interneurons
Effector
A violent argument broke out between the two men, but the Bell–Magendie law has gone down in history, reconciling them despite themselves.
YOU'RE GETTING ON MY LAST NERVE!

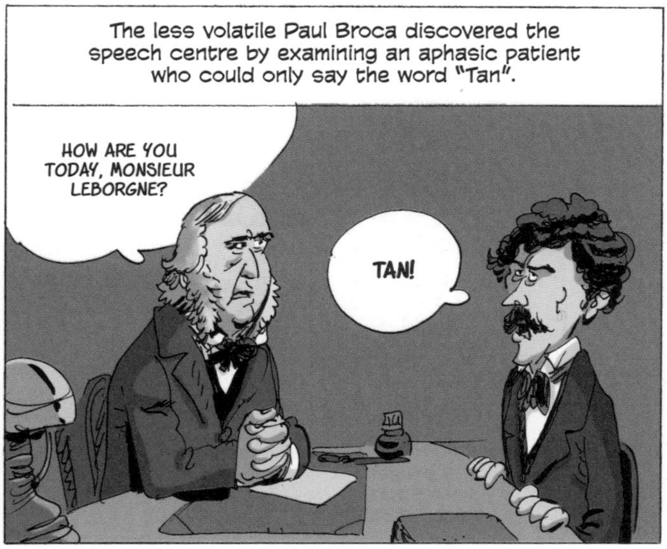
The less volatile Paul Broca discovered the speech centre by examining an aphasic patient who could only say the word "Tan".
HOW ARE YOU TODAY, MONSIEUR LEBORGNE?
TAN!

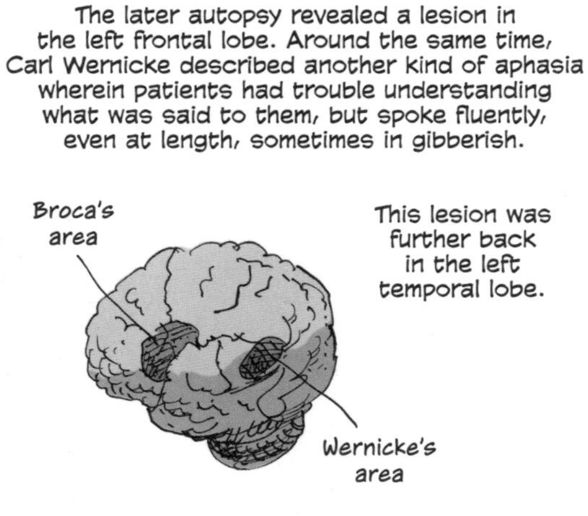
The later autopsy revealed a lesion in the left frontal lobe. Around the same time, Carl Wernicke described another kind of aphasia wherein patients had trouble understanding what was said to them, but spoke fluently, even at length, sometimes in gibberish.
Broca's area
This lesion was further back in the left temporal lobe.
Wernicke's area

* See pages 113 and 207.

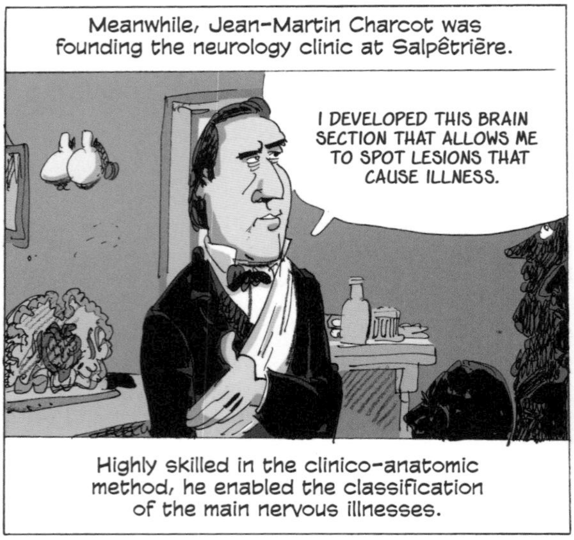
Meanwhile, Jean-Martin Charcot was founding the neurology clinic at Salpêtrière.
I DEVELOPED THIS BRAIN SECTION THAT ALLOWS ME TO SPOT LESIONS THAT CAUSE ILLNESS.
Highly skilled in the clinico-anatomic method, he enabled the classification of the main nervous illnesses.

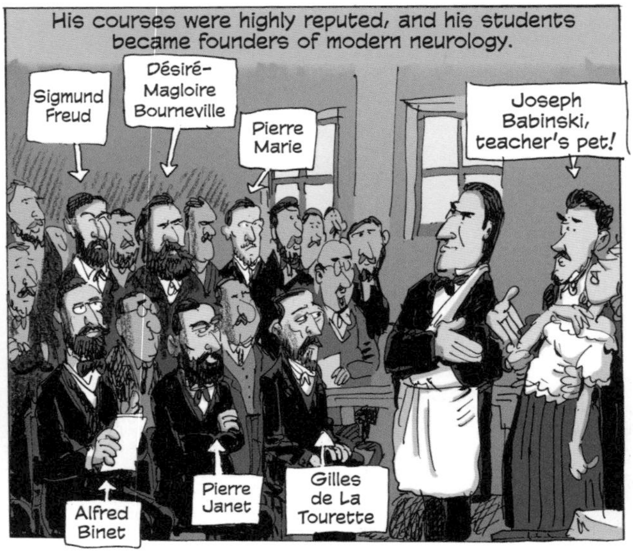
His courses were highly reputed, and his students became founders of modern neurology.
Sigmund Freud
Désiré-Magloire Bourneville
Pierre Marie
Joseph Babinski, teacher's pet!
Alfred Binet
Pierre Janet
Gilles de La Tourette

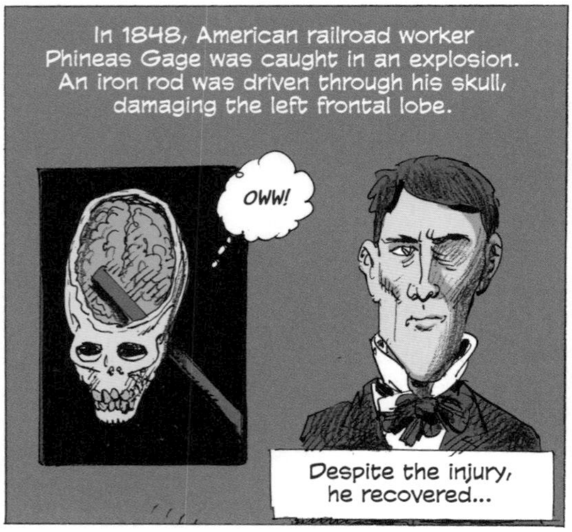
In 1848, American railroad worker Phineas Gage was caught in an explosion. An iron rod was driven through his skull, damaging the left frontal lobe.
OWW!
Despite the injury, he recovered...

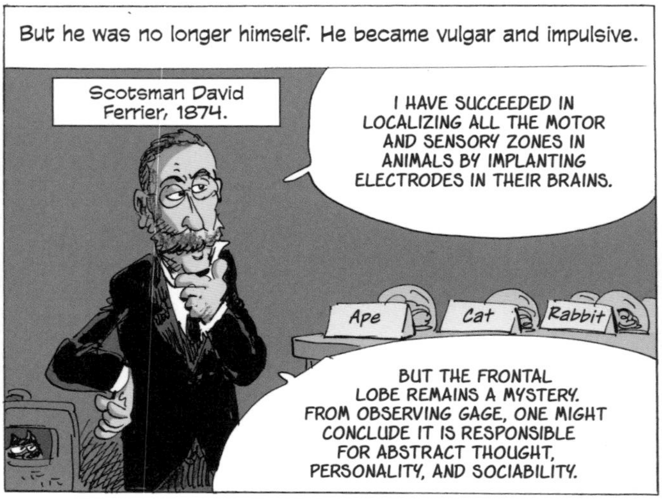
But he was no longer himself. He became vulgar and impulsive.
Scotsman David Ferrier, 1874.
I HAVE SUCCEEDED IN LOCALIZING ALL THE MOTOR AND SENSORY ZONES IN ANIMALS BY IMPLANTING ELECTRODES IN THEIR BRAINS.
Ape
Cat
Rabbit
BUT THE FRONTAL LOBE REMAINS A MYSTERY. FROM OBSERVING GAGE, ONE MIGHT CONCLUDE IT IS RESPONSIBLE FOR ABSTRACT THOUGHT, PERSONALITY, AND SOCIABILITY.

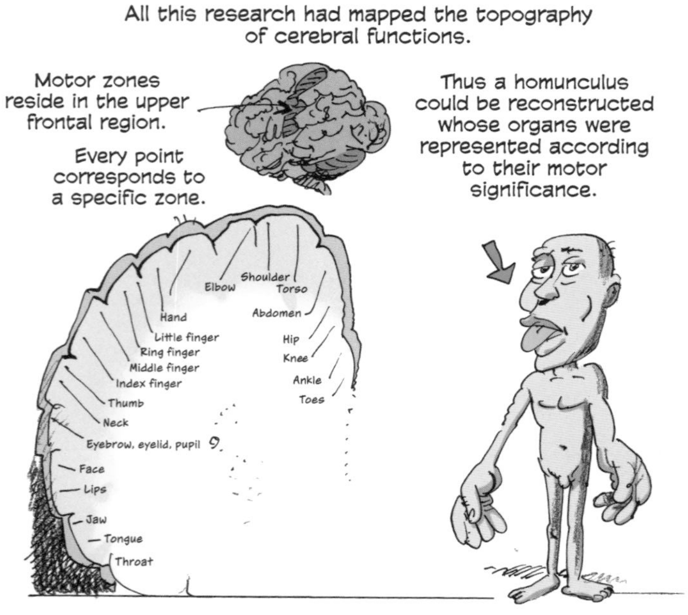
All this research had mapped the topography of cerebral functions.
Motor zones reside in the upper frontal region.
Every point corresponds to a specific zone.
Thus a homunculus could be reconstructed whose organs were represented according to their motor significance.
Shoulder
Elbow
Torso
Hand
Abdomen
Little finger
Hip
Ring finger
Knee
Middle finger
Index finger
Ankle
Toes
Thumb
Neck
Eyebrow, eyelid, pupil
Face
Lips
Jaw
Tongue
Throat

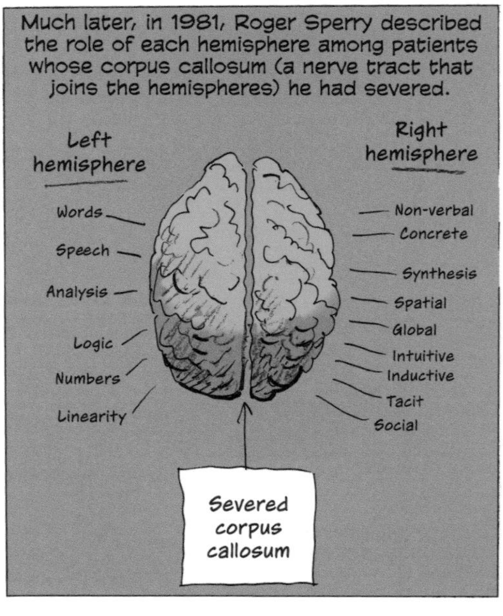
Much later, in 1981, Roger Sperry described the role of each hemisphere among patients whose corpus callosum (a nerve tract that joins the hemispheres) he had severed.
Left hemisphere
Right hemisphere
Words
Speech
Analysis
Logic
Numbers
Linearity
Non-verbal
Concrete
Synthesis
Spatial
Global
Intuitive
Inductive
Tacit
Social
Severed corpus callosum

NERVE CELLS

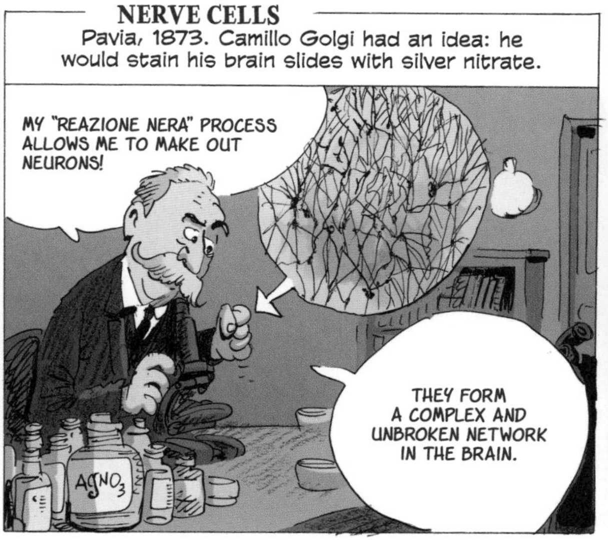
Pavia, 1873. Camillo Golgi had an idea: he would stain his brain slides with silver nitrate.
MY "REAZIONE NERA" PROCESS ALLOWS ME TO MAKE OUT NEURONS!
THEY FORM A COMPLEX AND UNBROKEN NETWORK IN THE BRAIN.
AgNO3

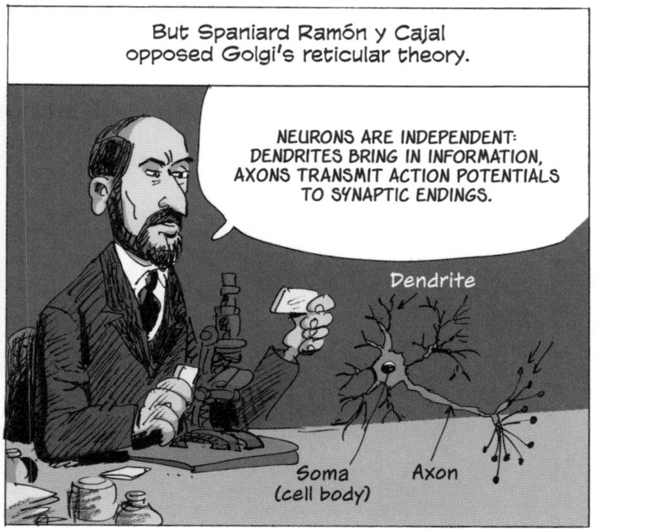
But Spaniard Ramón y Cajal opposed Golgi's reticular theory.
NEURONS ARE INDEPENDENT: DENDRITES BRING IN INFORMATION, AXONS TRANSMIT ACTION POTENTIALS TO SYNAPTIC ENDINGS.
Dendrite
Soma (cell body)
Axon

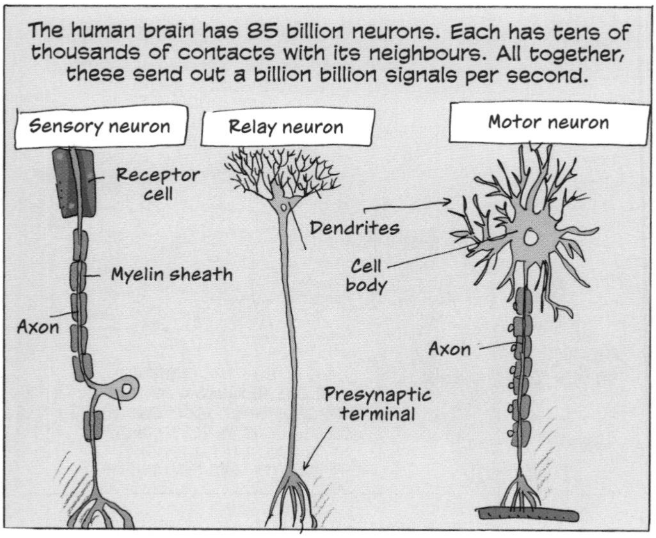
The human brain has 85 billion neurons. Each has tens of thousands of contacts with its neighbours. All together, these send out a billion billion signals per second.
Sensory neuron
Relay neuron
Motor neuron
Receptor cell
Myelin sheath
Axon
Dendrites
Cell body
Axon
Presynaptic terminal

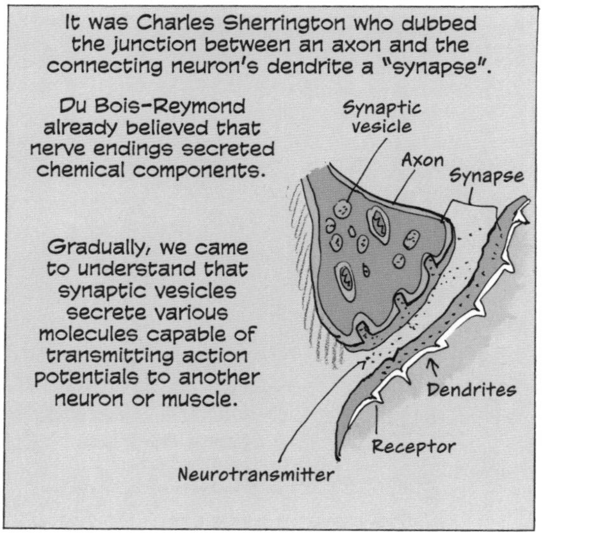
It was Charles Sherrington who dubbed the junction between an axon and the connecting neuron's dendrite a "synapse".
Du Bois-Reymond already believed that nerve endings secreted chemical components.
Gradually, we came to understand that synaptic vesicles secrete various molecules capable of transmitting action potentials to another neuron or muscle.
Synaptic vesicle
Axon
Synapse
Dendrites
Receptor
Neurotransmitter

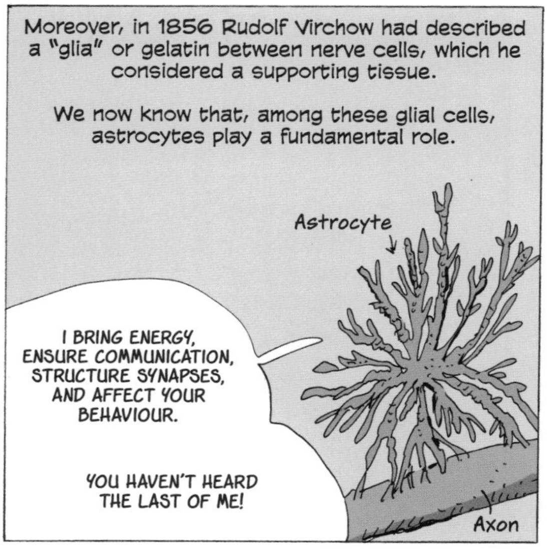
Moreover, in 1856 Rudolf Virchow had described a "glia" or gelatin between nerve cells, which he considered a supporting tissue.
We now know that, among these glial cells, astrocytes play a fundamental role.
Astrocyte
I BRING ENERGY, ENSURE COMMUNICATION, STRUCTURE SYNAPSES, AND AFFECT YOUR BEHAVIOUR.
YOU HAVEN'T HEARD THE LAST OF ME!
Axon

NEUROTRANSMITTERS

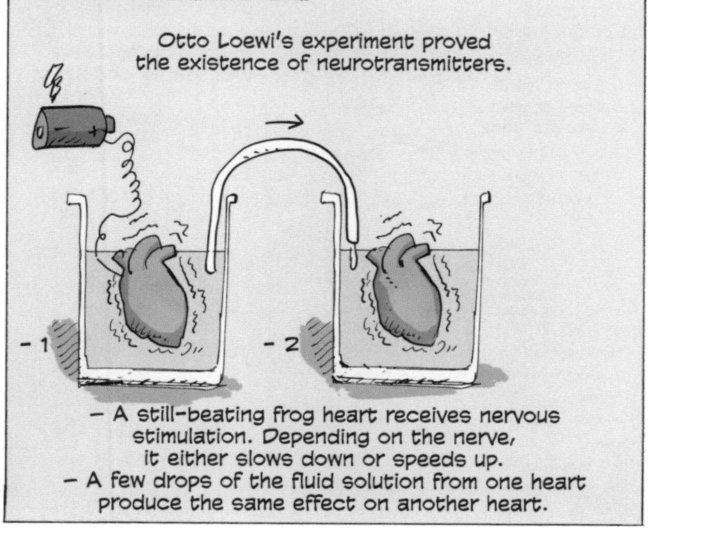
Otto Loewi's experiment proved the existence of neurotransmitters.
- 1
- 2
– A still-beating frog heart receives nervous stimulation. Depending on the nerve, it either slows down or speeds up.
– A few drops of the fluid solution from one heart produce the same effect on another heart.

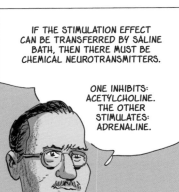

IF THE STIMULATION EFFECT CAN BE TRANSFERRED BY SALINE BATH, THEN THERE MUST BE CHEMICAL NEUROTRANSMITTERS.

ONE INHIBITS: ACETYLCHOLINE. THE OTHER STIMULATES: ADRENALINE.

Otto Loewi, 1921

Many substances have turned out to be neurotransmitters, such as serotonin, histamine, or dopamine (lack of which is responsible for Parkinson's disease).

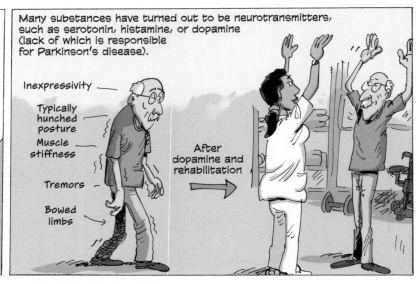

Inexpressivity

Typically hunched posture

Muscle stiffness

Tremors

Bowed limbs

After dopamine and rehabilitation

But the brain also makes transmitters in the form of neuropeptides (several hundred of them) synthesized in the hypothalamus.

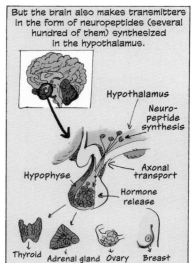

Hypothalamus

Neuro-peptide synthesis

Hypophyse

Axonal transport

Hormone release

Thyroid   Adrenal gland   Ovary   Breast

SURGERY AND IMAGING

In 1902, Halsted's student Harvey Cushing operated on a brain tumour.

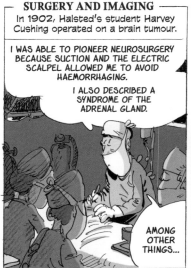

I WAS ABLE TO PIONEER NEUROSURGERY BECAUSE SUCTION AND THE ELECTRIC SCALPEL ALLOWED ME TO AVOID HAEMORRHAGING.

I ALSO DESCRIBED A SYNDROME OF THE ADRENAL GLAND.

AMONG OTHER THINGS...

Thierry de Martel and Clovis Vincent launched neurosurgery in France. Over the last half-century, progress has been considerable.

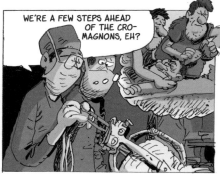

WE'RE A FEW STEPS AHEAD OF THE CRO-MAGNONS, EH?

Modern neurosurgery makes use of imaging, robotics, lasers, sterotaxis...

F.M.R.I.* and P.E.T.** scans have enabled significant advances in understanding lesions and brain functions.

These exams allow, respectively, for the recording of minute variations in localized cerebral bloodflow when specific zones are stimulated, and metabolic and molecular activity through positron emission.

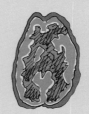 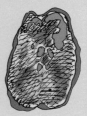

* Functional Magnetic Resonance Imaging.

** Positron Emission Tomography.

Due to their frequency and seriousness, C.V.A.s*** or strokes have been the object of several nationwide awareness campaigns in France. They may be due to haemorrhaging or else an interruption in cerebral blood circulation.

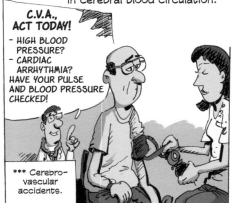

C.V.A., ACT TODAY!

- HIGH BLOOD PRESSURE?
- CARDIAC ARRHYTHMIA?
HAVE YOUR PULSE AND BLOOD PRESSURE CHECKED!

*** Cerebro-vascular accidents.

To sum up, neurology has taken massive strides in the last 20 years.

Understanding diseases of the brain and how to treat them are major issues for 21st-century medicine.

CHAPTER 13

OPHTHALMOLOGY

The eye is a magical organ. Throughout history, loss of sight has been one of the handicaps that has elicited the greatest compassion.

So it was that, upon returning from the Crusades, and inspired by what he had witnessed in Arab lands, Saint Louis IX, King of France, decided to found near Porte Saint-Honoré, "outside the walls" of the city of Paris, the Hospice des Quinze-Vingts, meant to house 300 ("15 times 20") blind paupers. By day, these men would beg for alms, dressed in a hospital uniform adorned with the fleur-de-lis, the stylized lily used as a royal emblem. Any money and food they received was turned over to the common treasury. Thus the blind were placed under the guardianship of the royal chaplain, but had a daily obligation to pray for the salvation of the King and Queen.

Call it well-ordered charity...

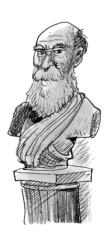

OPHTHALMOLOGY

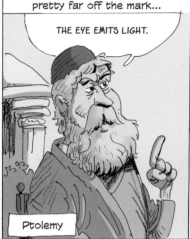

First of all, we had to understand what the eye was. And we started pretty far off the mark...

THE EYE EMITS LIGHT.

Ptolemy

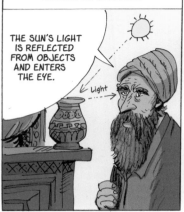

Alhazen discovered how the eye worked in 1021. But he believed the image formed on the lens.

THE SUN'S LIGHT IS REFLECTED FROM OBJECTS AND ENTERS THE EYE.

Light

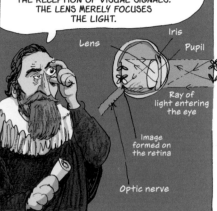

In 1610, Kepler finally solved the mystery.

THE RETINA IS THE SEAT OF THE RECEPTION OF VISUAL SIGNALS. THE LENS MERELY FOCUSES THE LIGHT.

Lens
Iris
Pupil
Ray of light entering the eye
Image formed on the retina
Optic nerve

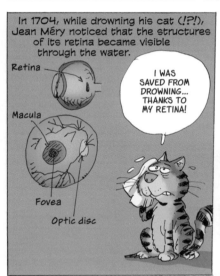

In 1704, while drowning his cat (!?!), Jean Méry noticed that the structures of its retina became visible through the water.

Retina
Macula
Fovea
Optic disc

I WAS SAVED FROM DROWNING... THANKS TO MY RETINA!

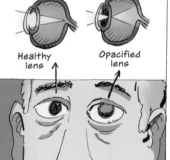

Actually, most cases of blindness worldwide have been caused by cataracts (opacification of the lens)...

Healthy lens
Opacified lens

...and still are today.

Arab physicians already knew how to treat cataracts by couching the lens.

This was historically the surgical technique used for cataracts. A sharp object is used to push the cloudy lens to the bottom of the eye with quick movements.

THE QUICKER THIS GOES, THE BETTER.

Some have always specialized in this operation, with varying degrees of success.

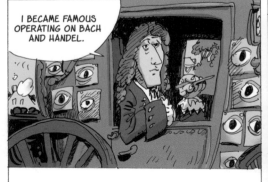

Around 1750, the self-styled "Chevalier" John Taylor roamed Europe, practising his art, in a coach painted with eyes.

I BECAME FAMOUS OPERATING ON BACH AND HANDEL.

Sadly, both composers went blind after his treatment.

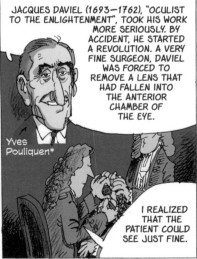

JACQUES DAVIEL (1693–1762), "OCULIST TO THE ENLIGHTENMENT", TOOK HIS WORK MORE SERIOUSLY. BY ACCIDENT, HE STARTED A REVOLUTION. A VERY FINE SURGEON, DAVIEL WAS FORCED TO REMOVE A LENS THAT HAD FALLEN INTO THE ANTERIOR CHAMBER OF THE EYE.

Yves Pouliquen*

I REALIZED THAT THE PATIENT COULD SEE JUST FINE.

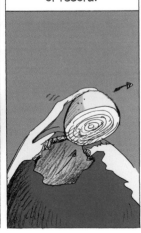

His extraction became the technique of record.

* Ophthalmologist, member of the French Academy, and author of *Un oculiste au temps des lumières* ("An Oculist in the Age of the Enlightenment"), 1999.

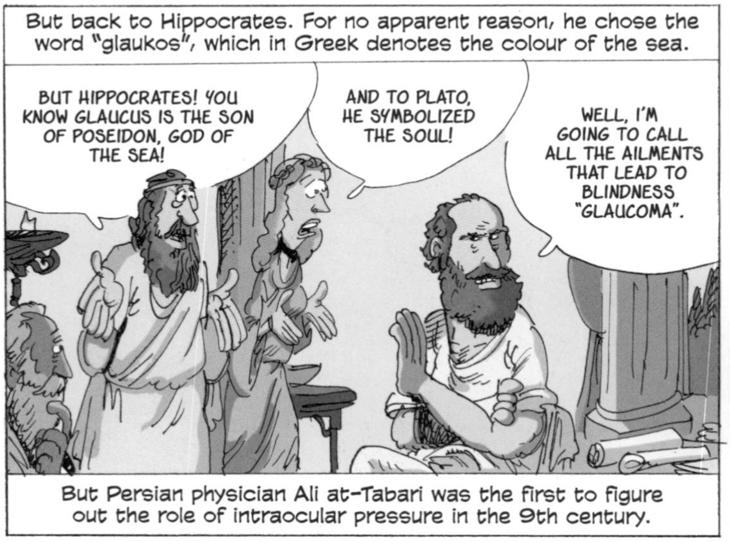
But back to Hippocrates. For no apparent reason, he chose the word "glaukos", which in Greek denotes the colour of the sea.
BUT HIPPOCRATES! YOU KNOW GLAUCUS IS THE SON OF POSEIDON, GOD OF THE SEA!
AND TO PLATO, HE SYMBOLIZED THE SOUL!
WELL, I'M GOING TO CALL ALL THE AILMENTS THAT LEAD TO BLINDNESS "GLAUCOMA".
But Persian physician Ali at-Tabari was the first to figure out the role of intraocular pressure in the 9th century.

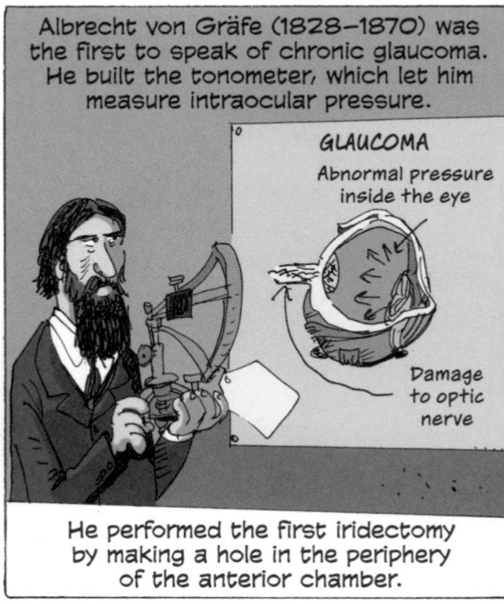
Albrecht von Gräfe (1828–1870) was the first to speak of chronic glaucoma. He built the tonometer, which let him measure intraocular pressure.
GLAUCOMA
Abnormal pressure inside the eye
Damage to optic nerve
He performed the first iridectomy by making a hole in the periphery of the anterior chamber.

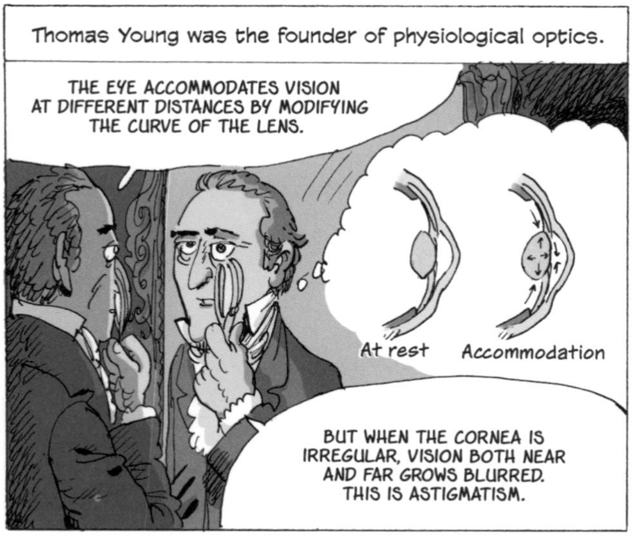
Thomas Young was the founder of physiological optics.
THE EYE ACCOMMODATES VISION AT DIFFERENT DISTANCES BY MODIFYING THE CURVE OF THE LENS.
At rest
Accommodation
BUT WHEN THE CORNEA IS IRREGULAR, VISION BOTH NEAR AND FAR GROWS BLURRED. THIS IS ASTIGMATISM.

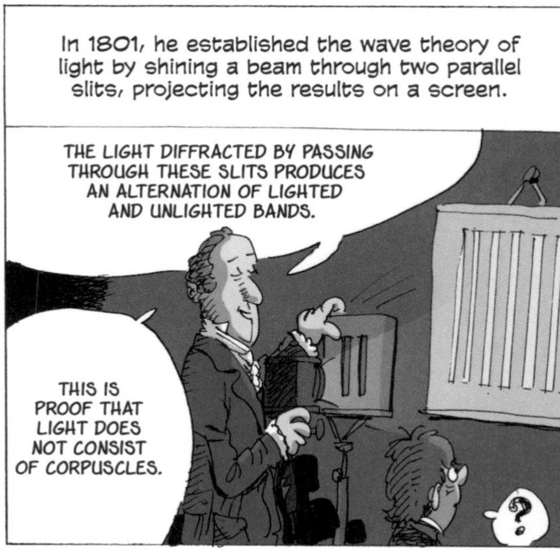
In 1801, he established the wave theory of light by shining a beam through two parallel slits, projecting the results on a screen.
THE LIGHT DIFFRACTED BY PASSING THROUGH THESE SLITS PRODUCES AN ALTERNATION OF LIGHTED AND UNLIGHTED BANDS.
THIS IS PROOF THAT LIGHT DOES NOT CONSIST OF CORPUSCLES.
?

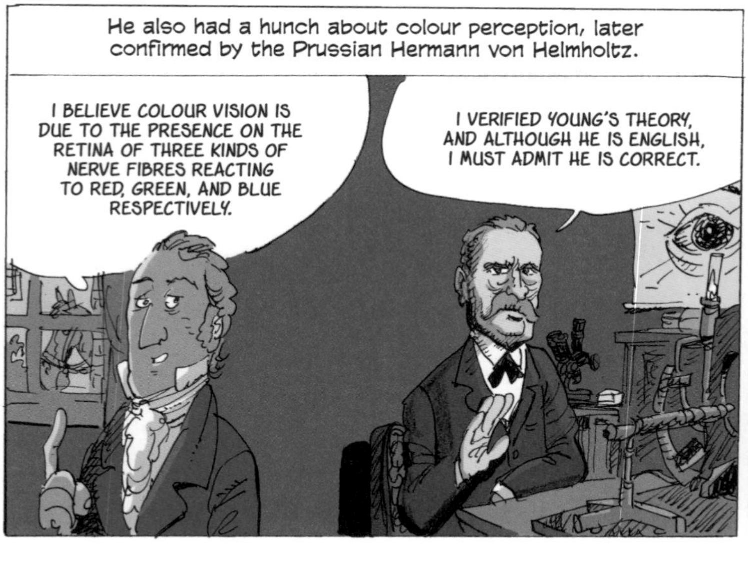
He also had a hunch about colour perception, later confirmed by the Prussian Hermann von Helmholtz.
I BELIEVE COLOUR VISION IS DUE TO THE PRESENCE ON THE RETINA OF THREE KINDS OF NERVE FIBRES REACTING TO RED, GREEN, AND BLUE RESPECTIVELY.
I VERIFIED YOUNG'S THEORY, AND ALTHOUGH HE IS ENGLISH, I MUST ADMIT HE IS CORRECT.

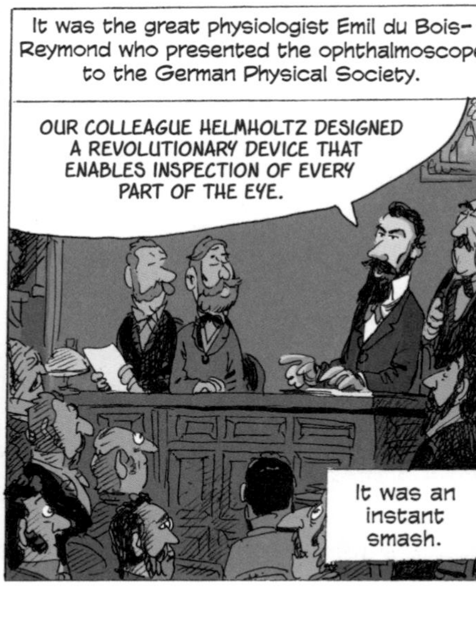
It was the great physiologist Emil du Bois-Reymond who presented the ophthalmoscope to the German Physical Society.
OUR COLLEAGUE HELMHOLTZ DESIGNED A REVOLUTIONARY DEVICE THAT ENABLES INSPECTION OF EVERY PART OF THE EYE.
It was an instant smash.

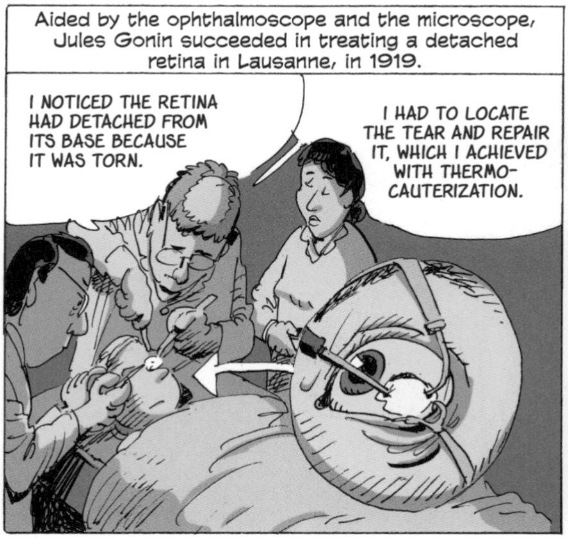
Aided by the ophthalmoscope and the microscope, Jules Gonin succeeded in treating a detached retina in Lausanne, in 1919.
I NOTICED THE RETINA HAD DETACHED FROM ITS BASE BECAUSE IT WAS TORN.
I HAD TO LOCATE THE TEAR AND REPAIR IT, WHICH I ACHIEVED WITH THERMO-CAUTERIZATION.

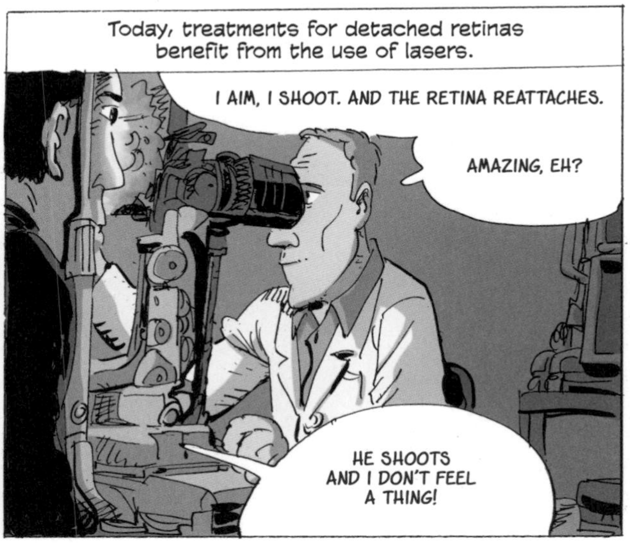
Today, treatments for detached retinas benefit from the use of lasers.
I AIM, I SHOOT. AND THE RETINA REATTACHES.
AMAZING, EH?
HE SHOOTS AND I DON'T FEEL A THING!

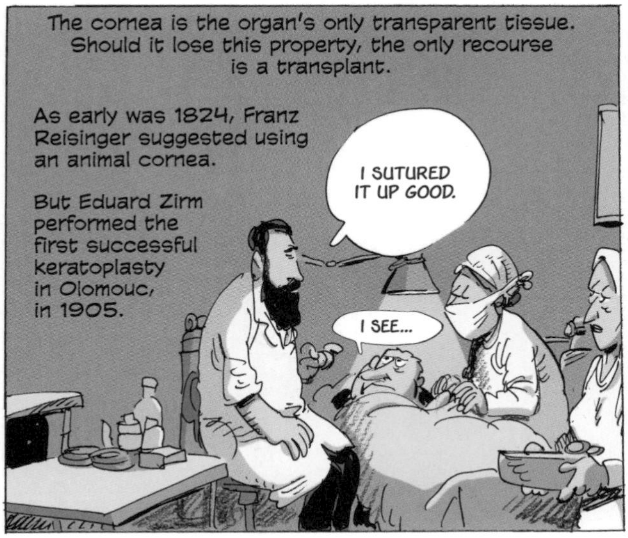
The cornea is the organ's only transparent tissue. Should it lose this property, the only recourse is a transplant.
As early was 1824, Franz Reisinger suggested using an animal cornea.
But Eduard Zirm performed the first successful keratoplasty in Olomouc, in 1905.
I SUTURED IT UP GOOD.
I SEE...

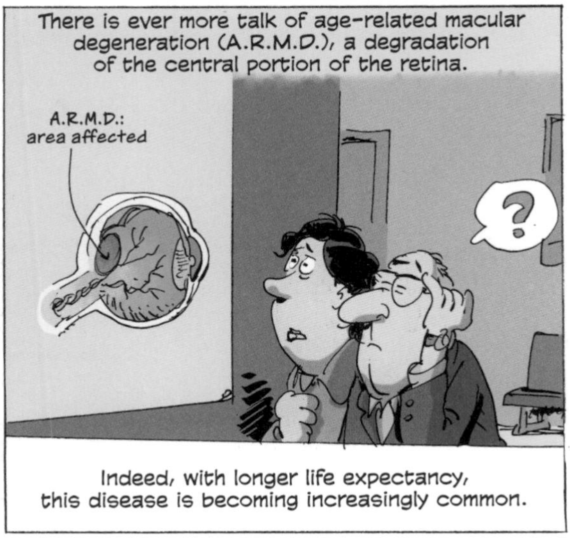
There is ever more talk of age-related macular degeneration (A.R.M.D.), a degradation of the central portion of the retina.
A.R.M.D.: area affected
?
Indeed, with longer life expectancy, this disease is becoming increasingly common.

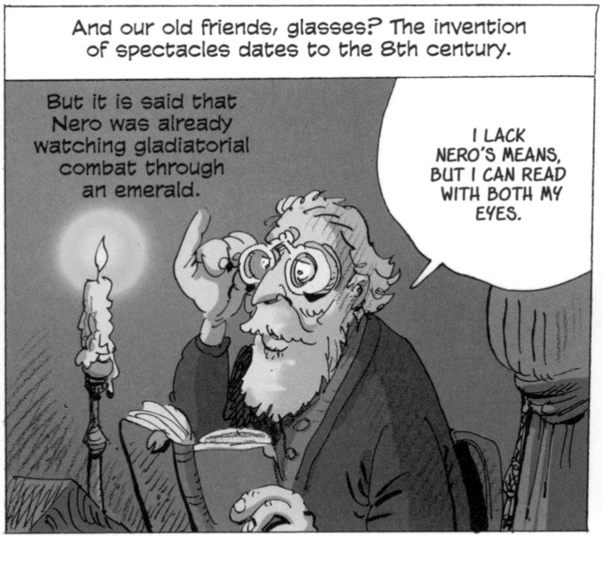
And our old friends, glasses? The invention of spectacles dates to the 8th century.
But it is said that Nero was already watching gladiatorial combat through an emerald.
I LACK NERO'S MEANS, BUT I CAN READ WITH BOTH MY EYES.

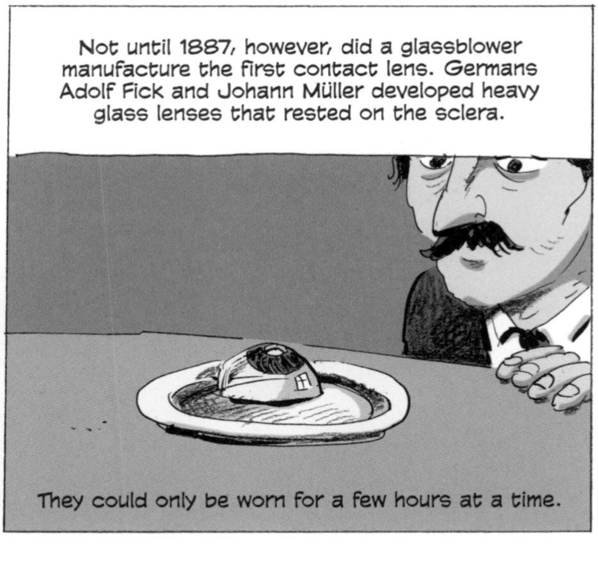
Not until 1887, however, did a glassblower manufacture the first contact lens. Germans Adolf Fick and Johann Müller developed heavy glass lenses that rested on the sclera.
They could only be worn for a few hours at a time.

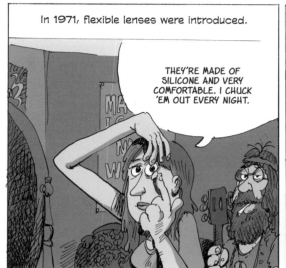

In 1971, flexible lenses were introduced.
THEY'RE MADE OF SILICONE AND VERY COMFORTABLE. I CHUCK 'EM OUT EVERY NIGHT.
But will the nearsighted ever be able to do without corrective lenses someday? In 1939, Tsutomo Sato invented refractive surgery. In Moscow, Fyodorov refined his method, which became "radial keratotomy" in 1974.
офтальм
I MAKE DEEP INCISIONS IN THE CORNEAL PERIPHERY, AND THEN THE INCISED AREAS WILL ARCH UNDER THE INFLUENCE OF INTRAOCULAR PRESSURE, WHILE THE CENTRAL AREA (OPTIC ZONE) WILL FLATTEN.
THIS REDUCES THE CORNEA'S REFRACTIVE POWER AND ALLOWS US TO CURE MYOPIA.
А Г Д И Я
Р Ю Ф Ъ
Э К Ж Ш
П Л В Ё Т
Х С Й З Ч Ы
And the eye itself: is it replaceable? For centuries, ocular prostheses have been merely cosmetic.
But in the last half-century, many systems for transmitting light to the brain have been studied.
1,500-microphotodiode implant transmitting an electric signal to the deep cells of the retina, to treat pigmentary retinitis.
We are headed towards the bionic eye...
Processing box
Cerebral implant
WE HAVE SUCCEEDED IN GIVING THE BLIND BACK THEIR SIGHT. BUT THE IMAGES THEY SEE ARE STILL NOT ENOUGH.
Dr. José-Alain Sahel, Director of the Vision Institute in Paris

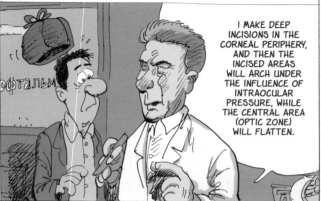

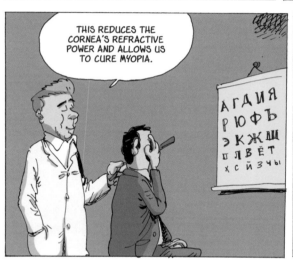

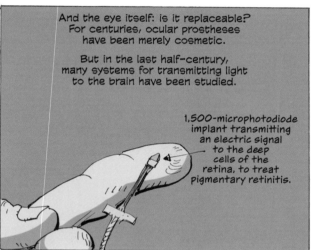

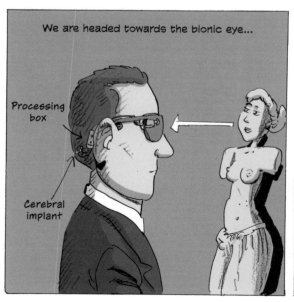

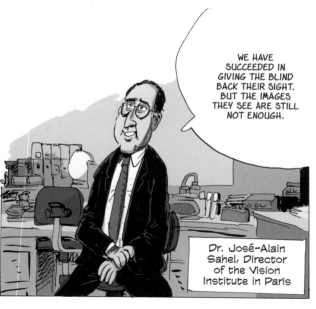

CHAPTER 14

THE FOUNDATIONS OF LIFE: CELLULAR BIOLOGY AND GENETICS

It took some time and quite a few microscope lenses to figure out that life consisted of minute fundamental units: cells.

In the 20th century, it was the great Rudolf Virchow in Berlin who demonstrated that all cells came from other cells, and that diseases originated in the body's cells. Today, he is still considered the "pope" of anatomical pathology.

But we were still a long way from understanding how living creatures passed on their traits.

And Virchow, in his ivory tower at Berlin's Charité Hospital, could not have known that even as he was setting forth his theories, in nearby Moravia a monk was fascinated by growing peas...

Nor could he have known that the discoveries to come would ask fundamental questions about the future of humankind.

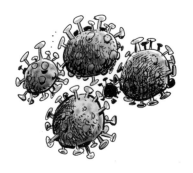

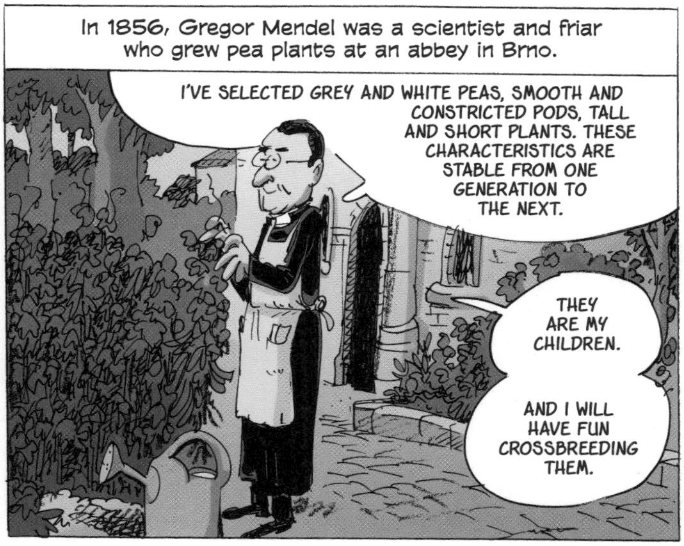
In 1856, Gregor Mendel was a scientist and friar who grew pea plants at an abbey in Brno.
I'VE SELECTED GREY AND WHITE PEAS, SMOOTH AND CONSTRICTED PODS, TALL AND SHORT PLANTS. THESE CHARACTERISTICS ARE STABLE FROM ONE GENERATION TO THE NEXT.
THEY ARE MY CHILDREN.
AND I WILL HAVE FUN CROSSBREEDING THEM.

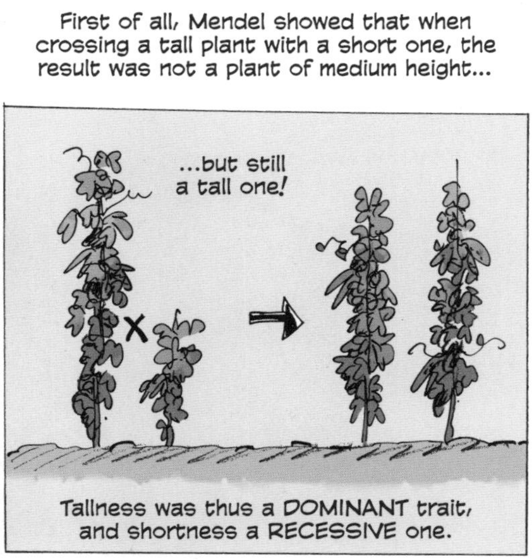
First of all, Mendel showed that when crossing a tall plant with a short one, the result was not a plant of medium height...
...but still a tall one!
Tallness was thus a DOMINANT trait, and shortness a RECESSIVE one.

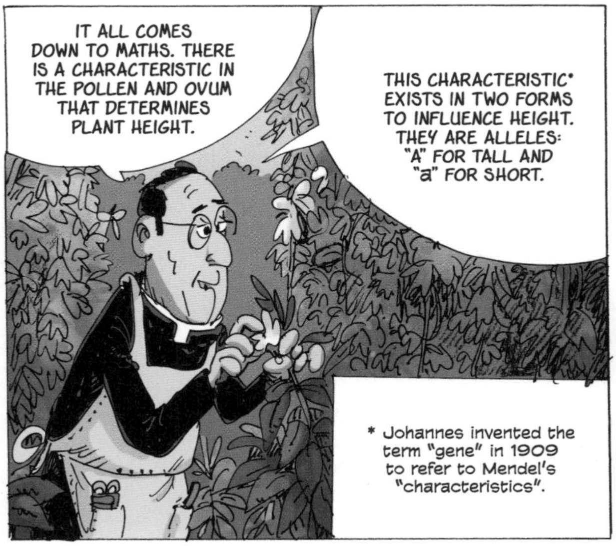
IT ALL COMES DOWN TO MATHS. THERE IS A CHARACTERISTIC IN THE POLLEN AND OVUM THAT DETERMINES PLANT HEIGHT.
THIS CHARACTERISTIC* EXISTS IN TWO FORMS TO INFLUENCE HEIGHT. THEY ARE ALLELES: "A" FOR TALL AND "a" FOR SHORT.
* Johannes invented the term "gene" in 1909 to refer to Mendel's "characteristics".

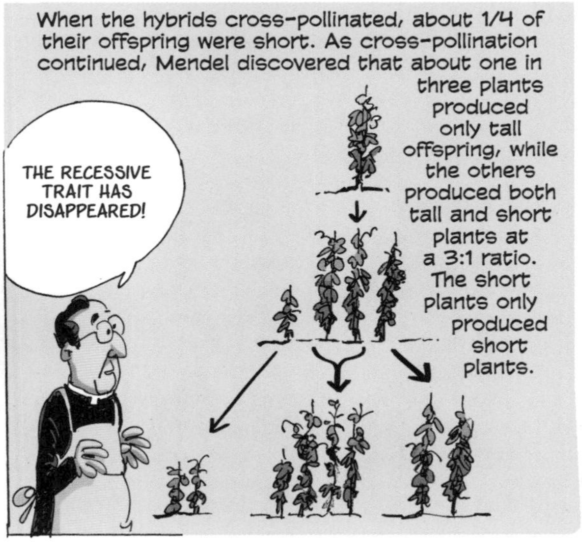
When the hybrids cross-pollinated, about 1/4 of their offspring were short. As cross-pollination continued, Mendel discovered that about one in three plants produced only tall offspring, while the others produced both tall and short plants at a 3:1 ratio. The short plants only produced short plants.
THE RECESSIVE TRAIT HAS DISAPPEARED!

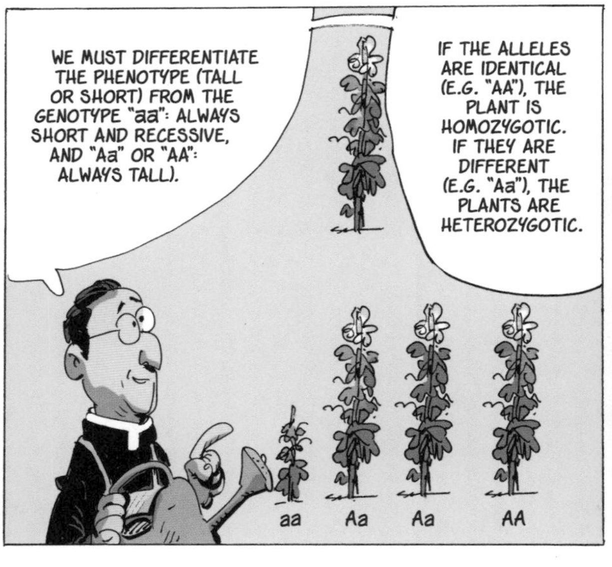
WE MUST DIFFERENTIATE THE PHENOTYPE (TALL OR SHORT) FROM THE GENOTYPE "aa": ALWAYS SHORT AND RECESSIVE, AND "Aa" OR "AA": ALWAYS TALL).
IF THE ALLELES ARE IDENTICAL (E.G. "AA"), THE PLANT IS HOMOZYGOTIC. IF THEY ARE DIFFERENT (E.G. "Aa"), THE PLANTS ARE HETEROZYGOTIC.
aa
Aa
Aa
AA

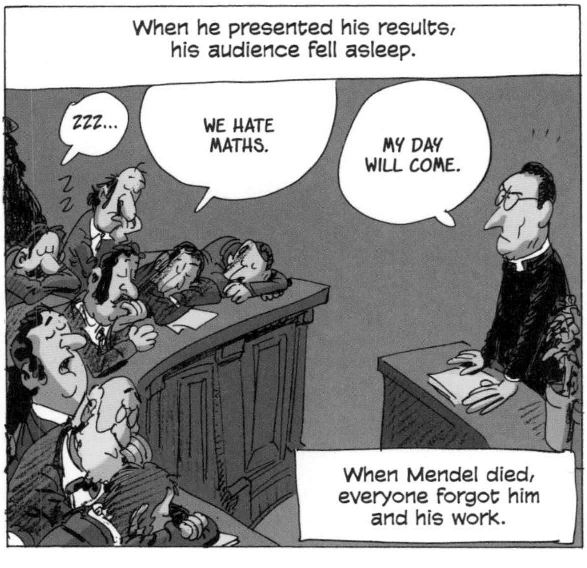
When he presented his results, his audience fell asleep.
ZZZ...
WE HATE MATHS.
MY DAY WILL COME.
When Mendel died, everyone forgot him and his work.

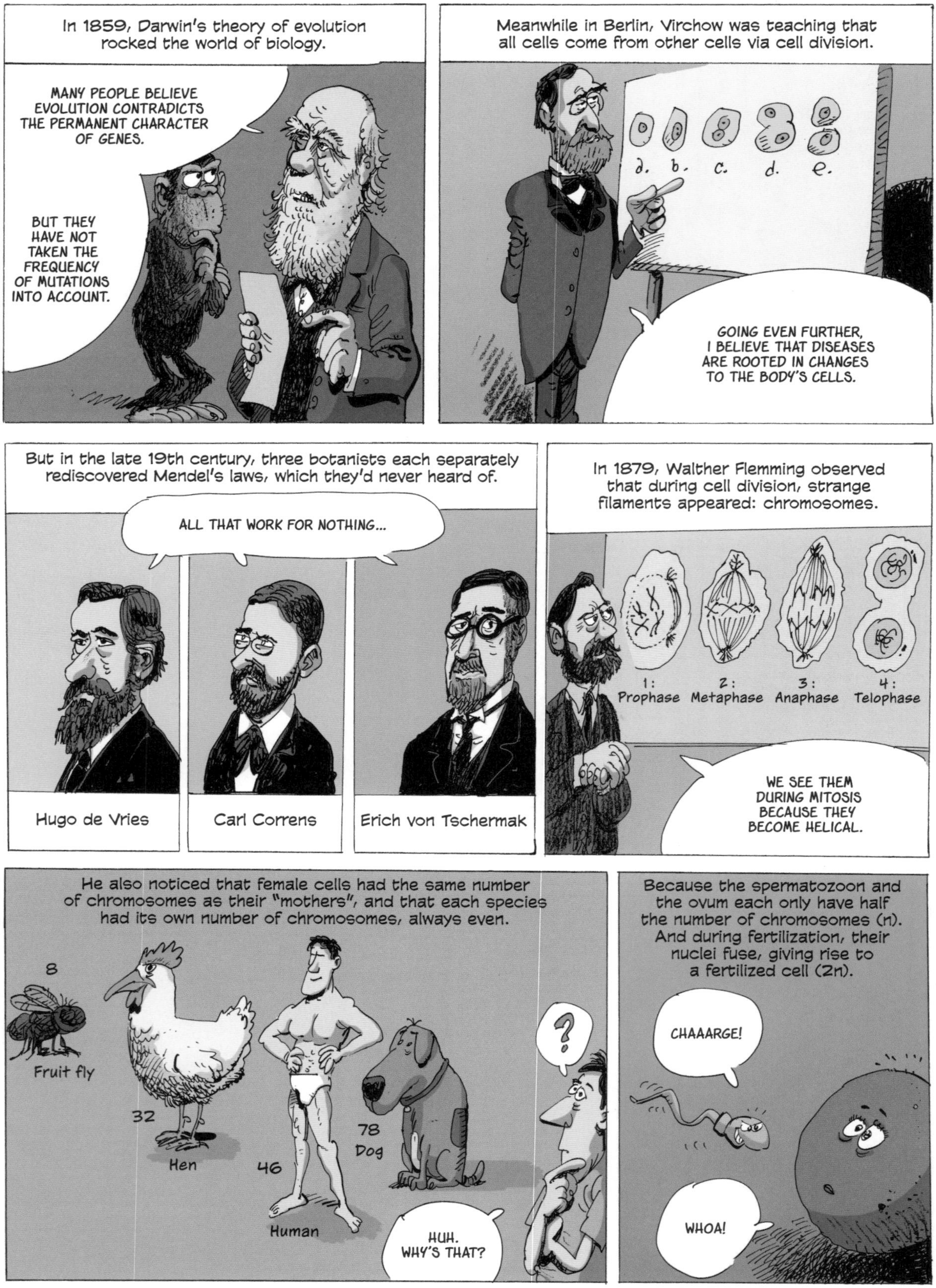
In 1859, Darwin's theory of evolution rocked the world of biology.
MANY PEOPLE BELIEVE EVOLUTION CONTRADICTS THE PERMANENT CHARACTER OF GENES.
BUT THEY HAVE NOT TAKEN THE FREQUENCY OF MUTATIONS INTO ACCOUNT.
Meanwhile in Berlin, Virchow was teaching that all cells come from other cells via cell division.
a. b. c. d. e.
GOING EVEN FURTHER, I BELIEVE THAT DISEASES ARE ROOTED IN CHANGES TO THE BODY'S CELLS.
But in the late 19th century, three botanists each separately rediscovered Mendel's laws, which they'd never heard of.
ALL THAT WORK FOR NOTHING...
Hugo de Vries
Carl Correns
Erich von Tschermak
In 1879, Walther Flemming observed that during cell division, strange filaments appeared: chromosomes.
1: Prophase
2: Metaphase
3: Anaphase
4: Telophase
WE SEE THEM DURING MITOSIS BECAUSE THEY BECOME HELICAL.
He also noticed that female cells had the same number of chromosomes as their "mothers", and that each species had its own number of chromosomes, always even.
8
Fruit fly
32
Hen
46
Human
78
Dog
?
HUH. WHY'S THAT?
Because the spermatozoon and the ovum each only have half the number of chromosomes (n). And during fertilization, their nuclei fuse, giving rise to a fertilized cell (2n).
CHAAARGE!
WHOA!

In 1902, Walter Sutton observed that each chromosome in the spermatozoon corresponded to one in the ovum.

A pair of homologous chromosomes (similar)

The same genes are present in the same place in each homologous chromosome

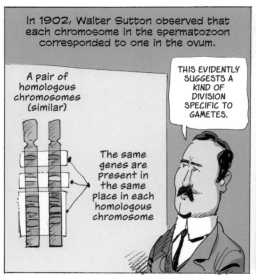

THIS EVIDENTLY SUGGESTS A KIND OF DIVISION SPECIFIC TO GAMETES.

The explanation was meiosis, which Edouard Van Beneden had described in 1887. And Sutton was able to put forth his chromosome theory of inheritance.

MEIOSIS IS, IN FACT, A DOUBLE DIVISION THAT PRODUCES FOUR CELLS EACH CONTAINING (N) CHROMOSOMES.

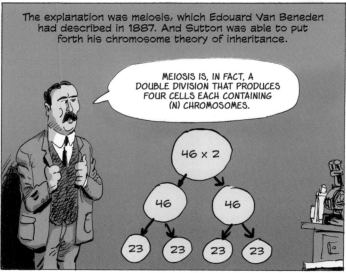

46 x 2

46   46

23   23   23   23

BY MATING, THE GAMETES PRODUCE A CELL WITH 2N CHROMOSOMES.

SUPER SIMPLE, RIGHT?

UH...

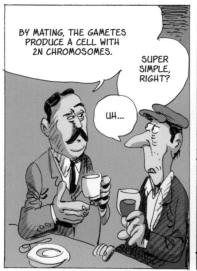

In 1911, geneticist Thomas Hunt Morgan decided to raise flies.

I'LL WORK WITH FRUIT FLIES.* SOME HAVE WHITE EYES, AND OTHERS RED.

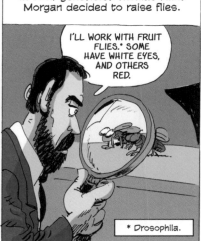

* Drosophila.

THEIR CHROMOSOMES ARE EASY TO STUDY, AND THEY REPRODUCE VERY QUICKLY.

ALL IN THE NAME OF SCIENCE!

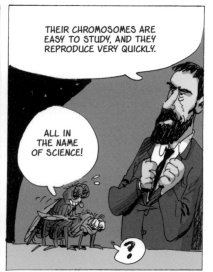

He proved Sutton's chromosome theory of inheritance and showed the existence of mutations, or "crossing over".

During meiosis, homologous chromosomes line up and the corresponding alleles touch.

P D
P D

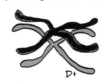

D+

Some segments recombine.

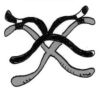

When they separate, there are new combinations of alleles...

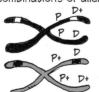

P   D+
P   D
P+   D
P+   D+

...with unexpected results.

ACTUALLY, I'M A MUTANT FRUIT FLY RECOMBINANT.

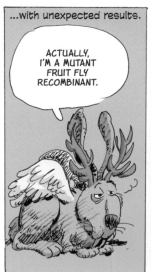

BUT WE STILL DIDN'T KNOW HOW INHERITED CHARACTERISTICS WERE TRANSMITTED.

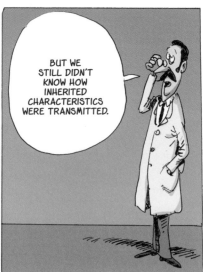

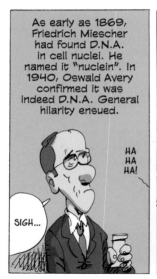

As early as 1869, Friedrich Miescher had found D.N.A. in cell nuclei. He named it "nuclein". In 1940, Oswald Avery confirmed it was indeed D.N.A. General hilarity ensued.
HA HA HA!
SIGH...
It was almost a century before James Watson, Francis Crick, and Rosalind Franklin discovered the molecule's structure: a double helix.
SUCH EXTRAORDINARY SIMPLICITY.
AND VERY STURDY!
In the double helix, every base always paired off with its complement.
THIS STRUCTURE ENSURES REPLICATION AND PROTEIN SYNTHESIS.
Sugar-phosphate backbone
Adenine
Base pair
Thymine
Guanine
Nitrogenous base
Cytosine
BUT TO UNDERSTAND HOW THIS ALL WORKS, LET'S GET DOWN TO BRASS TACKS.
Chromosomes are coiled-up D.N.A., which is itself the carrier of genetic information.
Chromosome
Centromere
Cell
Nucleus
Histone
D.N.A. DOUBLE HELIX
Coiled D.N.A.
BUT THE TRANSCRIPTION OF D.N.A.'S INFORMATION IS CARRIED OUT BY MESSENGER R.N.A., WHICH HEADS FOR THE CELLULAR CYTOPLASM.
TRANSFER R.N.A. (T.R.N.A.) TRANSPORTS AMINO ACIDS TO RIBOSOMES, WHERE THEY ARE ASSEMBLED ACCORDING TO THE GENETIC CODE.
FAIRLY SIMPLE, IN THE END.
D.N.A.
Messenger R.N.A. synthesis
m.R.N.A.
t.R.N.A.
Protein synthesis
Amino acids
The sequence of D.N.A. bases is a language coding for the fabrication of every protein in an organism.
D.N.A.: a unique 4-letter alphabet (A, T, G, C)
UNIVERSAL DICTIONARY OF LIVING BEINGS
PROTEIN: a chain of 20 amino acids
A GENE = A PROTEIN. AND A PROTEIN = AN ENZYME.
THIS APPLIES TO ALL LIVING THINGS, FROM BLUE ALGAE TO APES AND HUMANS.
Rosalind Franklin
In the early 1970s, everything seemed to be falling into place.
Cell
Nucleus
Chromosome
D.N.A. filament
D.N.A.
Nucleotides: Adenine Thymine Guanine Cytosine
All that remained was to map the human genome.
BY 12 FEBRUARY 2001, 95% OF THE HUMAN GENOME HAD BEEN SEQUENCED.
Double strand of D.N.A.
Gene
Sugar-phosphate backbone
Gene
The goal of the original Human Genome Project had been to sequence the 3 billion base pairs and identify all human genes (3% of the bases).

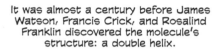

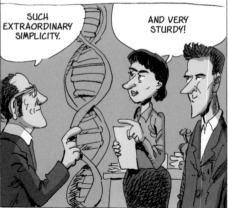

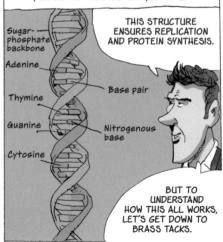

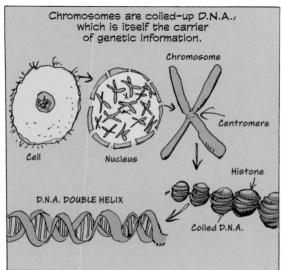

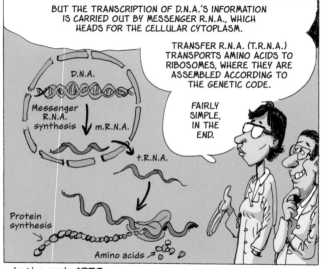

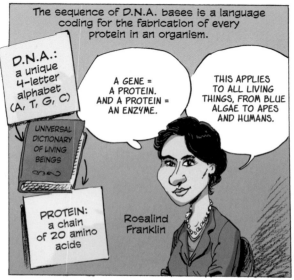

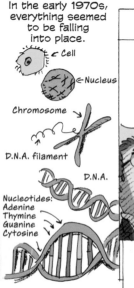

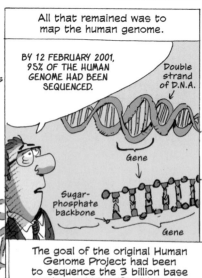

In 1952, Joshua Lederberg described "plasmids": a unit of D.N.A. distinct from a chromosome, able to replicate itself and non-essential to the survival of the cell.

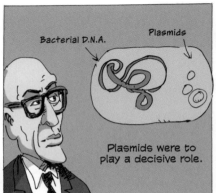

Bacterial D.N.A.   Plasmids

Plasmids were to play a decisive role.

Werner Arber went on to discover restriction endonucleases, which cut D.N.A. to isolate specific parts (for instance, a gene).

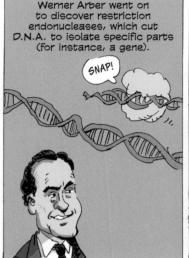

SNAP!

Herbert Boyer and Stanley Cohen would turn bacteria into genetic slaves, forcing them to fabricate human proteins (hormones, for example).

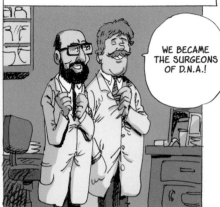

WE BECAME THE SURGEONS OF D.N.A.!

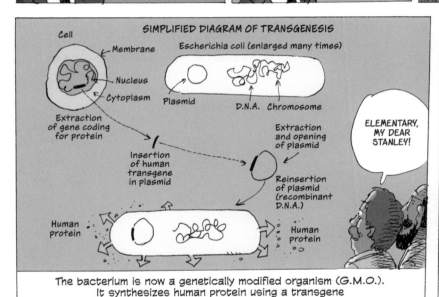

SIMPLIFIED DIAGRAM OF TRANSGENESIS

Cell
Membrane
Nucleus
Cytoplasm

Escherichia coli (enlarged many times)

Plasmid   D.N.A.   Chromosome

Extraction of gene coding for protein

Insertion of human transgene in plasmid

Extraction and opening of plasmid

Reinsertion of plasmid (recombinant D.N.A.)

Human protein

Human protein

ELEMENTARY, MY DEAR STANLEY!

The bacterium is now a genetically modified organism (G.M.O.). It synthesizes human protein using a transgene present in its recombinant D.N.A.

Gene therapy permits the treatment of conditions, inherited and otherwise, in which certain genes are defective or insufficient.

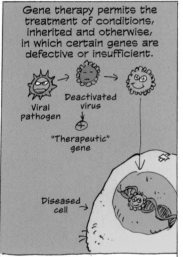

Viral pathogen

Deactivated virus

"Therapeutic" gene

Diseased cell

A deactivated virus is the vector used to penetrate the gene.

The principle is quite simple. Steven Rosenberg performed the first clinical trial in 1980.

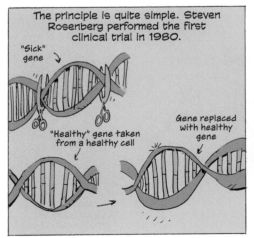

"Sick" gene

"Healthy" gene taken from a healthy cell

Gene replaced with healthy gene

Despite the success of Alain Fischer's procedure in 2000 on "bubble" babies, serious issues remained, like the risk of cancer or leukaemia.

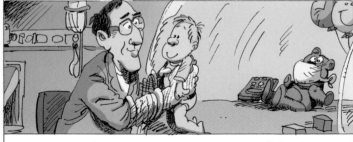

"Bubble" babies had a severe genetic deficiency that forced them to live in sterile bubbles lest they succumb to infection.

Cell therapy was developed around the same time.
1
2
Unused stem cells from an embryo fertilized in vitro
In a culture, they proliferate unchecked
3
4
At the lab, they are made to transform into any cell required – up to 200 different types
Implanted in a patient (for instance, a diabetic), they could replace diseased cells
Philippe Ménasché in Jean-Noël Fabiani's department in Paris ran trials to treat myocardial infarction.
1 Stem cell sample collected under local anaesthesia in a lab
...and a catheter into the previously unblocked coronary artery responsible for the infarction
Stem cells purified
2
3
Stem cells reinjected under local anaesthesia via syringe...
INFARCTION
4
Stem cells transform into cardiac muscle cells
Meanwhile, scientists were exploring cloning.
IN 1962, I MANAGED TO REMOVE THE NUCLEUS FROM A FROG EGG AND (1) REPLACE IT WITH THE NUCLEUS FROM A SPECIALIZED TADPOLE CELL (2). THE MODIFIED EGG DEVELOPED INTO A NORMAL TADPOLE, WHICH THEN BECAME A FROG (3).
1
2
3
John B. Gurdon
Cloning indeed turned out to be possible, even with mammals. In 1996, Dolly the sheep was born in Edinburgh.
Ewe A, nucleus donor
Nucleus extraction
Nucleus insertion
Transfer to breeder for gestation
Mammary gland cell
Ewe B, oocyte donor
Unfertilized oocyte
Ewe C, breeder
Oocyte enucleation
Birth of Dolly (1996)
BAA?
Another kind of cloning, aimed at replacing failing human organs, was also proposed.
AT FIRST, I WANTED TO BE AN ORTHOPAEDIC SURGEON, BUT I DECIDED TO RESEARCH HOW TO TURN PLURIPOTENT* STEM CELLS INTO ANY KIND OF CELL AT ALL!
* Capable of giving rise to several different cell types (e.g. neurons, myocardial cells).
In 2007, Shinya Yamanaka used a cocktail of genes to reprogramme cells into pluripotent cells.
Adult fibroblasts
Genetic reprogramming
Pluripotent cells
Heart
Fat
Neurons
Pancreas
Blood
This paved the way for therapeutic cloning.
WE WILL ALL BENEFIT FROM SUCH ADVANCES!

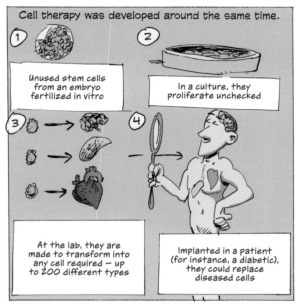

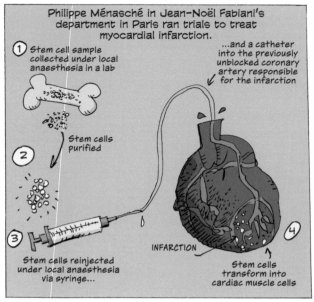

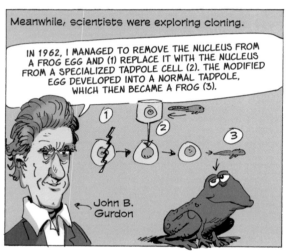

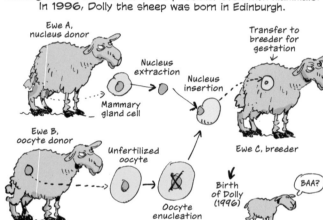

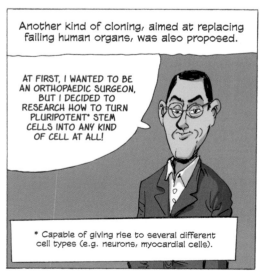

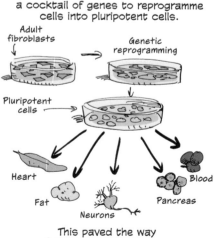

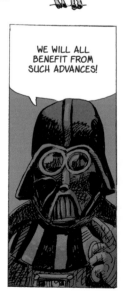

CHAPTER 15

PROCREATION, CONTRACEPTION... RECREATION

Sex has always fascinated humans as a species, and controlling birth has always been on women's minds. On the other hand, increasing fertility for struggling couples is a more recent concern, an offshoot of advances in cellular biology.

But when it comes to sex and procreation, morality and religion always have their tuppence-worth to put in, and the more medicine evolves, the louder their voices grow in the debate.

It must be acknowledged that the most recent progress opens up major moral questions for humanity. Panicked by our newfound power, we fear losing our traditional image of ourselves.

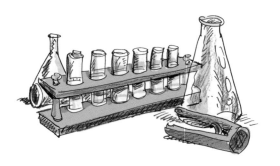

PROCREATION AND CONTRACEPTION

For centuries, no effective contraception existed, and abortion was forbidden.

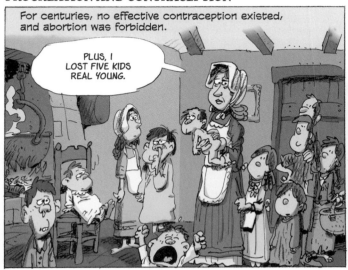

PLUS, I LOST FIVE KIDS REAL YOUNG.

While the 17th and 18th centuries were rather libertine...

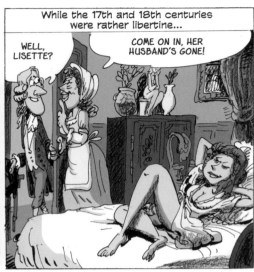

WELL, LISETTE?

COME ON IN, HER HUSBAND'S GONE!

In the 19th century, the desire for birth control went hand in hand with displays of prudishness.

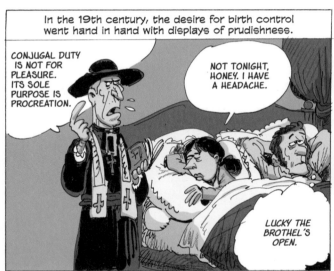

CONJUGAL DUTY IS NOT FOR PLEASURE. ITS SOLE PURPOSE IS PROCREATION.

NOT TONIGHT, HONEY. I HAVE A HEADACHE.

LUCKY THE BROTHEL'S OPEN.

Actually, contraception had been around for a long time, in the form of condoms.

In 3000 BCE, Egyptian soldiers used the intestinal membranes of lambs, or pig bladders.

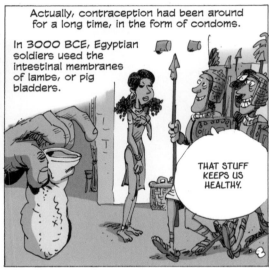

THAT STUFF KEEPS US HEALTHY.

But it was Charles Goodyear who began to mass-produce rubber condoms in 1844.

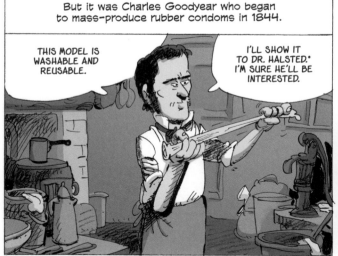

THIS MODEL IS WASHABLE AND REUSABLE.

I'LL SHOW IT TO DR. HALSTED.* I'M SURE HE'LL BE INTERESTED.

In 1928, Ernst Gräfenberg invented the Gräfenberg ring, an early intrauterine device (I.U.D.).

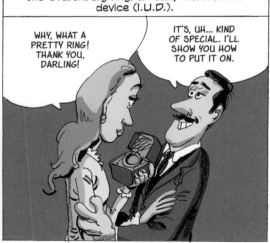

WHY, WHAT A PRETTY RING! THANK YOU, DARLING!

IT'S, UH... KIND OF SPECIAL. I'LL SHOW YOU HOW TO PUT IT ON.

* See page 107.

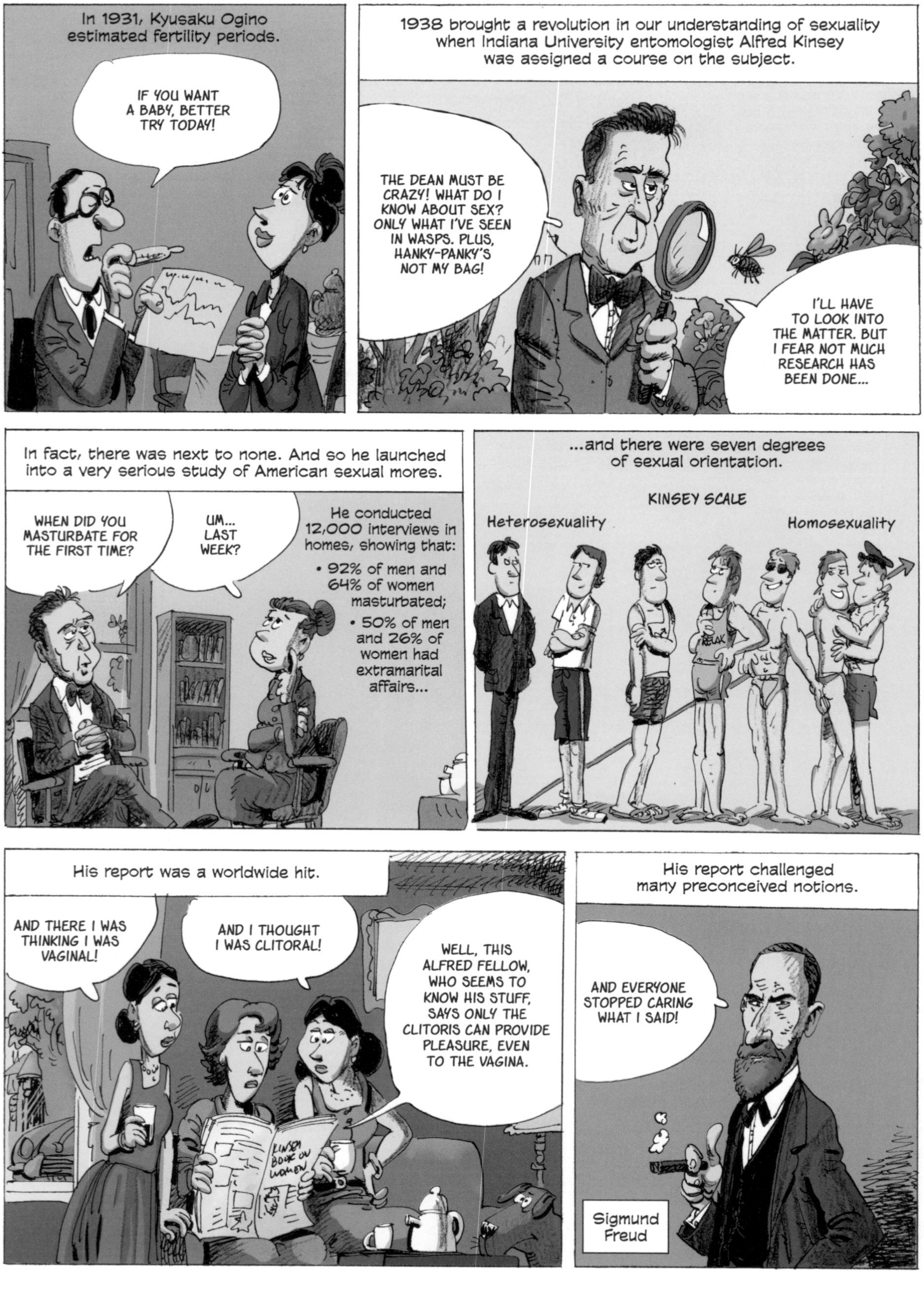
In 1931, Kyusaku Ogino estimated fertility periods.
IF YOU WANT A BABY, BETTER TRY TODAY!
1938 brought a revolution in our understanding of sexuality when Indiana University entomologist Alfred Kinsey was assigned a course on the subject.
THE DEAN MUST BE CRAZY! WHAT DO I KNOW ABOUT SEX? ONLY WHAT I'VE SEEN IN WASPS. PLUS, HANKY-PANKY'S NOT MY BAG!
I'LL HAVE TO LOOK INTO THE MATTER. BUT I FEAR NOT MUCH RESEARCH HAS BEEN DONE...
In fact, there was next to none. And so he launched into a very serious study of American sexual mores.
WHEN DID YOU MASTURBATE FOR THE FIRST TIME?
UM... LAST WEEK?
He conducted 12,000 interviews in homes, showing that:
• 92% of men and 64% of women masturbated;
• 50% of men and 26% of women had extramarital affairs...
...and there were seven degrees of sexual orientation.
KINSEY SCALE
Heterosexuality
Homosexuality
RELAX
His report was a worldwide hit.
AND THERE I WAS THINKING I WAS VAGINAL!
AND I THOUGHT I WAS CLITORAL!
WELL, THIS ALFRED FELLOW, WHO SEEMS TO KNOW HIS STUFF, SAYS ONLY THE CLITORIS CAN PROVIDE PLEASURE, EVEN TO THE VAGINA.
KINSEY BOOK ON WOMEN
His report challenged many preconceived notions.
AND EVERYONE STOPPED CARING WHAT I SAID!
Sigmund Freud

Another study into human sexual behaviour made a big splash in the 1960s: Masters and Johnson used volunteers monitored with electrodes, whom they observed through one-way glass.

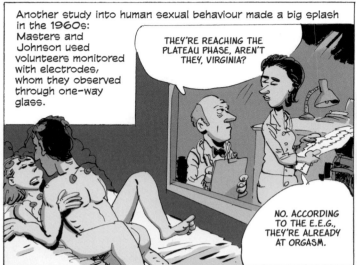

THEY'RE REACHING THE PLATEAU PHASE, AREN'T THEY, VIRGINIA?

NO. ACCORDING TO THE E.E.G., THEY'RE ALREADY AT ORGASM.

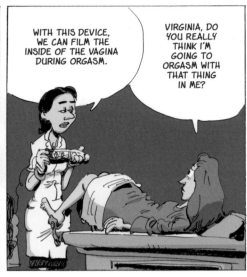

WITH THIS DEVICE, WE CAN FILM THE INSIDE OF THE VAGINA DURING ORGASM.

VIRGINIA, DO YOU REALLY THINK I'M GOING TO ORGASM WITH THAT THING IN ME?

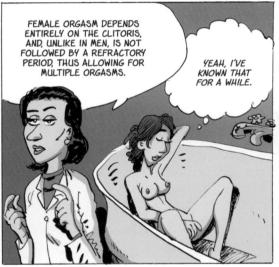

FEMALE ORGASM DEPENDS ENTIRELY ON THE CLITORIS, AND, UNLIKE IN MEN, IS NOT FOLLOWED BY A REFRACTORY PERIOD, THUS ALLOWING FOR MULTIPLE ORGASMS.

YEAH, I'VE KNOWN THAT FOR A WHILE.

Their book was also a worldwide success. They opened a clinic to treat couples with sexual problems.

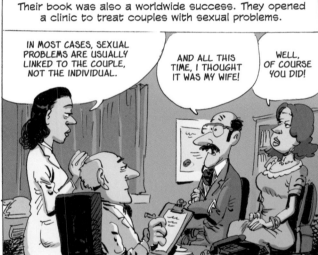

IN MOST CASES, SEXUAL PROBLEMS ARE USUALLY LINKED TO THE COUPLE, NOT THE INDIVIDUAL.

AND ALL THIS TIME, I THOUGHT IT WAS MY WIFE!

WELL, OF COURSE YOU DID!

The same era saw Gregory Pincus' research into sexual hormones (1951).

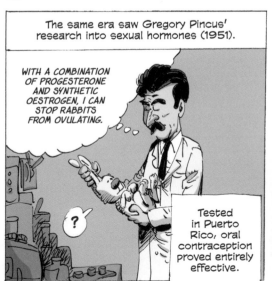

WITH A COMBINATION OF PROGESTERONE AND SYNTHETIC OESTROGEN, I CAN STOP RABBITS FROM OVULATING.

?

Tested in Puerto Rico, oral contraception proved entirely effective.

The pill was available in Germany in 1956, but was banned in France until the Neuwirth Law in 1967.

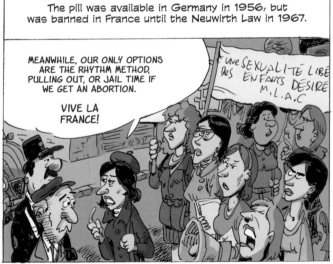

MEANWHILE, OUR ONLY OPTIONS ARE THE RHYTHM METHOD, PULLING OUT, OR JAIL TIME IF WE GET AN ABORTION.

VIVE LA FRANCE!

UNE SEXUALITÉ LIBRE DES ENFANTS DÉSIRÉS M.L.A.C

The law of 17 January 1975 concerning the voluntary interruption of pregnancy made abortion legal in France.
GENTLEMEN OF CONGRESS, ABORTION MUST REMAIN AN EXCEPTION, A LAST RESORT FOR SITUATIONS DEVOID OF OTHER OPTIONS.
Simone Veil
With advances in medically assisted procreation (M.A.P.), many cases of sterility could be examined. But as early as 1789, John Hunter had deposited a husband's sperm in his wife's uterus, resulting in pregnancy. And in Philadelphia in 1884, William Pancoast performed the first artificial insemination from a donor.
AHEM!
WHAT HAPPENED? I FEEL PREGNANT.
In 1968, the first sperm banks opened. And 1969 saw the first pregnancy from ovary stimulation by gonadotropin injection.*
OVER HERE, BOYS!
* Hormone secreted by the hypophyse that stimulates ovarian activity.
Artificial insemination consists of introducing sperm into a woman's uterine cavity.
Spermatozoa
Uterus
Fallopian tube
Oocyte
Ovarian follicle
Ovary
Cervix
Vagina
Insemination catheter
The work of Patrick Steptoe and Robert Edwards enabled the first test-tube baby to be born in 1978, in the UK.
IN VITRO FERTILIZATION (I.V.F.)
1. Stimulation: hormone injection
2. Collect egg and fluid from follicles
3. Fertilization pipette
Embryo
Stimulated ovary
Spermatozoa
Oocyte
4. Embryo development
5. Embryo transfer
CALL ME TUBIE!
CURRENTLY, I.V.F. HAS A 70% SUCCESS RATE.
René Frydman, the "father" of I.V.F. in France
These developments led to a number of ethical and religious debates.
THE ONLY JUSTIFICATION FOR THE ACT OF LOVE IS THE DESIRE TO PROCREATE.
THE CHURCH FORBIDS ARTIFICIAL INSEMINATION AND ALL FORMS OF IN VITRO FERTILIZATION, EVEN FOR MARRIED COUPLES.
Surrogacy is still banned in France.
LUCKILY, WE FOUND SOMEONE ABROAD TO BEAR OUR CHILD FOR US. OTHERWISE...
BEING A SURROGATE KEEPS ME IN CIGGIES AND WHISKY.
As for what to do with frozen embryos... in 1984, Linda Mohr and Alan Trounson pulled off the first human pregnancy following cryopreservation.
-196°
Frozen embryo
Vial in liquid nitrogen
But the future of unused human embryos remains an unresolved issue.

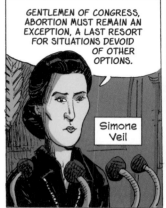

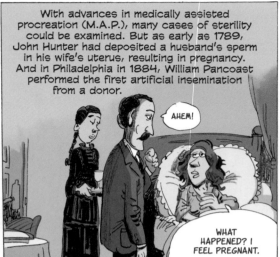

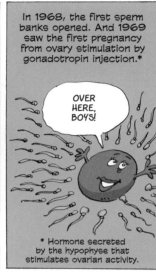

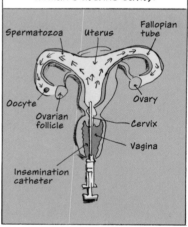

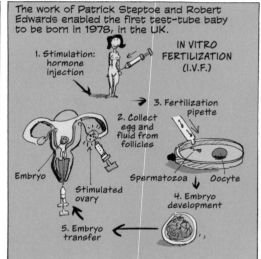

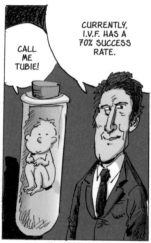

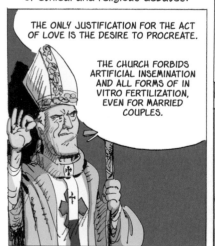

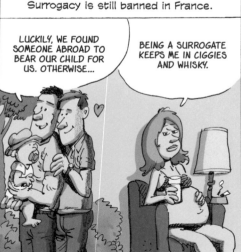

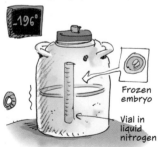

CHAPTER 16

AS GOOD AS NEW

Another of the great adventures in medicine was the possibility of replacing organs or tissues with transplants or prostheses.

Time and again, surgeons were driven to attempt what was first a dream and then a mad hope, to no avail. Not until the 20th century did we understand at last what was part of the self and what was not. Through tireless labour and discoveries in which chance played a large part, we finally succeeded in making transplants "take".

Prostheses, too, have made great strides, from the peglegs of yore to the artificial heart. We are no longer a far cry from the artificial human of recent science-fiction movies. An entirely bioprosthetic body in the service of a computer-enhanced brain no longer seems unbelievable.

In the end, Darth Vader may be but a rough draft for the humans of tomorrow!

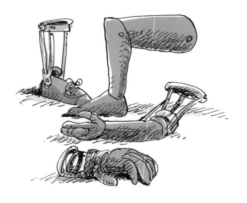

TISSUE GRAFTS AND ORGAN TRANSPLANTS

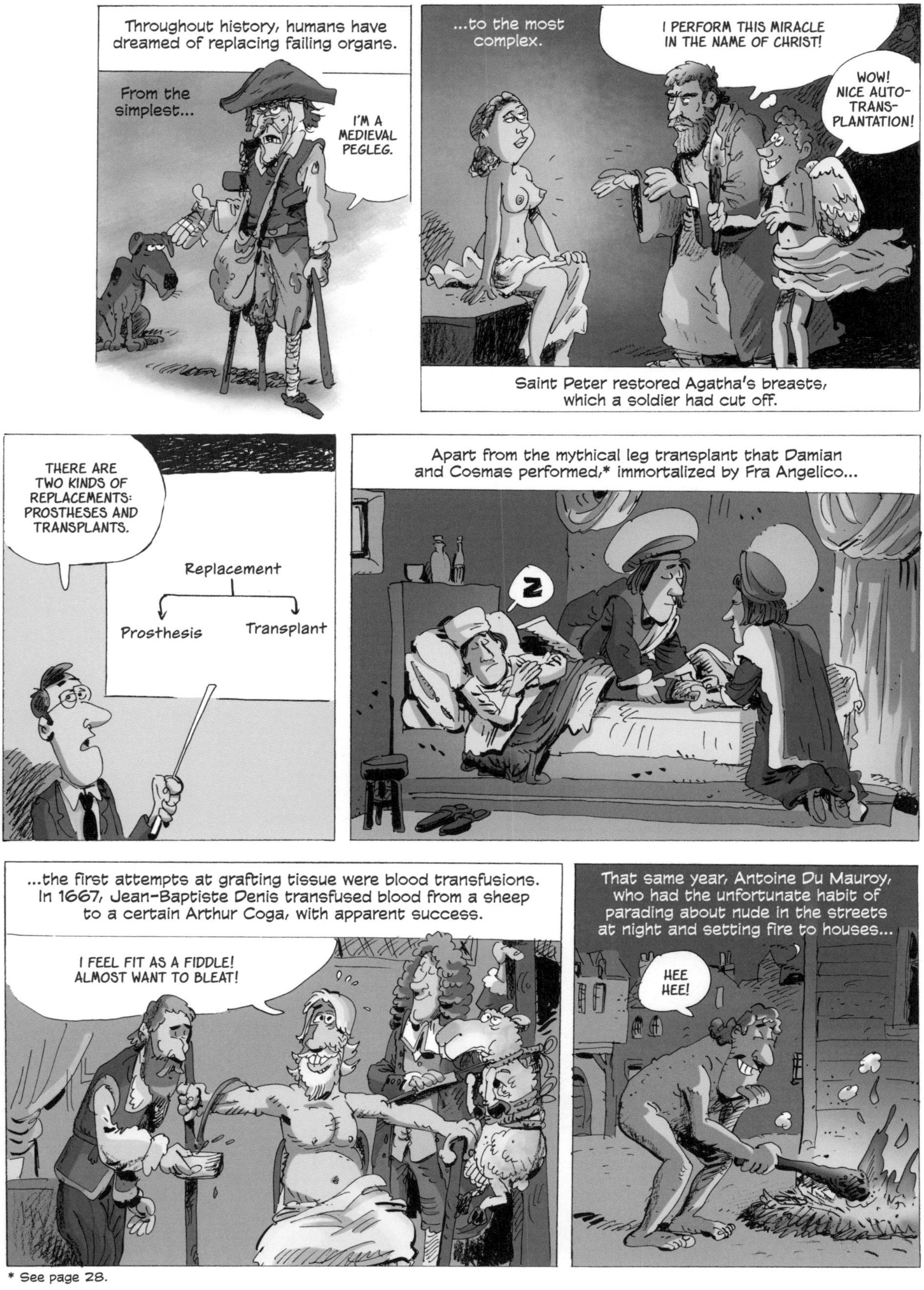

Throughout history, humans have dreamed of replacing failing organs.
From the simplest...
I'M A MEDIEVAL PEGLEG.
...to the most complex.
I PERFORM THIS MIRACLE IN THE NAME OF CHRIST!
WOW! NICE AUTO-TRANS-PLANTATION!
Saint Peter restored Agatha's breasts, which a soldier had cut off.
THERE ARE TWO KINDS OF REPLACEMENTS: PROSTHESES AND TRANSPLANTS.
Replacement
Prosthesis
Transplant
Apart from the mythical leg transplant that Damian and Cosmas performed,* immortalized by Fra Angelico...
Z
...the first attempts at grafting tissue were blood transfusions. In 1667, Jean-Baptiste Denis transfused blood from a sheep to a certain Arthur Coga, with apparent success.
I FEEL FIT AS A FIDDLE! ALMOST WANT TO BLEAT!
That same year, Antoine Du Mauroy, who had the unfortunate habit of parading about nude in the streets at night and setting fire to houses...
HEE HEE!

* See page 28.

...was taken to Paris by his wife to see the great Jean-Baptiste Denis. Denis chose a calf for the transfusion.

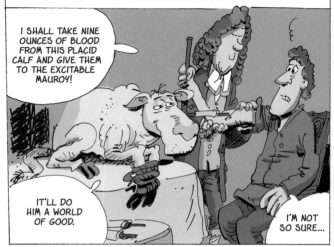

I SHALL TAKE NINE OUNCES OF BLOOD FROM THIS PLACID CALF AND GIVE THEM TO THE EXCITABLE MAUROY!

IT'LL DO HIM A WORLD OF GOOD.

I'M NOT SO SURE...

The first transfusion went well. But a few months later, Madame Du Mauroy came knocking.

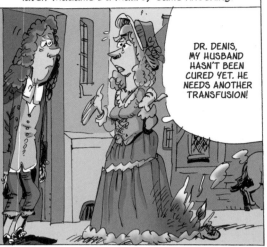

DR. DENIS, MY HUSBAND HASN'T BEEN CURED YET. HE NEEDS ANOTHER TRANSFUSION!

During this transfusion, however...

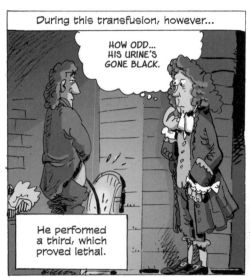

HOW ODD... HIS URINE'S GONE BLACK.

He performed a third, which proved lethal.

Madame Du Mauroy filed a suit, the first ever case involving infected blood. Denis Diderot recounts it in his *Encyclopedia*.

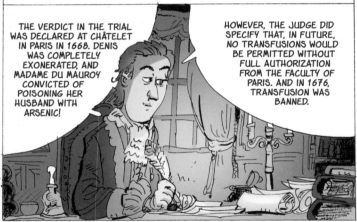

THE VERDICT IN THE TRIAL WAS DECLARED AT CHÂTELET IN PARIS IN 1668. DENIS WAS COMPLETELY EXONERATED, AND MADAME DU MAUROY CONVICTED OF POISONING HER HUSBAND WITH ARSENIC!

HOWEVER, THE JUDGE DID SPECIFY THAT, IN FUTURE, NO TRANSFUSIONS WOULD BE PERMITTED WITHOUT FULL AUTHORIZATION FROM THE FACULTY OF PARIS. AND IN 1676, TRANSFUSION WAS BANNED.

James Blundell attempted the first human-to-human blood transfusions in 1829 to save patients with postpartum haemorrhage.

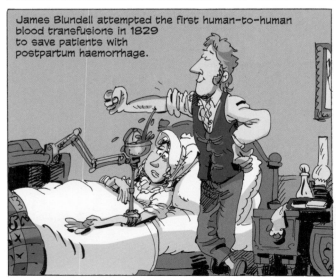

All these transfusions were done with no regard to donor or receiver.

BLOOD GROUPS

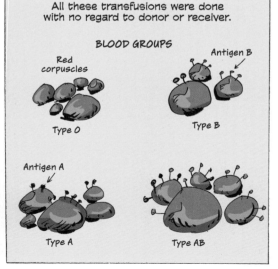

Red corpuscles

Antigen B

Type O

Type B

Antigen A

Type A

Type AB

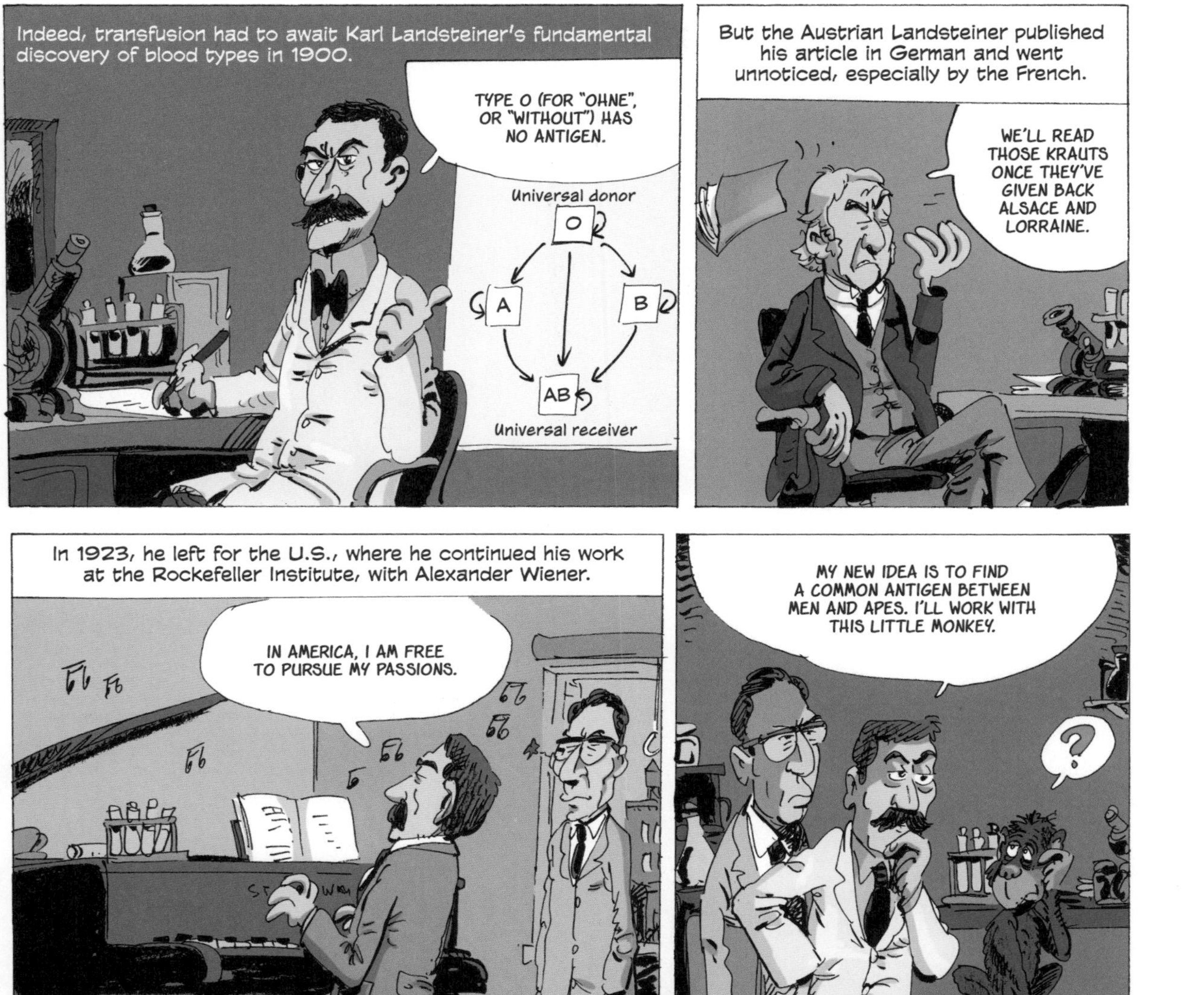

Indeed, transfusion had to await Karl Landsteiner's fundamental discovery of blood types in 1900.
TYPE O (FOR "OHNE", OR "WITHOUT") HAS NO ANTIGEN.
Universal donor
O
A
B
AB
Universal receiver
But the Austrian Landsteiner published his article in German and went unnoticed, especially by the French.
WE'LL READ THOSE KRAUTS ONCE THEY'VE GIVEN BACK ALSACE AND LORRAINE.
In 1923, he left for the U.S., where he continued his work at the Rockefeller Institute, with Alexander Wiener.
IN AMERICA, I AM FREE TO PURSUE MY PASSIONS.
MY NEW IDEA IS TO FIND A COMMON ANTIGEN BETWEEN MEN AND APES. I'LL WORK WITH THIS LITTLE MONKEY.
?
In so doing, they discovered another blood group: rhesus (1940). They observed that 85% of white subjects had antibodies against macaque blood (Rh+). Which could explain haemolytic disease in newborn babies.
I'M A RHESUS MACAQUE, AND THOSE TWO JOKERS PUT ME THROUGH TWO EXPERIMENTS. NO FUN AT ALL!
The Great War marked the true beginning of transfusion. On 16 October 1914, Corporal Legrain had just arrived at the hospital in Biarritz. During shelling at the Somme, he had lost a leg. The surgeons had amputated just five inches from his hip. Obviously, there was great blood loss.
BAOUM

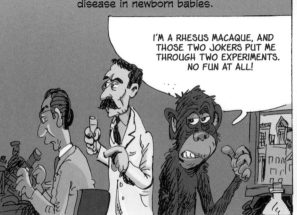

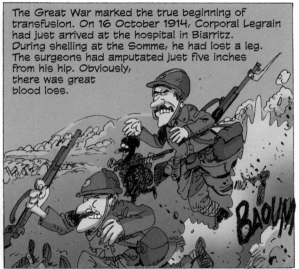

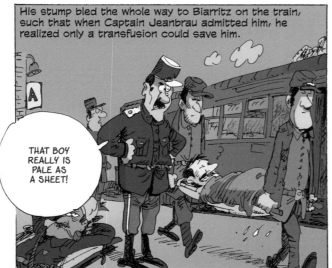

His stump bled the whole way to Biarritz on the train, such that when Captain Jeanbrau admitted him, he realized only a transfusion could save him.

THAT BOY REALLY IS PALE AS A SHEET!

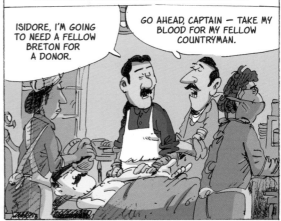

The only method they could use was arm to arm: from the donor's artery to the receiver's vein. There was no discussion of blood groups, which most doctors still hadn't heard of.

ISIDORE, I'M GOING TO NEED A FELLOW BRETON FOR A DONOR.

GO AHEAD, CAPTAIN — TAKE MY BLOOD FOR MY FELLOW COUNTRYMAN.

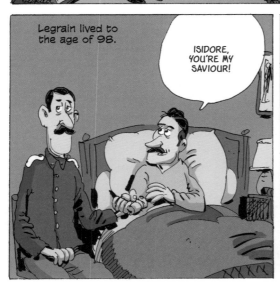

Legrain lived to the age of 98.

ISIDORE, YOU'RE MY SAVIOUR!

In 1916, Albert Hustin discovered the anticoagulant properties of citrate, allowing him to preserve blood for four days, and thus transfuse in combat zones.

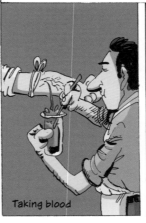

Taking blood

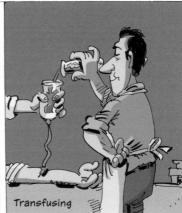

Transfusing

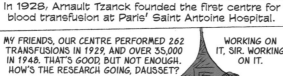

In 1928, Arnault Tzanck founded the first centre for blood transfusion at Paris' Saint Antoine Hospital.

MY FRIENDS, OUR CENTRE PERFORMED 262 TRANSFUSIONS IN 1929, AND OVER 35,000 IN 1948. THAT'S GOOD, BUT NOT ENOUGH. HOW'S THE RESEARCH GOING, DAUSSET?

WORKING ON IT, SIR. WORKING ON IT.

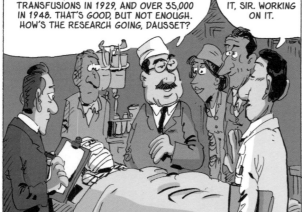

In 1940, the American Edwin Cohn developed a technique for fractionating blood into its component proteins, enabling the preparation of albumin.

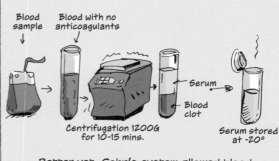

Blood sample

Blood with no anticoagulants

Centrifugation 1200G for 10-15 mins.

Serum

Blood clot

Serum stored at -20°

Better yet, Cohn's system allowed blood cells to be separated. Their use became essential in transfusion.

EARLY SOLID TISSUE GRAFTS

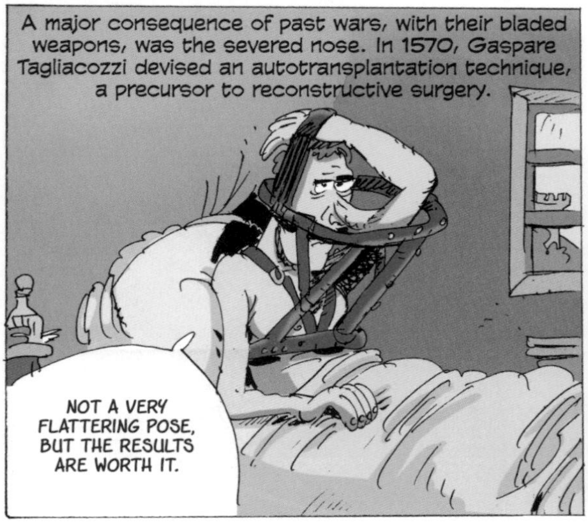
A major consequence of past wars, with their bladed weapons, was the severed nose. In 1570, Gaspare Tagliacozzi devised an autotransplantation technique, a precursor to reconstructive surgery.
NOT A VERY FLATTERING POSE, BUT THE RESULTS ARE WORTH IT.

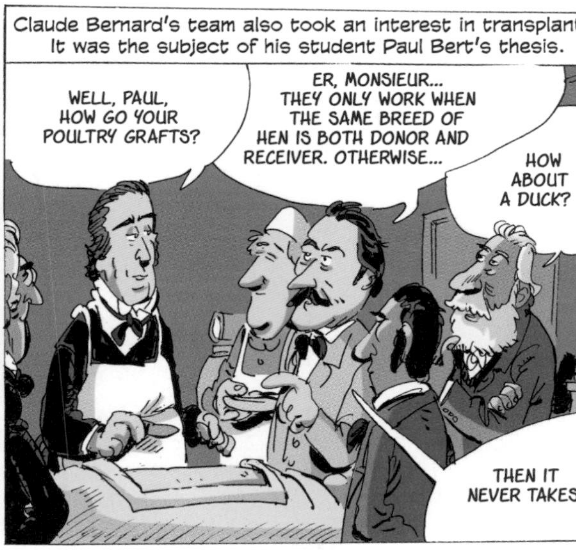
Claude Bernard's team also took an interest in transplants. It was the subject of his student Paul Bert's thesis.
WELL, PAUL, HOW GO YOUR POULTRY GRAFTS?
ER, MONSIEUR... THEY ONLY WORK WHEN THE SAME BREED OF HEN IS BOTH DONOR AND RECEIVER. OTHERWISE...
HOW ABOUT A DUCK?
THEN IT NEVER TAKES.

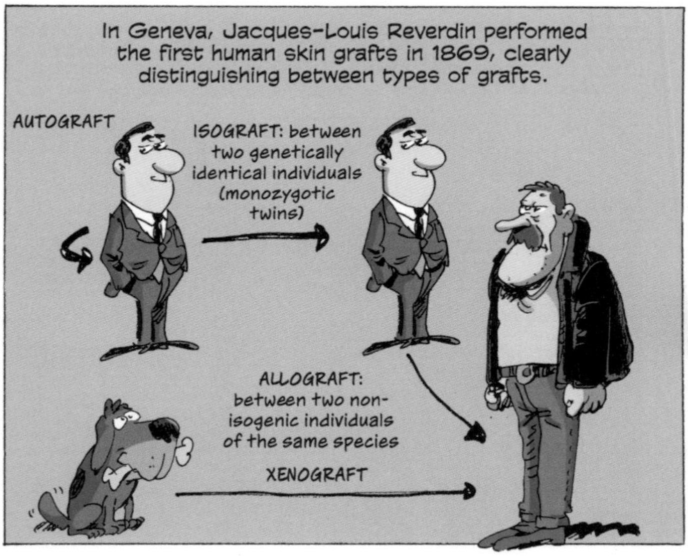
In Geneva, Jacques-Louis Reverdin performed the first human skin grafts in 1869, clearly distinguishing between types of grafts.
AUTOGRAFT
ISOGRAFT: between two genetically identical individuals (monozygotic twins)
ALLOGRAFT: between two non-isogenic individuals of the same species
XENOGRAFT

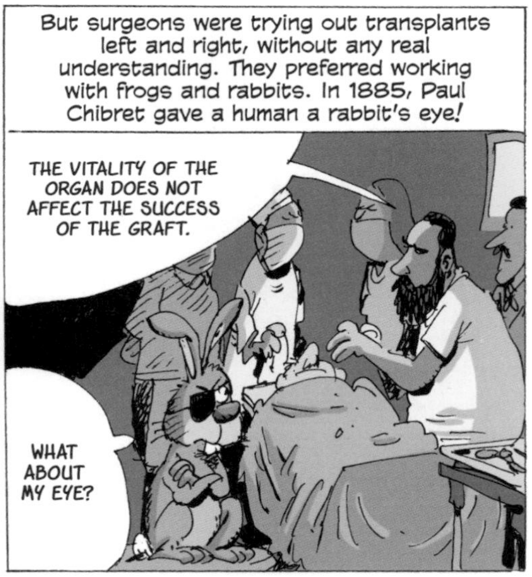
But surgeons were trying out transplants left and right, without any real understanding. They preferred working with frogs and rabbits. In 1885, Paul Chibret gave a human a rabbit's eye!
THE VITALITY OF THE ORGAN DOES NOT AFFECT THE SUCCESS OF THE GRAFT.
WHAT ABOUT MY EYE?

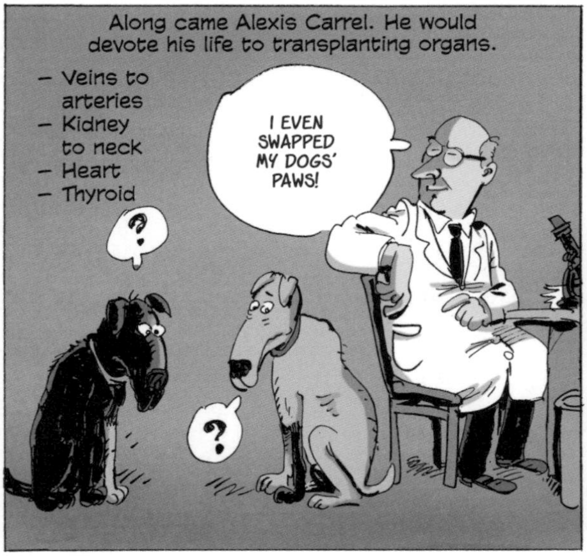
Along came Alexis Carrel. He would devote his life to transplanting organs.
– Veins to arteries
– Kidney to neck
– Heart
– Thyroid
I EVEN SWAPPED MY DOGS' PAWS!
?
?

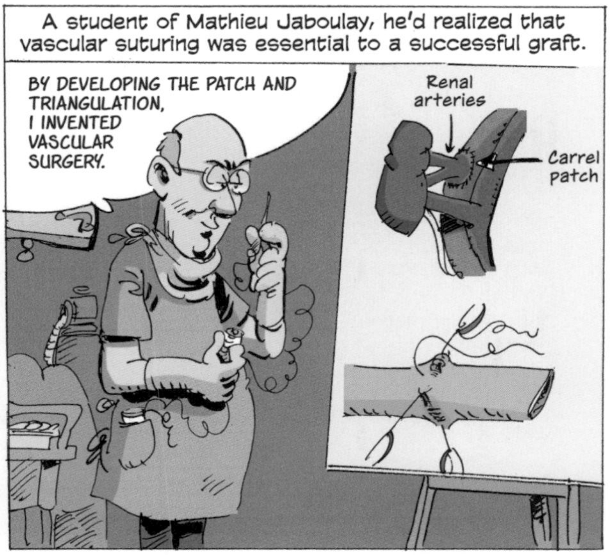
A student of Mathieu Jaboulay, he'd realized that vascular suturing was essential to a successful graft.
BY DEVELOPING THE PATCH AND TRIANGULATION, I INVENTED VASCULAR SURGERY.
Renal arteries
Carrel patch

To perfect his technique, he worked with Lyons lacemaker Madame Leroudier.

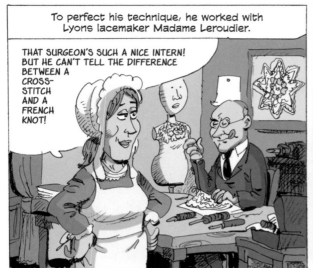

THAT SURGEON'S SUCH A NICE INTERN! BUT HE CAN'T TELL THE DIFFERENCE BETWEEN A CROSS-STITCH AND A FRENCH KNOT!

He started out by performing every kind of transplant possible on every kind of animal.

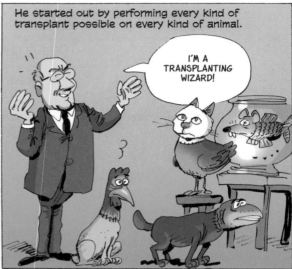

I'M A TRANSPLANTING WIZARD!

But Carrel was forced to leave for America, since the Lyons authorities found it hard to square his work with his Catholicism. He continued his work with Charles Guthrie at the Rockefeller Institute and won the Nobel Prize in 1912.

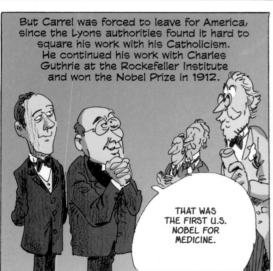

THAT WAS THE FIRST U.S. NOBEL FOR MEDICINE.

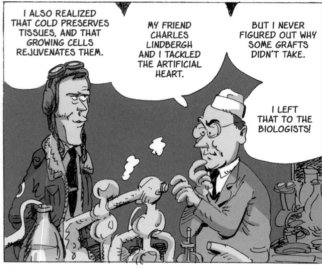

I ALSO REALIZED THAT COLD PRESERVES TISSUES, AND THAT GROWING CELLS REJUVENATES THEM.

MY FRIEND CHARLES LINDBERGH AND I TACKLED THE ARTIFICIAL HEART.

BUT I NEVER FIGURED OUT WHY SOME GRAFTS DIDN'T TAKE.

I LEFT THAT TO THE BIOLOGISTS!

And yet the biologist James Murphy worked alongside Carrel at the Rockefeller.

In 1912, while transplanting tumours, he discovered three basic things:

- rejection eliminated grafted tissue, except in embryos;
- small white corpuscles were responsible;
- X-rays diminished rejection.

But his visionary work made no impact.

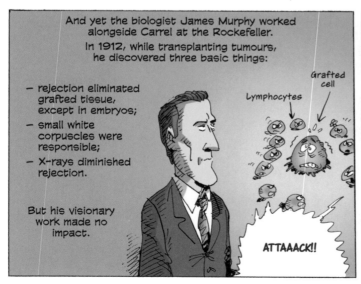

Lymphocytes

Grafted cell

ATTAAACK!!

That the body considered grafts an invasive attack was also known. In 1926, E. Holman showed that skin grafts could provoke specific defence reactions involving white blood cells and antibodies.

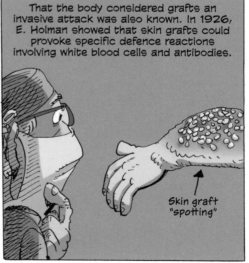

Skin graft "spotting"

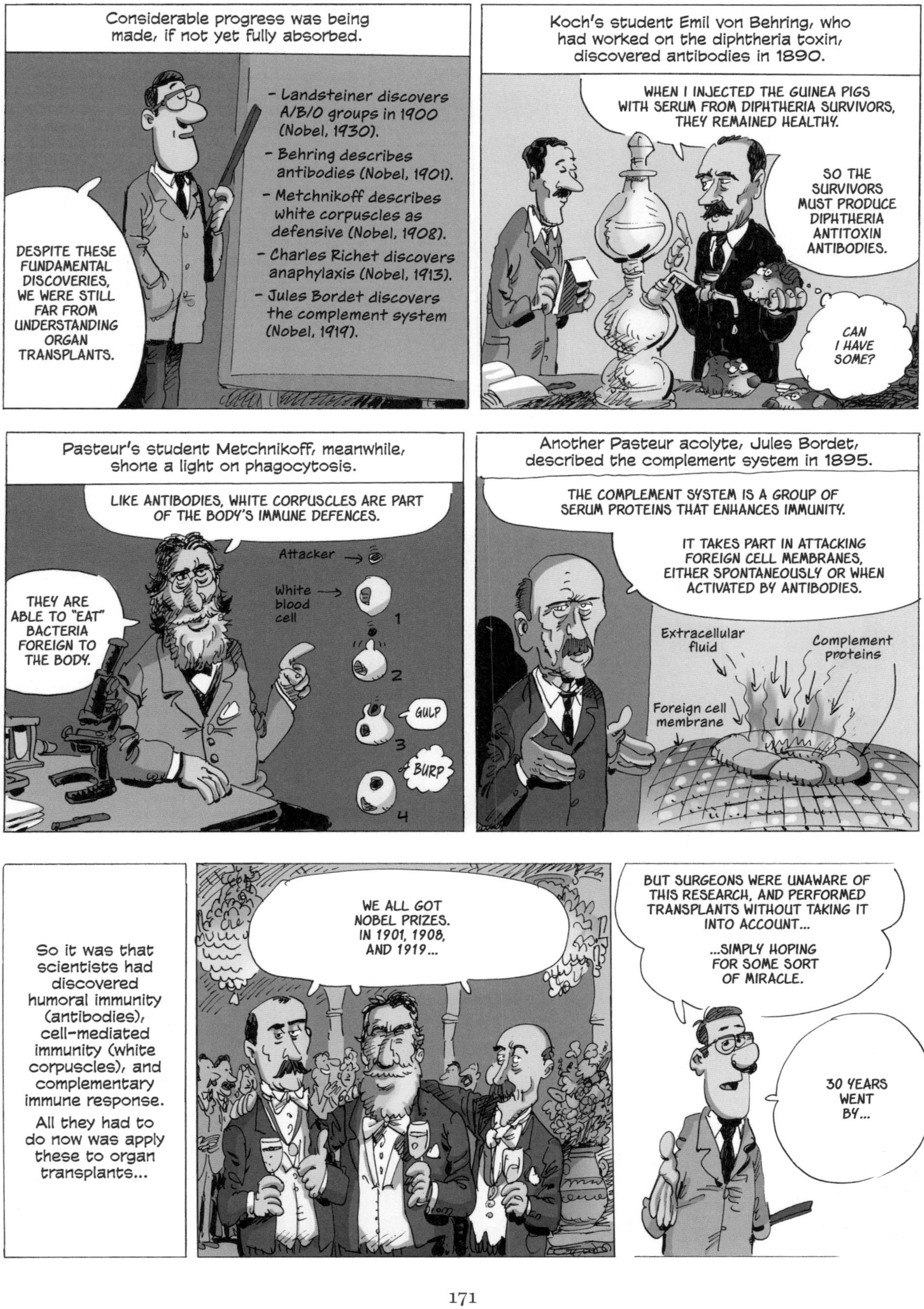
Considerable progress was being made, if not yet fully absorbed.
- Landsteiner discovers A/B/O groups in 1900 (Nobel, 1930).
- Behring describes antibodies (Nobel, 1901).
- Metchnikoff describes white corpuscles as defensive (Nobel, 1908).
- Charles Richet discovers anaphylaxis (Nobel, 1913).
- Jules Bordet discovers the complement system (Nobel, 1919).
DESPITE THESE FUNDAMENTAL DISCOVERIES, WE WERE STILL FAR FROM UNDERSTANDING ORGAN TRANSPLANTS.
Koch's student Emil von Behring, who had worked on the diphtheria toxin, discovered antibodies in 1890.
WHEN I INJECTED THE GUINEA PIGS WITH SERUM FROM DIPHTHERIA SURVIVORS, THEY REMAINED HEALTHY.
SO THE SURVIVORS MUST PRODUCE DIPHTHERIA ANTITOXIN ANTIBODIES.
CAN I HAVE SOME?
Pasteur's student Metchnikoff, meanwhile, shone a light on phagocytosis.
LIKE ANTIBODIES, WHITE CORPUSCLES ARE PART OF THE BODY'S IMMUNE DEFENCES.
THEY ARE ABLE TO "EAT" BACTERIA FOREIGN TO THE BODY.
Attacker
White blood cell
1
2
GULP
3
BURP
4
Another Pasteur acolyte, Jules Bordet, described the complement system in 1895.
THE COMPLEMENT SYSTEM IS A GROUP OF SERUM PROTEINS THAT ENHANCES IMMUNITY.
IT TAKES PART IN ATTACKING FOREIGN CELL MEMBRANES, EITHER SPONTANEOUSLY OR WHEN ACTIVATED BY ANTIBODIES.
Extracellular fluid
Complement proteins
Foreign cell membrane
So it was that scientists had discovered humoral immunity (antibodies), cell-mediated immunity (white corpuscles), and complementary immune response.
All they had to do now was apply these to organ transplants...
WE ALL GOT NOBEL PRIZES. IN 1901, 1908, AND 1919...
BUT SURGEONS WERE UNAWARE OF THIS RESEARCH, AND PERFORMED TRANSPLANTS WITHOUT TAKING IT INTO ACCOUNT...
...SIMPLY HOPING FOR SOME SORT OF MIRACLE.
30 YEARS WENT BY...

ORGAN TRANSPLANTS

In 1947, Boston doctor David Hume received a young woman with acute kidney failure resulting from an abortion. He asked permission to attempt a kidney transplant, but was denied.

So he performed it secretly, at night, in the patient's room.

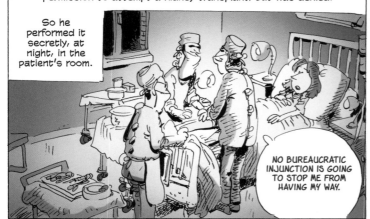

NO BUREAUCRATIC INJUNCTION IS GOING TO STOP ME FROM HAVING MY WAY.

The kidney began producing urine right away. Over the next few days, the patient's own kidney started working again, while the transplant was rejected and taken out. But it had helped her through a critical juncture.

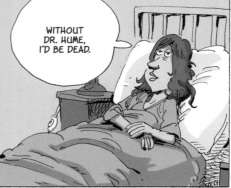

WITHOUT DR. HUME, I'D BE DEAD.

Kidney transplants became all the rage: Lawler, 1950; Dubost, Servelle, and Küss, 1951.

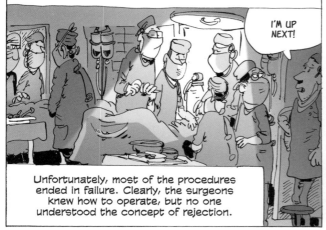

I'M UP NEXT!

Unfortunately, most of the procedures ended in failure. Clearly, the surgeons knew how to operate, but no one understood the concept of rejection.

In 1951, prisoners on death row became kidney donors.

DR. OEKONOMOS, KEEP THAT KIDNEY WARM WHEN YOU BRING IT OVER FROM PRISON!*

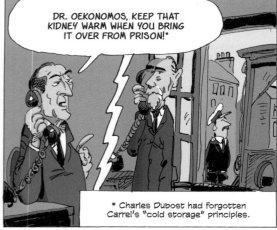

* Charles Dubost had forgotten Carrel's "cold storage" principles.

As for René Küss, he simplified things by leaving the diseased kidneys in place.

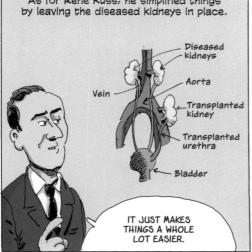

Diseased kidneys

Vein

Aorta

Transplanted kidney

Transplanted urethra

Bladder

IT JUST MAKES THINGS A WHOLE LOT EASIER.

In December 1952, Marius Renard, a 16-year-old carpenter, fell from some scaffolding. Uncontrollable haemorrhaging forced the surgeon to remove a kidney. Unfortunately, he only had one. The artificial kidney did not yet exist. It was a death sentence.

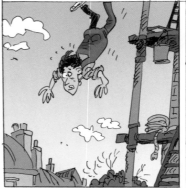

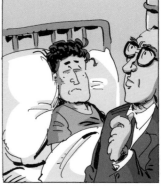

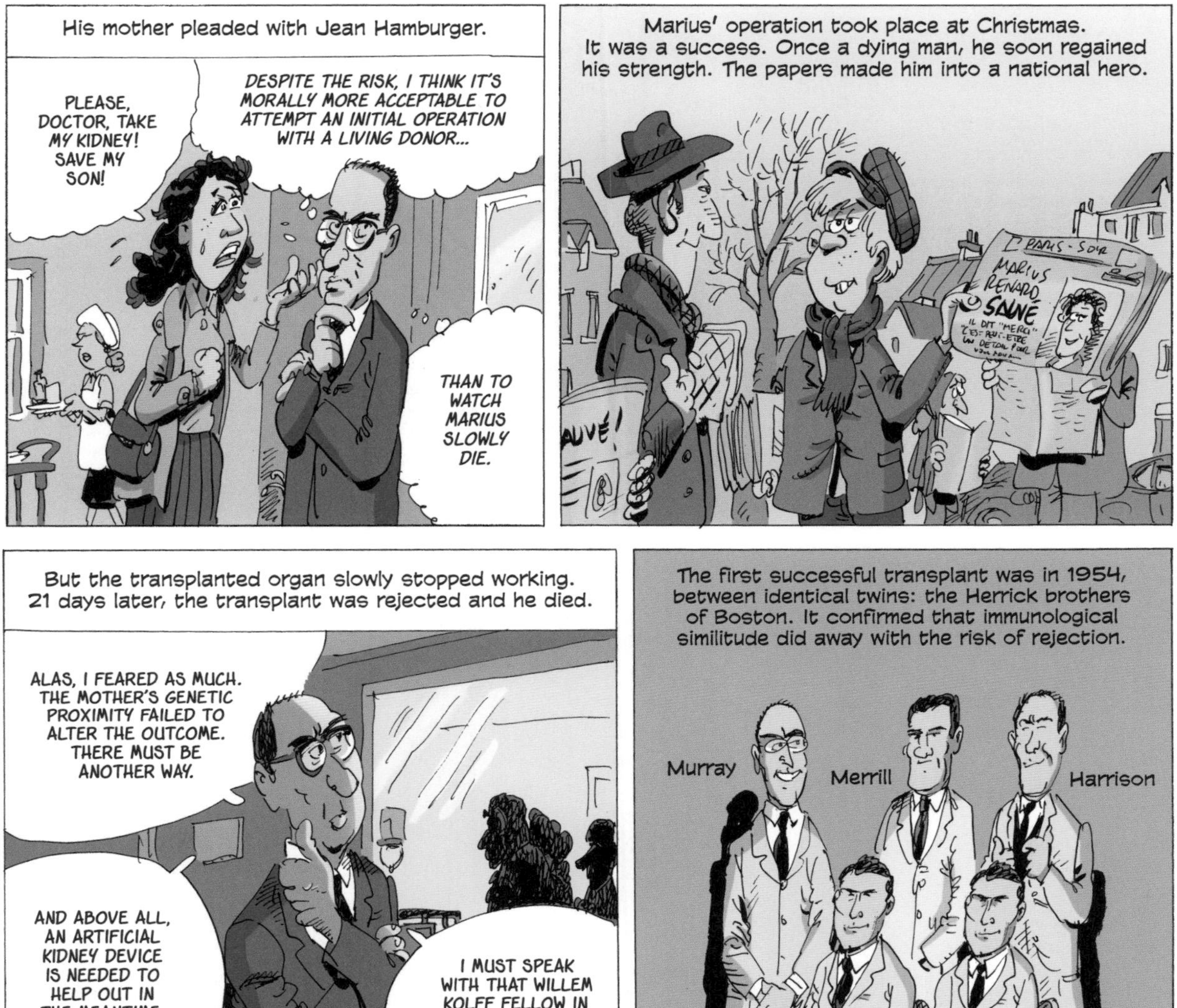
His mother pleaded with Jean Hamburger.
PLEASE, DOCTOR, TAKE MY KIDNEY! SAVE MY SON!
DESPITE THE RISK, I THINK IT'S MORALLY MORE ACCEPTABLE TO ATTEMPT AN INITIAL OPERATION WITH A LIVING DONOR...
THAN TO WATCH MARIUS SLOWLY DIE.
Marius' operation took place at Christmas. It was a success. Once a dying man, he soon regained his strength. The papers made him into a national hero.
PARIS-SOIR
MARIUS RENARD SAUVÉ
But the transplanted organ slowly stopped working. 21 days later, the transplant was rejected and he died.
ALAS, I FEARED AS MUCH. THE MOTHER'S GENETIC PROXIMITY FAILED TO ALTER THE OUTCOME. THERE MUST BE ANOTHER WAY.
AND ABOVE ALL, AN ARTIFICIAL KIDNEY DEVICE IS NEEDED TO HELP OUT IN THE MEANTIME.
I MUST SPEAK WITH THAT WILLEM KOLFF FELLOW IN HOLLAND.
The first successful transplant was in 1954, between identical twins: the Herrick brothers of Boston. It confirmed that immunological similitude did away with the risk of rejection.
Murray
Merrill
Harrison
As Hamburger suspected, other solutions to prevent rejection were still needed.
In 1958, he had an idea: to irradiate future recipients in order to temporarily suppress bone marrow from making lymphocytes, which were the agents of rejection.
Beam of cobalt 80
THIS RADIATION TREATMENT WILL LET ME KEEP MY KIDNEY AND LEAVE ME OPEN TO EVERY PASSING GERM!
The treatment carried a very high risk of infection, but transplants between fraternal twins were successful.
EVERYONE SMILE FOR THE DOCTOR!

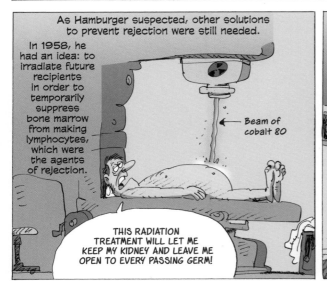

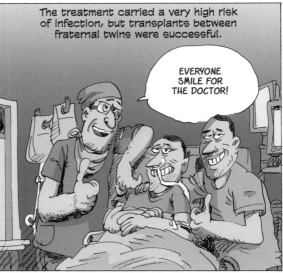

At the same time, biologists were making great strides. In 1959, the Australian Frank Macfarlane Burnet set forth a hypothesis that during embryonic development, cells acquired the capacity to recognize foreign cells.
THE BODY IS ABLE TO IDENTIFY ITS OWN TISSUES. THIS IS THE BASIS OF THE IMMUNE RESPONSE, AND THE BIOLOGICAL DEFINITION OF SELFHOOD.
SO IF WE COULD TRANSPLANT A FOETUS OR AN EMBRYO, THERE'D BE NO REJECTION?
In 1943, Peter Medawar had already confirmed that a second skin graft was rejected more swiftly than the first.
THE REJECTION IS IMMUNOGENIC IN ORIGIN, TIED TO IMMUNOCOMPETENT CELLS.*
* T cells, in fact.
MEDAWAR'S EXPERIMENT
Skin graft
Leucocytes
Rejection 10 days
Rejection 5 days
Rejection 5 days
Medawar had understood that antigens on the white corpuscles' surface were responsible for rejecting the rabbits' skin grafts.
But the major find belonged to Jean Dausset.
AT FIRST, I HANDLED BLOOD TRANSFUSIONS...
Dausset's first question was: are there blood groups for white blood cells just as there are for red?
After some remarkable research, Dausset discovered in 1958 that each individual possesses specific proteins on the surface of cells with nuclei (thus including white corpuscles).
Molecule of self
M.H.C. marker
Cell
The major histocompatibility complex (M.H.C.) is fundamental to transplant rejection.
People were starting to understand the phenomenon of rejection: macrophages identify the transplanted organ's antigens...
WE MACROPHAGES ARE THE BODY'S BORDER PATROL, DEMANDING PAPERS FROM ALL FOREIGNERS.
Then they present significant fragments to B cells and T cells. Each antigen leads to the proliferation of a specific clone (1, 2, 3) directed against the transplanted organ's antibodies.
Macrophages
B cell clones
B1
B2
B3
T cell clones
T1
T2
T3
T2
T2
T2
Killer cells
B2 antibodies
Rejection summons these killer cells and antibodies to intervene.
Recognition
Liquidation
T cell attack
A
B
T cell recognizes a foreign cell
Release of chemical signals, leading to death of cell
Release of proteins able to create pores in cell membrane
Antibodies attack
Cell ruptures

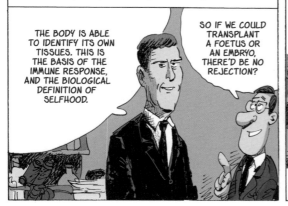

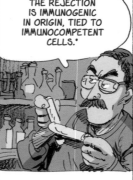

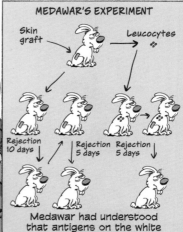

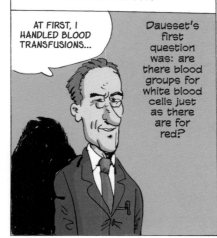

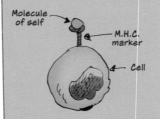

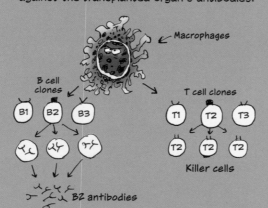

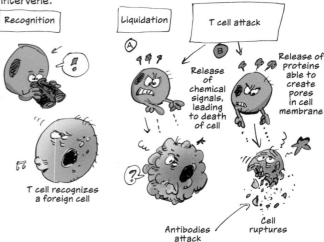

Naturally, the same mechanism fights off infection.

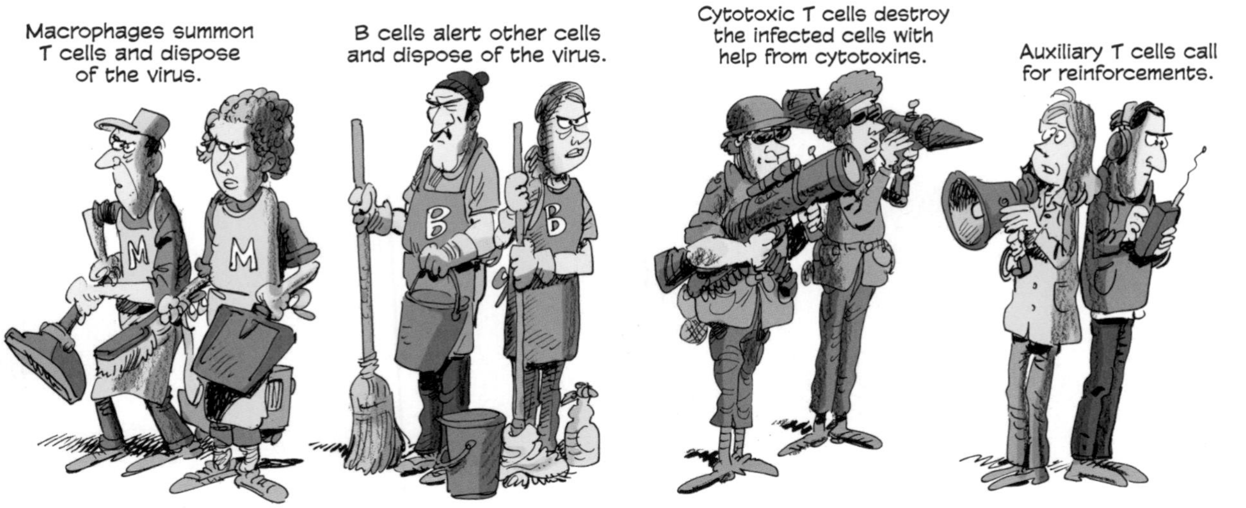
Macrophages summon T cells and dispose of the virus.
M
M
B cells alert other cells and dispose of the virus.
B
B
Cytotoxic T cells destroy the infected cells with help from cytotoxins.
Auxiliary T cells call for reinforcements.

This means that any treatment against rejection decreases the body's resistance to infection.

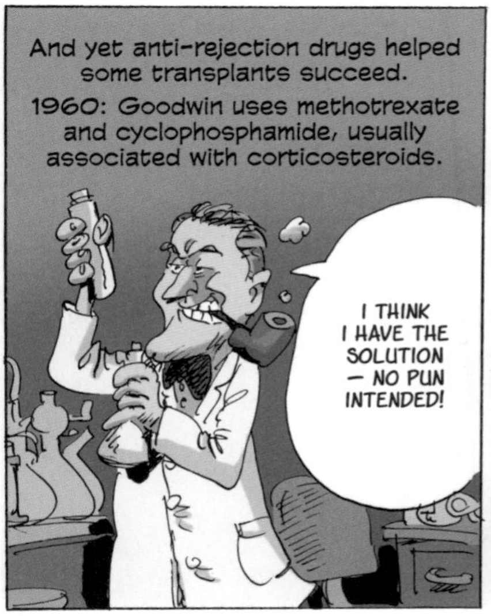
And yet anti-rejection drugs helped some transplants succeed.
1960: Goodwin uses methotrexate and cyclophosphamide, usually associated with corticosteroids.
I THINK I HAVE THE SOLUTION — NO PUN INTENDED!

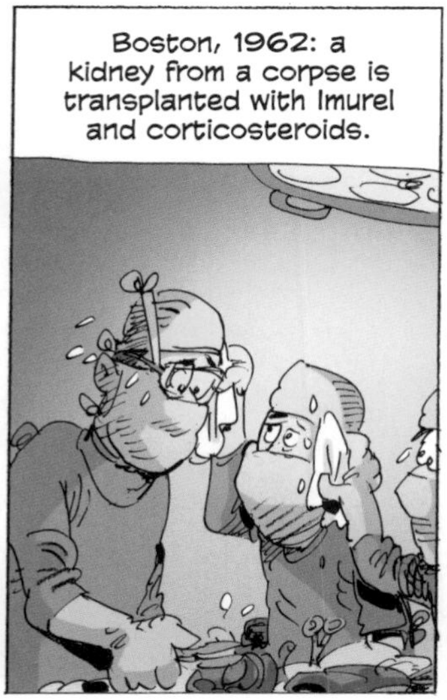
Boston, 1962: a kidney from a corpse is transplanted with Imurel and corticosteroids.

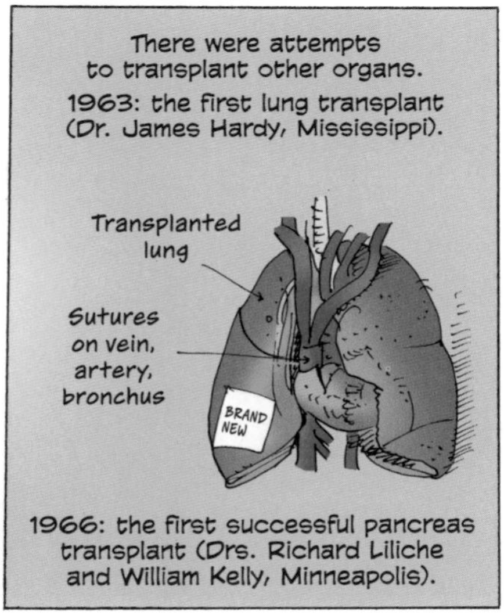
There were attempts to transplant other organs.
1963: the first lung transplant (Dr. James Hardy, Mississippi).
Transplanted lung
Sutures on vein, artery, bronchus
BRAND NEW
1966: the first successful pancreas transplant (Drs. Richard Liliche and William Kelly, Minneapolis).

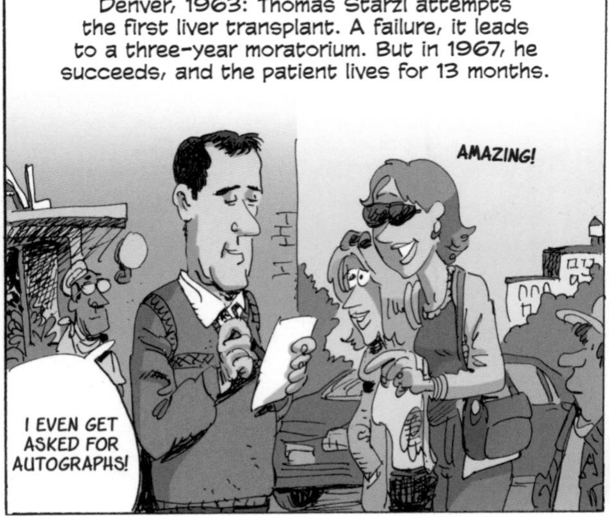
Denver, 1963: Thomas Starzl attempts the first liver transplant. A failure, it leads to a three-year moratorium. But in 1967, he succeeds, and the patient lives for 13 months.
AMAZING!
I EVEN GET ASKED FOR AUTOGRAPHS!

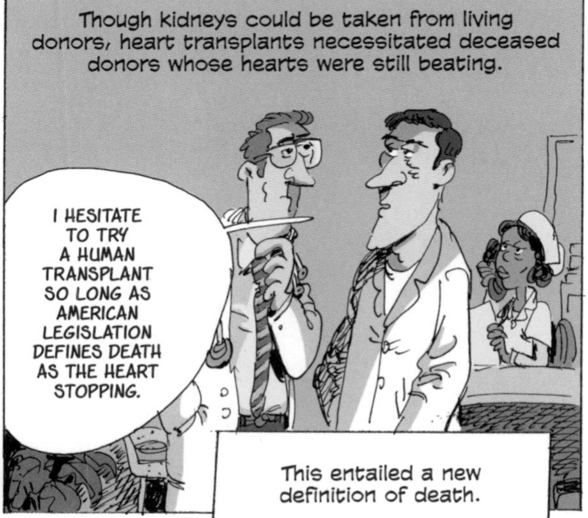
Though kidneys could be taken from living donors, heart transplants necessitated deceased donors whose hearts were still beating.
I HESITATE TO TRY A HUMAN TRANSPLANT SO LONG AS AMERICAN LEGISLATION DEFINES DEATH AS THE HEART STOPPING.
This entailed a new definition of death.

WHAT IS DEATH?

In Antiquity, the difference between the living and the dead was clear: the body's warmth.

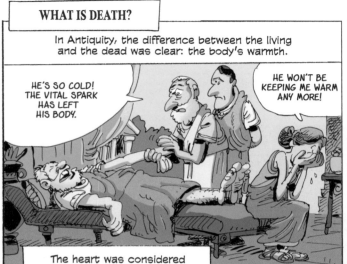

HE'S SO COLD! THE VITAL SPARK HAS LEFT HIS BODY.

HE WON'T BE KEEPING ME WARM ANY MORE!

The heart was considered the body's furnace.

Such that nature itself had provided two bellows — the lungs — to fan its flames should they dwindle.

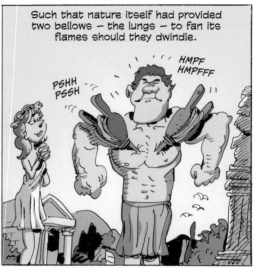

PSHH PSSH

HMPF HMPFFF

At least, that was what Aristotle thought.

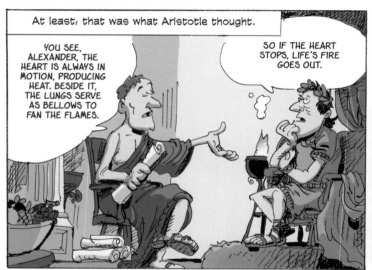

YOU SEE, ALEXANDER, THE HEART IS ALWAYS IN MOTION, PRODUCING HEAT. BESIDE IT, THE LUNGS SERVE AS BELLOWS TO FAN THE FLAMES.

SO IF THE HEART STOPS, LIFE'S FIRE GOES OUT.

Later, people were considered dead when they stopped breathing.

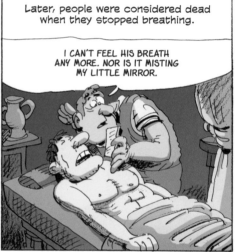

I CAN'T FEEL HIS BREATH ANY MORE. NOR IS IT MISTING MY LITTLE MIRROR.

Such that cardiorespiratory arrest was long synonymous with death.

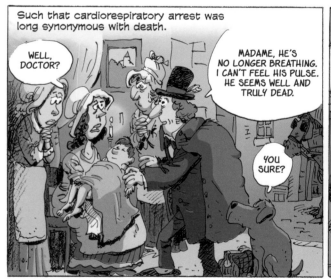

WELL, DOCTOR?

MADAME, HE'S NO LONGER BREATHING. I CAN'T FEEL HIS PULSE. HE SEEMS WELL AND TRULY DEAD.

YOU SURE?

But in the absence of a clear definition, society entrusted undertakers with the task of confirming death.

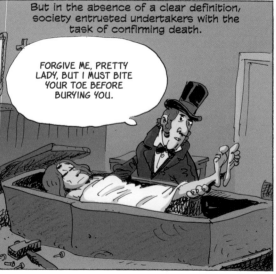

FORGIVE ME, PRETTY LADY, BUT I MUST BITE YOUR TOE BEFORE BURYING YOU.

Resuscitation would turn these old rules upside down.

First came Kouwenhoven's closed-chest cardiac massage, in 1960...

Then mouth-to-mouth...

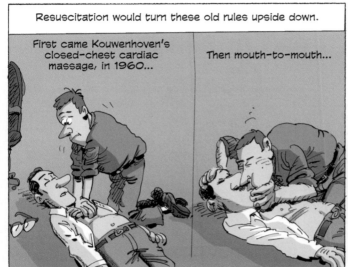

And then the ability to keep patients alive by using artificial organs.

ALL MY PATIENT'S ORGANS ARE OUTSIDE OF HIM, EXCEPT HIS BRAIN, WHICH IS WORKING JUST FINE.

BUT WE KNOCKED HIM OUT, TO SPARE HIM PAIN.

Artificial respirator

Dialysis machine

Artificial heart

I.V. drip

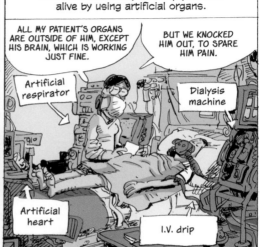

Actually, we owe the idea of resuscitation to two Parisian doctors from the 1950s.

Jean Hamburger, Necker Hospital, 1953

THANKS TO MY ARTIFICIAL KIDNEY, I CAN NOW ENSURE INTERNAL EQUILIBRIUM.

Pierre Mollaret, Claude-Bernard Hospital, 1954

THANKS TO MY MACHINES, I CAN ENSURE MY POLIO PATIENTS WILL STILL BE ABLE TO BREATHE.

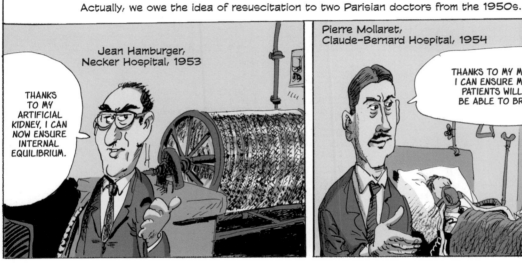
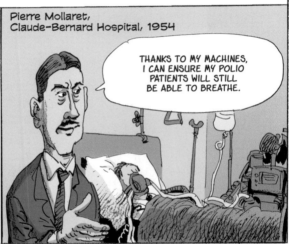

From this rather specific context, a new definition of death emerged: brain death.

In 1959, Goulon and Mollaret published a groundbreaking article: "Beyond Coma".

I REGRET TO INFORM YOU THAT YOUR FATHER IS DEAD. HE CONTINUES TO BREATHE AND URINATE, BUT ONLY ARTIFICIALLY. HIS HEART IS STILL BEATING, BUT HIS BRAIN IS DEAD.

HE IS NOW AN ORGAN DONOR, IF HE GAVE PERMISSION FOR THAT IN HIS LIFETIME.

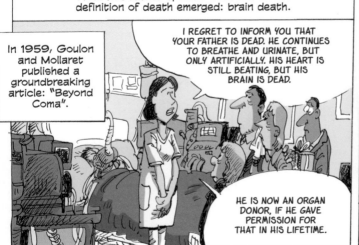

Proof of irreversible brain death is entrusted to two doctors and two E.E.G. flatlines of 30 minutes, each done four hours apart, or by angiography.

Normal M.R.I.

Brain death

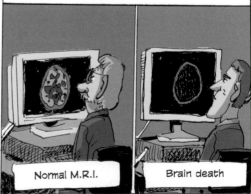

HEART TRANSPLANTS

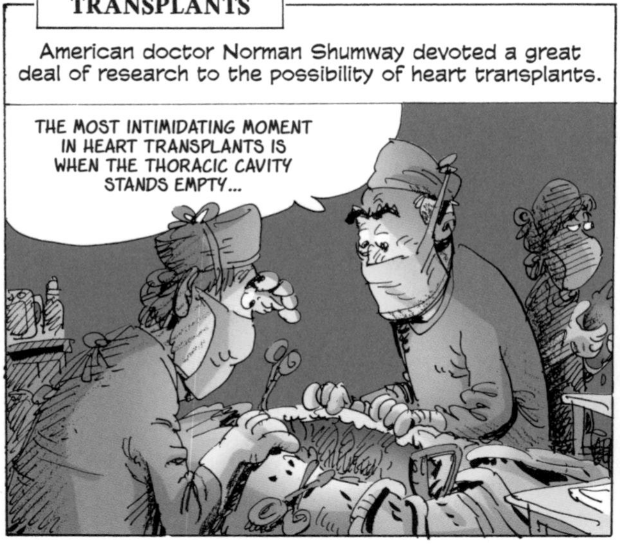
American doctor Norman Shumway devoted a great deal of research to the possibility of heart transplants.
THE MOST INTIMIDATING MOMENT IN HEART TRANSPLANTS IS WHEN THE THORACIC CAVITY STANDS EMPTY...

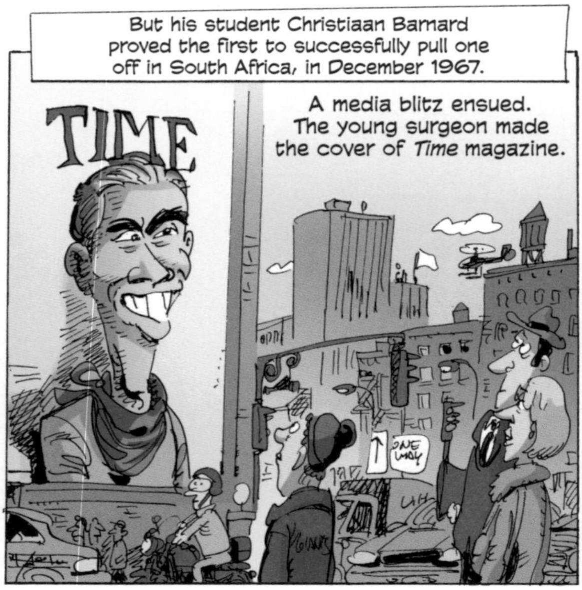
But his student Christiaan Barnard proved the first to successfully pull one off in South Africa, in December 1967.
TIME
A media blitz ensued. The young surgeon made the cover of *Time* magazine.
ONE WAY

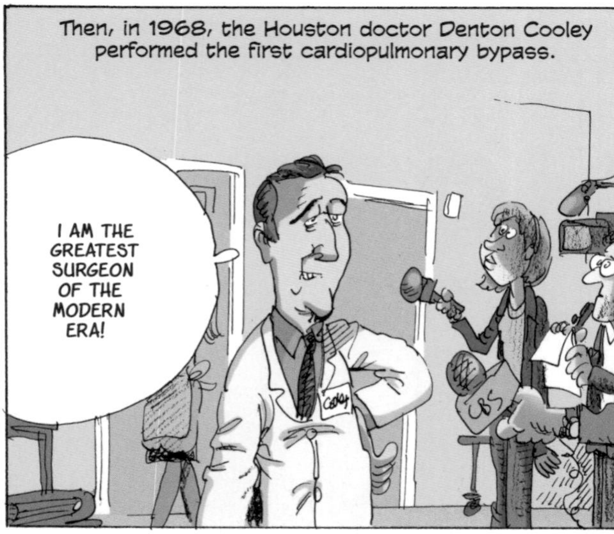
Then, in 1968, the Houston doctor Denton Cooley performed the first cardiopulmonary bypass.
I AM THE GREATEST SURGEON OF THE MODERN ERA!
CBS

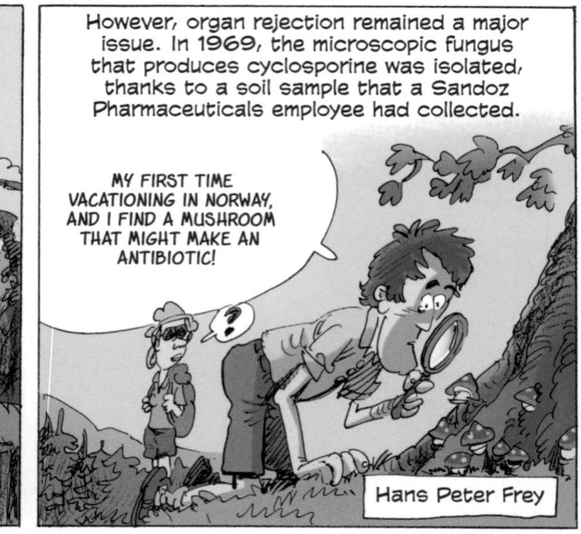
However, organ rejection remained a major issue. In 1969, the microscopic fungus that produces cyclosporine was isolated, thanks to a soil sample that a Sandoz Pharmaceuticals employee had collected.
MY FIRST TIME VACATIONING IN NORWAY, AND I FIND A MUSHROOM THAT MIGHT MAKE AN ANTIBIOTIC!
?
Hans Peter Frey

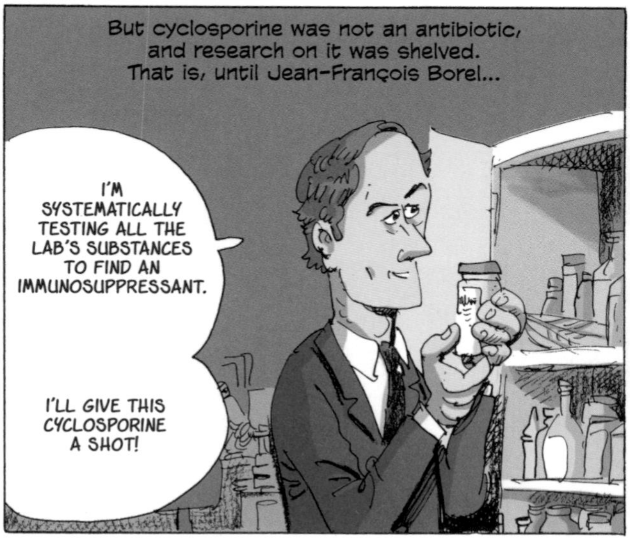
But cyclosporine was not an antibiotic, and research on it was shelved. That is, until Jean-François Borel...
I'M SYSTEMATICALLY TESTING ALL THE LAB'S SUBSTANCES TO FIND AN IMMUNOSUPPRESSANT.
I'LL GIVE THIS CYCLOSPORINE A SHOT!

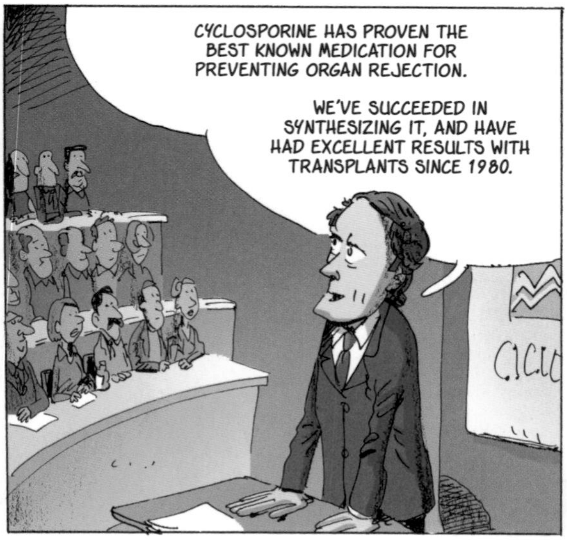
CYCLOSPORINE HAS PROVEN THE BEST KNOWN MEDICATION FOR PREVENTING ORGAN REJECTION.
WE'VE SUCCEEDED IN SYNTHESIZING IT, AND HAVE HAD EXCELLENT RESULTS WITH TRANSPLANTS SINCE 1980.

Starting in 1980, there was an explosion in organ transplants, limited only by the number of donors.
700 600 500 400 300 200 100
632 559 525 430 408 397 368 370 321 328 316 319 283 317 339 358 366 360
Heart transplants level off in France
In 1968, Marseilles native Emmanuel Vitria received a transplant and lived for over 18 years.
THERE WASN'T ANY CYCLOSPORINE BACK THEN.
I THINK MY SURGEON PUT A TWIN BROTHER'S HEART IN ME BY MISTAKE.
Aside from organ transplants, some tissues can be transplanted without immunosuppressant treatment.
The aorta and valve from a cadaver are preserved in liquid nitrogen...
...and used by a surgeon when needed.
In New Zealand, Sir Brian Barratt-Boyes pioneered homograft cardiac valve replacement. He was immortalized on a stamp in his native land.
THE LESS VASCULAR A TISSUE, THE MORE EASILY IT IS ACCEPTED.
FOR INSTANCE, CARDIAC VALVES, BLOOD VESSELS, OR THE CORNEA.
NEW ZEALAND
But early arterial operations in 1951 were already using homografts. Charles Dubost had been the first to treat an aortic aneurysm in just such a fashion.
JACQUES OUDOT PREPPED AN AORTIC GRAFT, AND I STITCHED IT IN PLACE.
Open aneurysm
Homograft from cadaver
Corneal transplants, too, were yielding fine results.

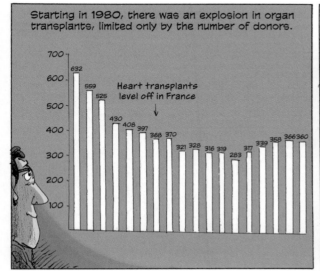

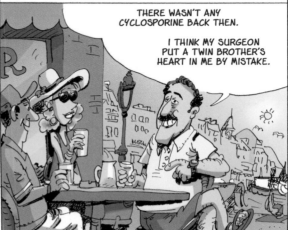

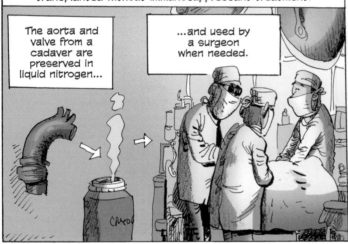

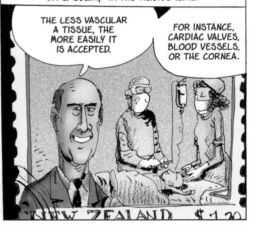

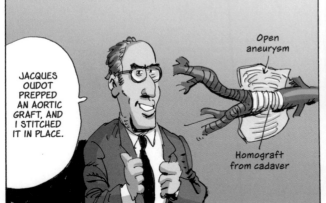

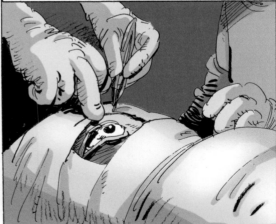

Bone marrow transplants allow stem cells to be used in for cases of blood cancer.

Marrow can be found in every bone in the body.

It is what produces haematopoietic stem cells...

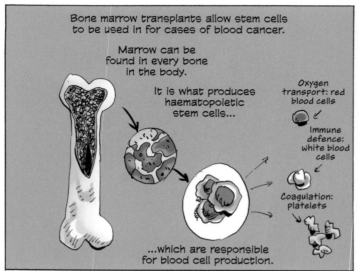

Oxygen transport: red blood cells

Immune defence: white blood cells

Coagulation: platelets

...which are responsible for blood cell production.

Meanwhile, Alain Carpentier was looking into heterografts (from animals).

Heart valves must be treated with glutaraldehyde to suppress their antigen sites.

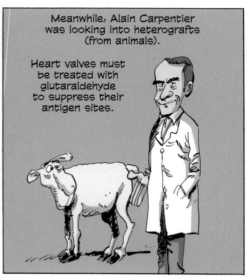

In 1968, he proposed replacing the heart's diseased valves with porcine heterografts.

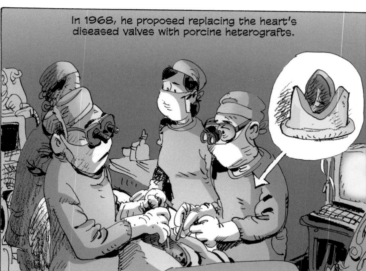

Unlike tissues, however, organs were systematically rejected, for animals have genes that humans do not.

I NEED AN INGENIOUS IDEA...

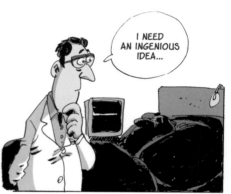

Plans were made to create genetically modified animals on biological farms.

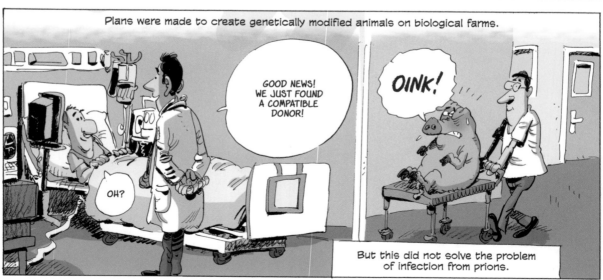

GOOD NEWS! WE JUST FOUND A COMPATIBLE DONOR!

OH?

OINK!

But this did not solve the problem of infection from prions.

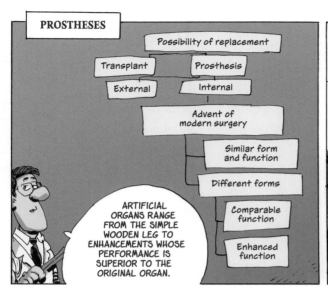

PROSTHESES

Possibility of replacement

Transplant — Prosthesis

External — Internal

Advent of modern surgery

Similar form and function

Different forms

Comparable function

Enhanced function

ARTIFICIAL ORGANS RANGE FROM THE SIMPLE WOODEN LEG TO ENHANCEMENTS WHOSE PERFORMANCE IS SUPERIOR TO THE ORIGINAL ORGAN.

EXTERNAL PROSTHESES

The Egyptians were already able to amputate and design prostheses: the mummy of a woman who died 3,000 years ago was found with an amputated big toe on her right foot. It had been replaced with a prosthesis of sculpted wood.

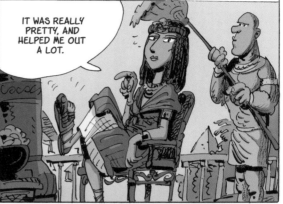

IT WAS REALLY PRETTY, AND HELPED ME OUT A LOT.

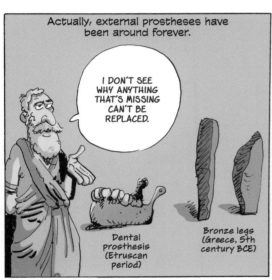

Actually, external prostheses have been around forever.

I DON'T SEE WHY ANYTHING THAT'S MISSING CAN'T BE REPLACED.

Dental prosthesis (Etruscan period)

Bronze legs (Greece, 5th century BCE)

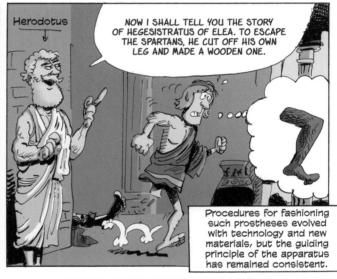

Herodotus

NOW I SHALL TELL YOU THE STORY OF HEGESISTRATUS OF ELEA. TO ESCAPE THE SPARTANS, HE CUT OFF HIS OWN LEG AND MADE A WOODEN ONE.

Procedures for fashioning such prostheses evolved with technology and new materials, but the guiding principle of the apparatus has remained consistent.

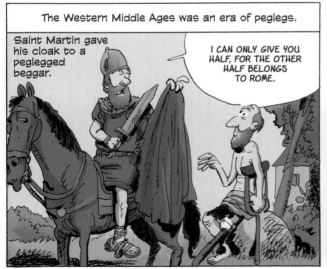

The Western Middle Ages was an era of peglegs.

Saint Martin gave his cloak to a peglegged beggar.

I CAN ONLY GIVE YOU HALF, FOR THE OTHER HALF BELONGS TO ROME.

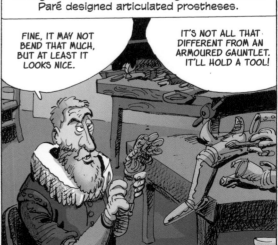

During the Renaissance, the ingenious Ambroise Paré designed articulated prostheses.

FINE, IT MAY NOT BEND THAT MUCH, BUT AT LEAST IT LOOKS NICE.

IT'S NOT ALL THAT DIFFERENT FROM AN ARMOURED GAUNTLET. IT'LL HOLD A TOOL!

INTERNAL PROSTHESES

Artificial noses had been around since ancient times, but not until World War One were there any significant advances.
I CERTAINLY NEEDED A PROSTHESIS TO FIX MY SHATTERED FACE AND MAKE ME LOOK HUMAN AGAIN.
Artificial joints were developed during the 20th century.
Fingers
Hip
Knee
Jaw
In 1947, Robert Judet in France and Austin Moore in the U.S.A. conceived of hip replacement prostheses.
MY GOAL WAS TO HAVE ELDERLY PEOPLE WITH FEMUR FRACTURES BACK ON THEIR FEET AGAIN, IN ORDER TO AVOID COMPLICATIONS DUE TO EXTENDED BED REST.
Robert Judet
Moore prosthesis
Artificial limbs have evolved tremendously, and wooden legs have transformed into high-tech products.
Carbon-fibre prostheses
Myoelectric articulated prostheses
The pegleg in Antiquity, 4th century BCE
For now, these prostheses are body-powered, but in the future, they could well respond to mental commands.
HNGH!
The goal is to connect sensory receptors at nerve endings along the residual limb that will react to electrical impulses to move the prosthesis.
Among paraplegics, software-controlled exoskeletons are increasingly common.
Rehabilitation combines intensive immersion in virtual reality with physical exercises, so that the exoskeleton can enable mind-controlled locomotion.
A HELMET WITH ELECTRODES ALLOWS US TO RECEIVE SIGNALS ASSOCIATED WITH MOVEMENTS THAT THE BRAIN SENDS OUT, USING SOFTWARE THAT CAN DECODE THEM.
THE SURGEONS HAVE REALLY TRANSFORMED ME — ONE BIT AT A TIME.
BUS
CHOOSING A PROSTHESIS

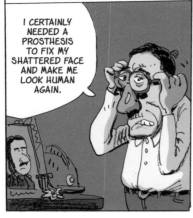

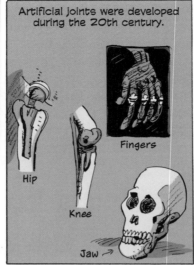

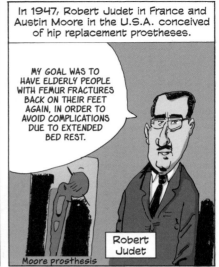

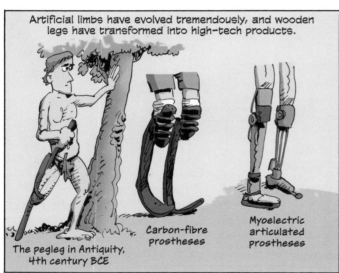

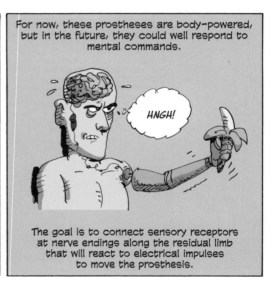

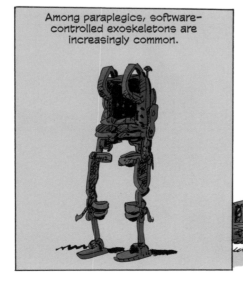

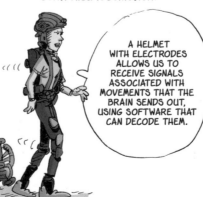

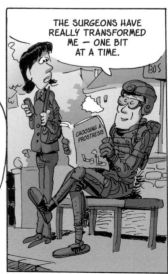

ARTIFICIAL ORGANS

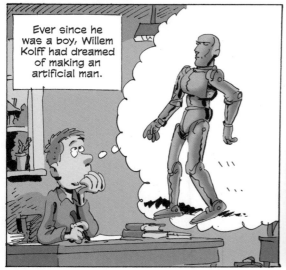

Ever since he was a boy, Willem Kolff had dreamed of making an artificial man.

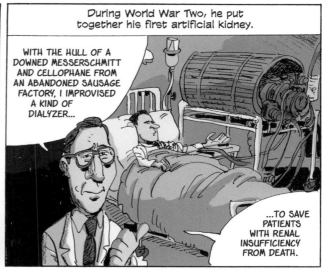

During World War Two, he put together his first artificial kidney.

WITH THE HULL OF A DOWNED MESSERSCHMITT AND CELLOPHANE FROM AN ABANDONED SAUSAGE FACTORY, I IMPROVISED A KIND OF DIALYZER...

...TO SAVE PATIENTS WITH RENAL INSUFFICIENCY FROM DEATH.

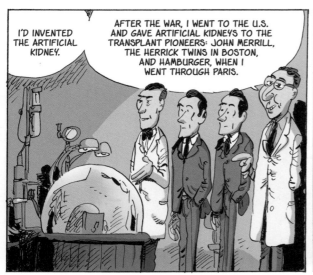

I'D INVENTED THE ARTIFICIAL KIDNEY.

AFTER THE WAR, I WENT TO THE U.S. AND GAVE ARTIFICIAL KIDNEYS TO THE TRANSPLANT PIONEERS: JOHN MERRILL, THE HERRICK TWINS IN BOSTON, AND HAMBURGER, WHEN I WENT THROUGH PARIS.

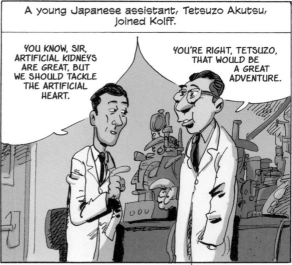

A young Japanese assistant, Tetsuzo Akutsu, joined Kolff.

YOU KNOW, SIR, ARTIFICIAL KIDNEYS ARE GREAT, BUT WE SHOULD TACKLE THE ARTIFICIAL HEART.

YOU'RE RIGHT, TETSUZO, THAT WOULD BE A GREAT ADVENTURE.

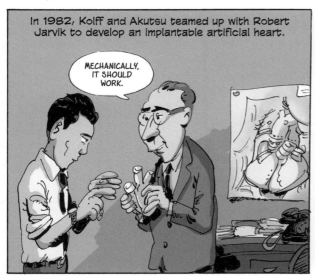

In 1982, Kolff and Akutsu teamed up with Robert Jarvik to develop an implantable artificial heart.

MECHANICALLY, IT SHOULD WORK.

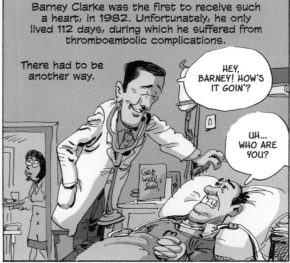

Barney Clarke was the first to receive such a heart, in 1982. Unfortunately, he only lived 112 days, during which he suffered from thromboembolic complications.

There had to be another way.

HEY, BARNEY! HOW'S IT GOIN'?

UH... WHO ARE YOU?

Faced with these difficulties, and the complexity of the operation, doctors opted for external artificial hearts while patients waited for a transplant.

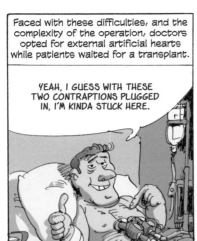

YEAH, I GUESS WITH THESE TWO CONTRAPTIONS PLUGGED IN, I'M KINDA STUCK HERE.

But things were about to get better...

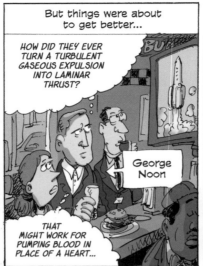

HOW DID THEY EVER TURN A TURBULENT GASEOUS EXPULSION INTO LAMINAR THRUST?

George Noon

THAT MIGHT WORK FOR PUMPING BLOOD IN PLACE OF A HEART...

Noon and Michael DeBakey introduced a turbine to replace a failing heart.

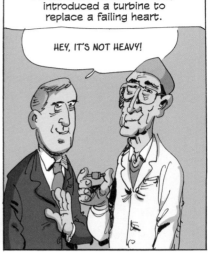

HEY, IT'S NOT HEAVY!

Noon and J.-N. Fabiani implanted the first turbine in France in 1999.

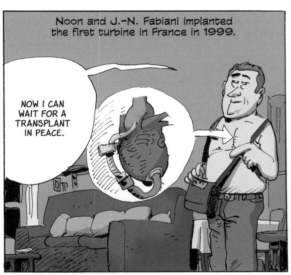

NOW I CAN WAIT FOR A TRANSPLANT IN PEACE.

Meanwhile, in Paris, Alain Carpentier met Jean-Luc Lagardère.

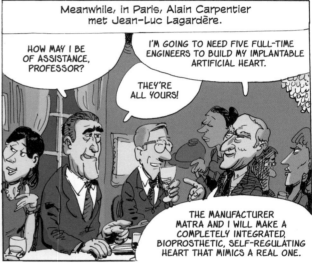

HOW MAY I BE OF ASSISTANCE, PROFESSOR?

I'M GOING TO NEED FIVE FULL-TIME ENGINEERS TO BUILD MY IMPLANTABLE ARTIFICIAL HEART.

THEY'RE ALL YOURS!

THE MANUFACTURER MATRA AND I WILL MAKE A COMPLETELY INTEGRATED, BIOPROSTHETIC, SELF-REGULATING HEART THAT MIMICS A REAL ONE.

The CARMAT heart* was designed to be the perfect implant.

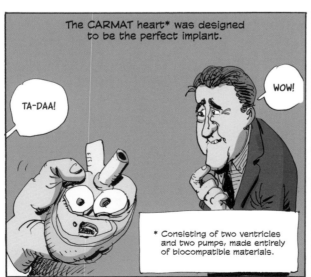

TA-DAA!

WOW!

* Consisting of two ventricles and two pumps, made entirely of biocompatible materials.

Such that today, any part of the human cardiovascular system can be replaced with prostheses or transplants.

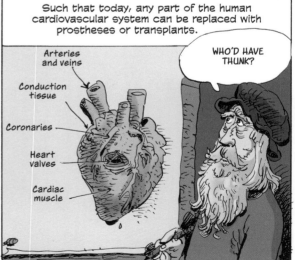

WHO'D HAVE THUNK?

Arteries and veins

Conduction tissue

Coronaries

Heart valves

Cardiac muscle

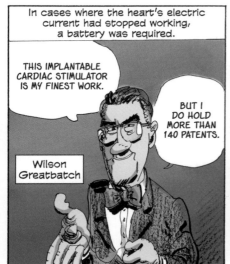

In cases where the heart's electric current had stopped working, a battery was required.

THIS IMPLANTABLE CARDIAC STIMULATOR IS MY FINEST WORK.

BUT I DO HOLD MORE THAN 140 PATENTS.

Wilson Greatbatch

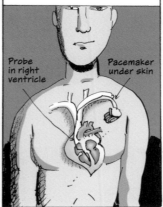

Ake Senning implanted the first pacemaker in Sweden in October 1958.

Probe in right ventricle

Pacemaker under skin

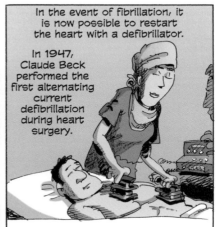

In the event of fibrillation, it is now possible to restart the heart with a defibrillator.

In 1947, Claude Beck performed the first alternating current defibrillation during heart surgery.

Michel Mirowski developed the first implantable cardiac defibrillator in 1970.

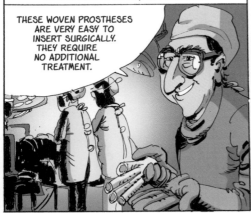

Homografts were the first arterial replacements to be used, but soon prostheses made of Dacron became the norm, thanks to Michael DeBakey in Houston.

THESE WOVEN PROSTHESES ARE VERY EASY TO INSERT SURGICALLY. THEY REQUIRE NO ADDITIONAL TREATMENT.

Arterial stents, meanwhile, can be introduced into arteries without surgical intervention, via remote control.

Ⓐ Ⓑ

Introduction of prosthesis

Abdominal aortic aneurysm

Cholesterol build-up

Iliac artery

Prosthesis in place in aorta and iliac arteries

Albert Starr fabricated the first artificial heart valve in 1960.

I WAS INSPIRED BY THE WINE BOTTLE STOPPER...

CARDIAC VALVE

...TO MAKE THE FIRST MITRAL VALVE!

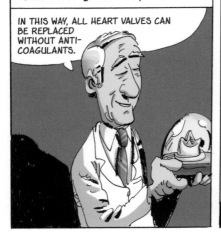

In 1968, Carpentier introduced the concept of bioprosthesis (half heterograft, half prosthesis).

IN THIS WAY, ALL HEART VALVES CAN BE REPLACED WITHOUT ANTI-COAGULANTS.

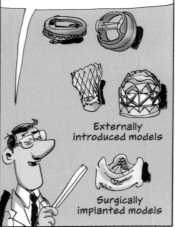

MANY OTHER VALVE MODELS WERE DEVELOPED, BOTH MECHANICAL AND BIOLOGICAL.

Externally introduced models

Surgically implanted models

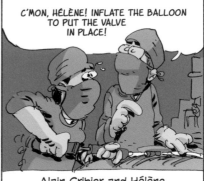

It is now possible to replace the heart's valves under local anaesthesia, without open heart surgery.

C'MON, HÉLÈNE! INFLATE THE BALLOON TO PUT THE VALVE IN PLACE!

Alain Cribier and Hélène Eltchaninoff in Rouen, 2002

CHAPTER 17

FROM HERBS TO PILLS

From "simples"—the medicinal herbs monks grew in monastery gardens—to the pills of today: what a story!

Every plant tells its own tale, every drug recounts an adventure.

For centuries, the trade in herbal remedies has been a success story—one that continues to this day, though sometimes at the expense of more industrialized pharmaceutical medications. Why, it's almost as if the pharma companies, despite two centuries of groundbreaking research, still haven't managed to win the trust of their patients...

And yet, what a mistake that is, in light of the revolution that modern medication presents!

Let's take a closer look at this world, where brilliant, groundbreaking research and seductive charlatanism can too often be indistinguishable.

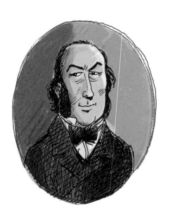

PLANTS HAVE BEEN AROUND FOREVER

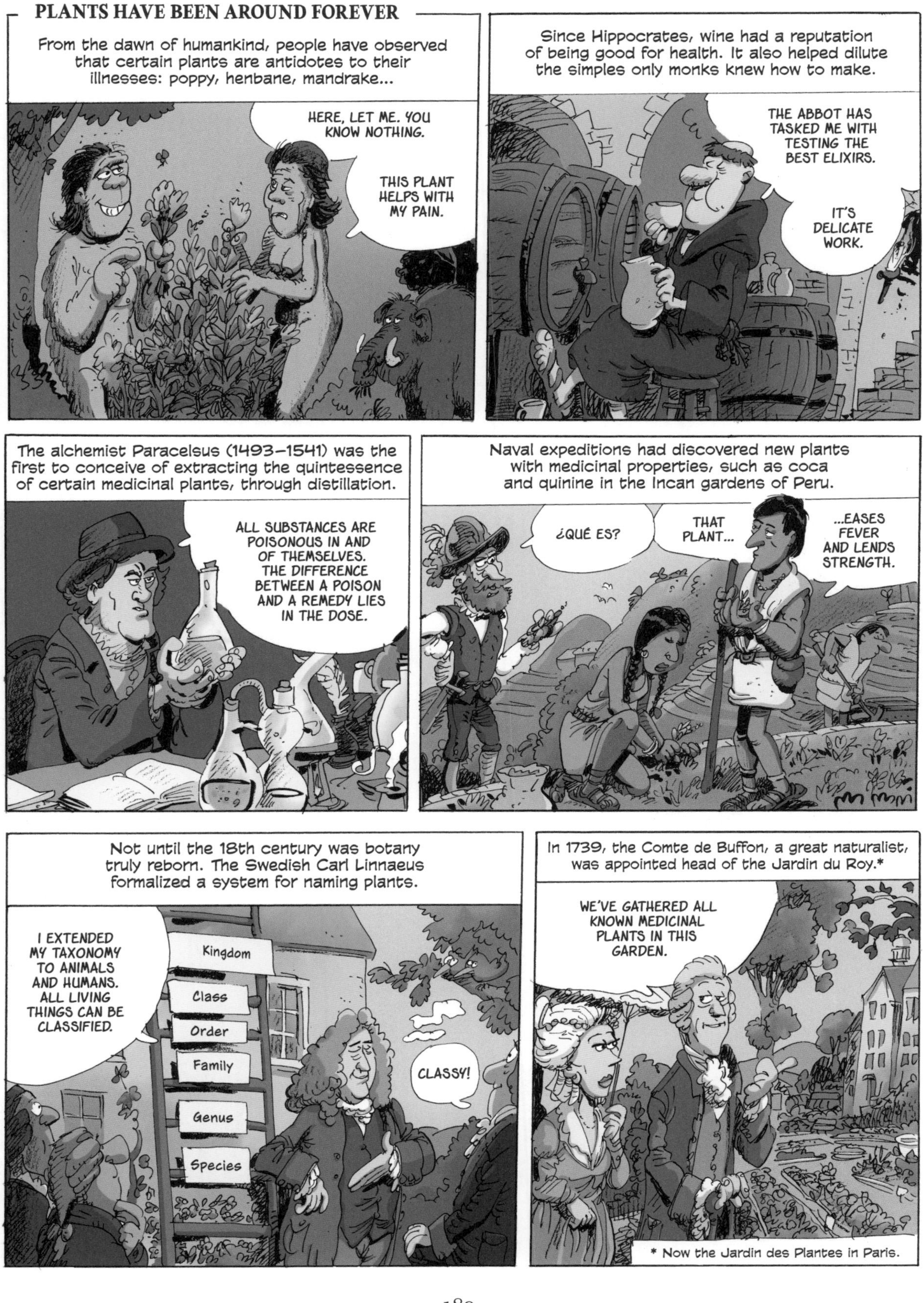
From the dawn of humankind, people have observed that certain plants are antidotes to their illnesses: poppy, henbane, mandrake...
HERE, LET ME. YOU KNOW NOTHING.
THIS PLANT HELPS WITH MY PAIN.
Since Hippocrates, wine had a reputation of being good for health. It also helped dilute the simples only monks knew how to make.
THE ABBOT HAS TASKED ME WITH TESTING THE BEST ELIXIRS.
IT'S DELICATE WORK.
The alchemist Paracelsus (1493–1541) was the first to conceive of extracting the quintessence of certain medicinal plants, through distillation.
ALL SUBSTANCES ARE POISONOUS IN AND OF THEMSELVES. THE DIFFERENCE BETWEEN A POISON AND A REMEDY LIES IN THE DOSE.
Naval expeditions had discovered new plants with medicinal properties, such as coca and quinine in the Incan gardens of Peru.
¿QUÉ ES?
THAT PLANT...
...EASES FEVER AND LENDS STRENGTH.
Not until the 18th century was botany truly reborn. The Swedish Carl Linnaeus formalized a system for naming plants.
I EXTENDED MY TAXONOMY TO ANIMALS AND HUMANS. ALL LIVING THINGS CAN BE CLASSIFIED.
Kingdom
Class
Order
Family
Genus
Species
CLASSY!
In 1739, the Comte de Buffon, a great naturalist, was appointed head of the Jardin du Roy.*
WE'VE GATHERED ALL KNOWN MEDICINAL PLANTS IN THIS GARDEN.
* Now the Jardin des Plantes in Paris.

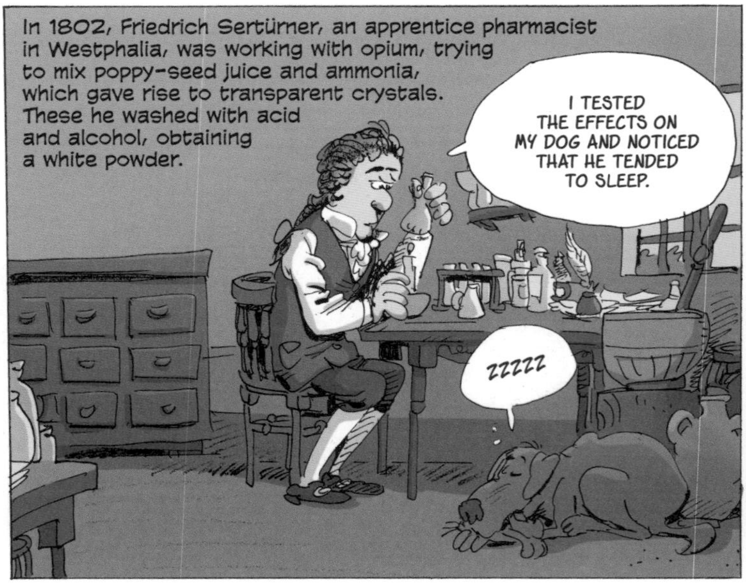
In 1802, Friedrich Sertürner, an apprentice pharmacist in Westphalia, was working with opium, trying to mix poppy-seed juice and ammonia, which gave rise to transparent crystals. These he washed with acid and alcohol, obtaining a white powder.
I TESTED THE EFFECTS ON MY DOG AND NOTICED THAT HE TENDED TO SLEEP.
ZZZZZ

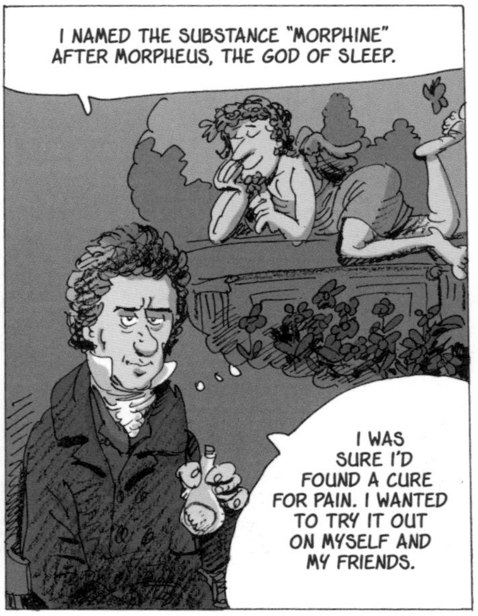
I NAMED THE SUBSTANCE "MORPHINE" AFTER MORPHEUS, THE GOD OF SLEEP.
I WAS SURE I'D FOUND A CURE FOR PAIN. I WANTED TO TRY IT OUT ON MYSELF AND MY FRIENDS.

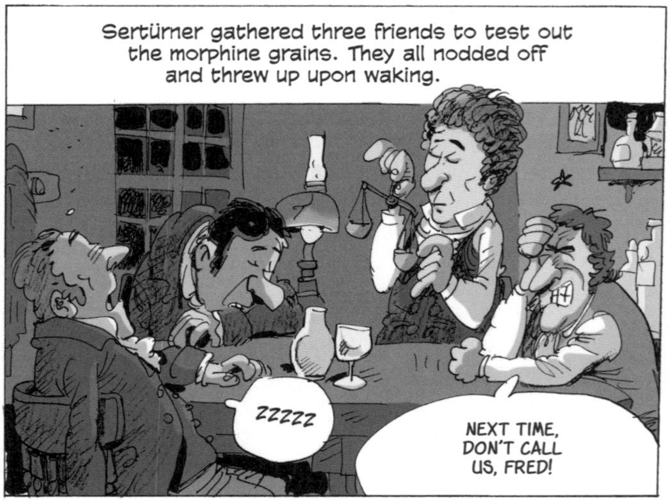
Sertürner gathered three friends to test out the morphine grains. They all nodded off and threw up upon waking.
ZZZZZ
NEXT TIME, DON'T CALL US, FRED!

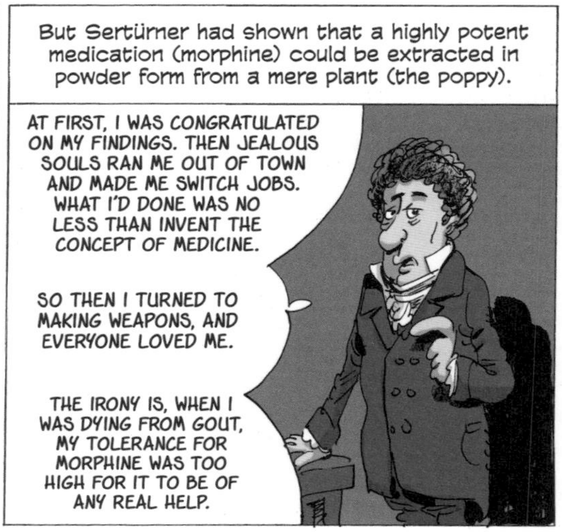
But Sertürner had shown that a highly potent medication (morphine) could be extracted in powder form from a mere plant (the poppy).
AT FIRST, I WAS CONGRATULATED ON MY FINDINGS. THEN JEALOUS SOULS RAN ME OUT OF TOWN AND MADE ME SWITCH JOBS. WHAT I'D DONE WAS NO LESS THAN INVENT THE CONCEPT OF MEDICINE.
SO THEN I TURNED TO MAKING WEAPONS, AND EVERYONE LOVED ME.
THE IRONY IS, WHEN I WAS DYING FROM GOUT, MY TOLERANCE FOR MORPHINE WAS TOO HIGH FOR IT TO BE OF ANY REAL HELP.

Inspired by Sertürner's discovery, pharmacists set to work seeking the therapeutic secrets of plants.

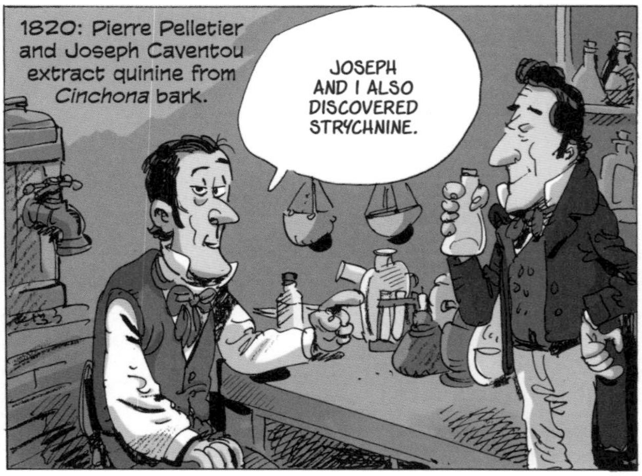
1820: Pierre Pelletier and Joseph Caventou extract quinine from *Cinchona* bark.
JOSEPH AND I ALSO DISCOVERED STRYCHNINE.

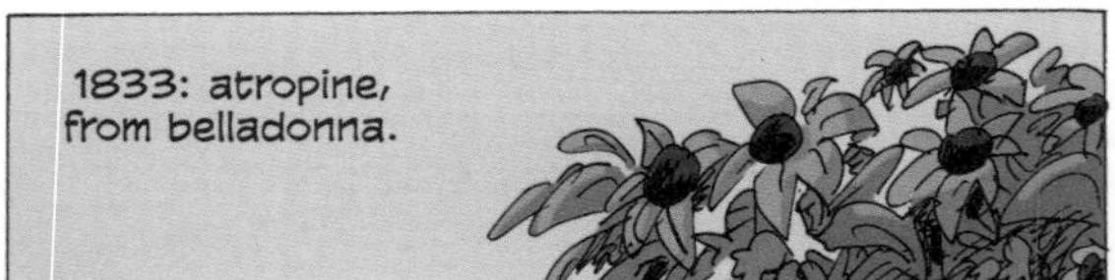
1833: atropine, from belladonna.

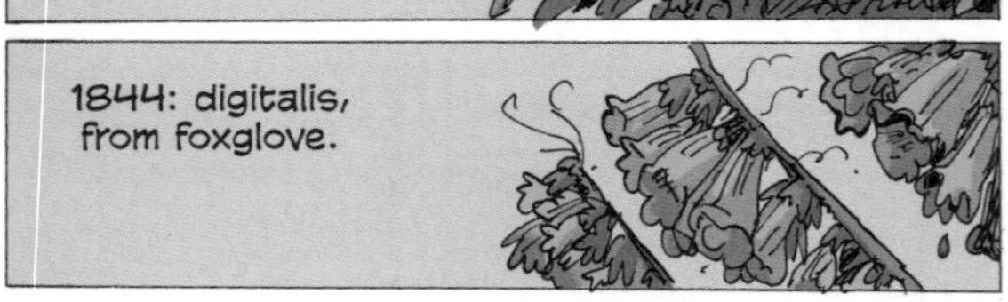
1844: digitalis, from foxglove.

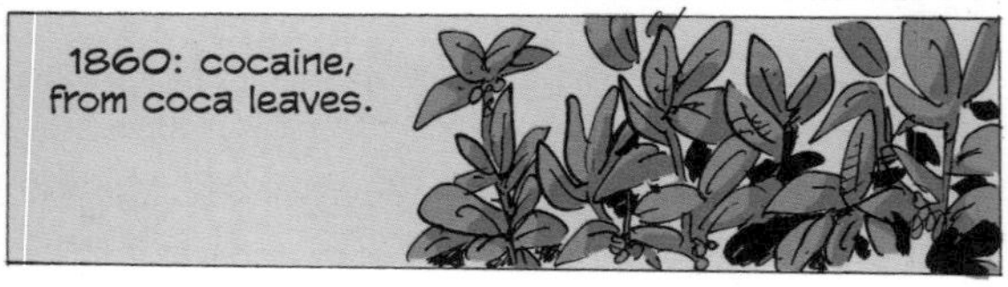
1860: cocaine, from coca leaves.

Most of these plants were known to be dangerous.

Indeed, *Digitalis purpurea* had long been considered poisonous, a magical plant used by witches.
WITH FLOWERS FROM THESE FOXGLOVES, I'LL MAKE A PASTE TO PUT ON HOUSES AS A PROTECTION AGAINST EVIL FORCES FROM UNDERGROUND.
In 1844, the French pharmacist Claude Nativelle isolated digitalis in crystalline form from *Digitalis* leaves in an alcoholic solution.
DIGITALIS IS A WONDERFUL DRUG. IT SLOWS OR HASTENS THE HEARTBEAT.
CAREFUL, THOUGH! THE LINE BETWEEN THE THERAPEUTIC AND TOXIC DOSES IS VERY THIN.
IT CAN BECOME A POISON THAT KILLS VIA HEART ATTACK.
The name "atropine" comes from Atropos, one of the Fates, who cut the thread of life. What an introduction! But for a long time, it was also called belladonna (literally "beautiful lady"), for in the past, ladies used drops of *Atropia belladonna* to enhance their beauty...
...by dilating the pupils of their eyes. Ophthalmologists still use it in eye examinations.
Atropine was isolated in 1833. It is found in belladonna, henbane, and mandrake. It inhibits parasympathetic effects and is an acetylcholine antagonist. In high doses, it becomes a poison.
HEY, MUM, CAN I EAT THESE BERRIES HERE?
ABSOLUTELY NOT, DARLING. THAT'S DEADLY NIGHTSHADE. IT'LL KILL YOU!
In 1885, the pharmacist John Pemberton invented "French Wine Coca".
LADIES AND GENTLEMEN, COME AND TRY MY NEW HEALTHFUL AND INVIGORATING PLANT-BASED BEVERAGE! IT'S GOT A GREAT FUTURE!
ORIGINAL TASTE
WINE 5¢ COCA
WINE 5¢ COC
It was an alcoholic mixture of coca, kola nut, and damiana inspired by "Mariani's wine", created by French chemist Angelo Mariani.
Later, slightly modified, the formula proved a hit. A famous ad featuring Santa Claus made it the world's number one drink.
Coca-Cola
TO THINK THIS STUFF USED TO BE ALCOHOLIC... HIC!

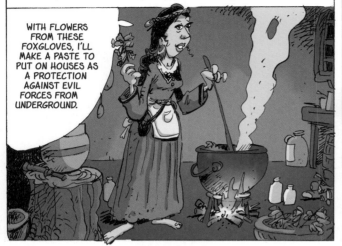

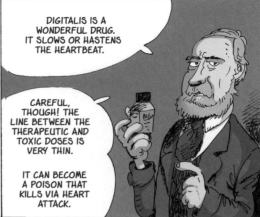

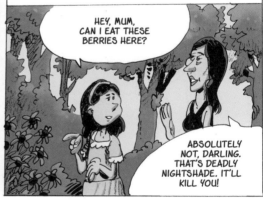

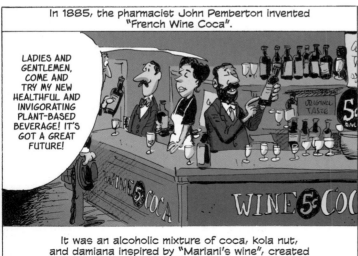

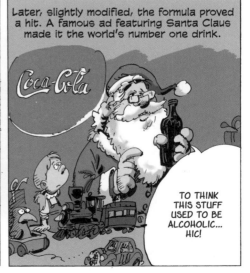

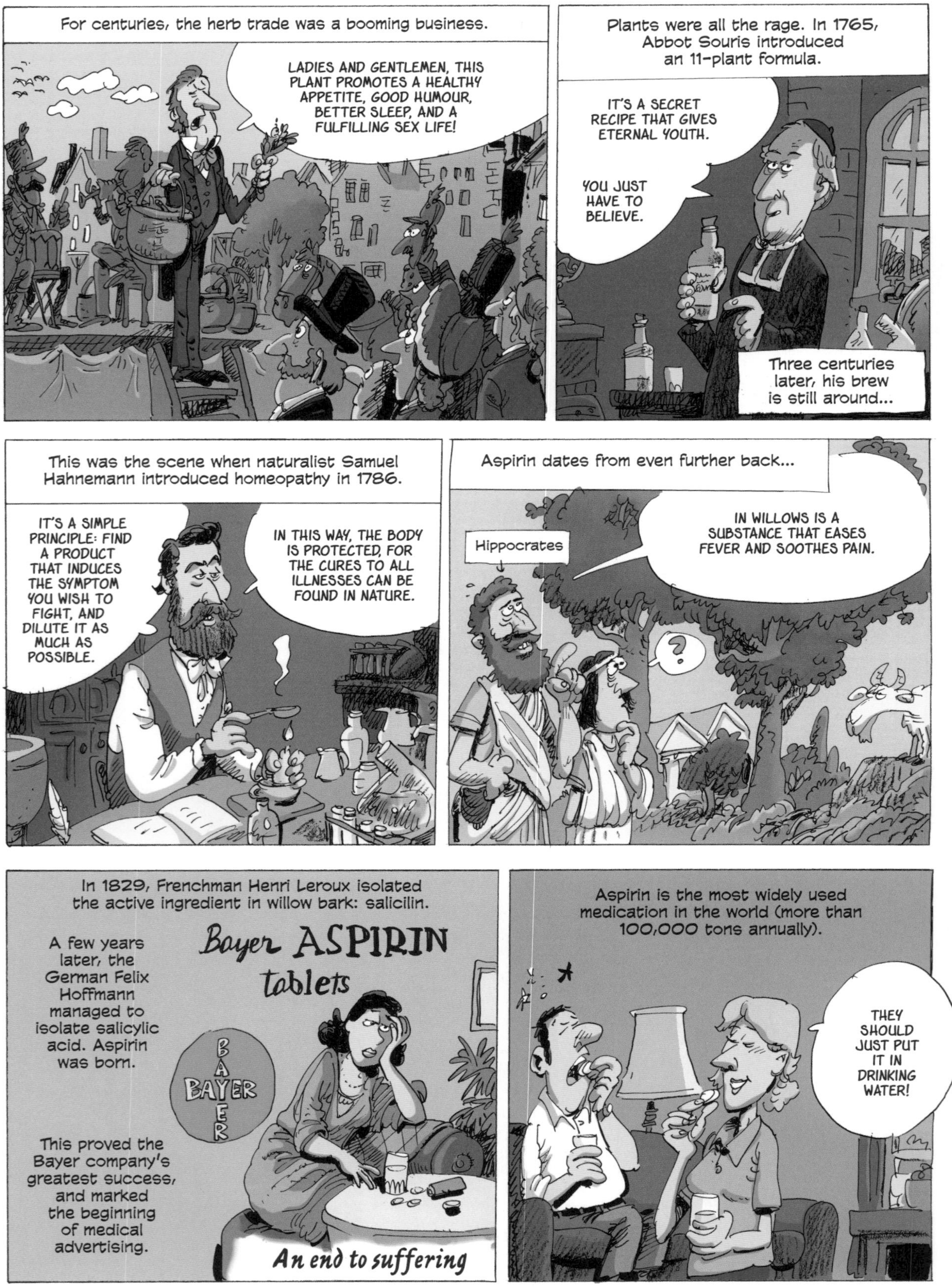
For centuries, the herb trade was a booming business.
LADIES AND GENTLEMEN, THIS PLANT PROMOTES A HEALTHY APPETITE, GOOD HUMOUR, BETTER SLEEP, AND A FULFILLING SEX LIFE!
Plants were all the rage. In 1765, Abbot Souris introduced an 11-plant formula.
IT'S A SECRET RECIPE THAT GIVES ETERNAL YOUTH.
YOU JUST HAVE TO BELIEVE.
Three centuries later, his brew is still around...
This was the scene when naturalist Samuel Hahnemann introduced homeopathy in 1786.
IT'S A SIMPLE PRINCIPLE: FIND A PRODUCT THAT INDUCES THE SYMPTOM YOU WISH TO FIGHT, AND DILUTE IT AS MUCH AS POSSIBLE.
IN THIS WAY, THE BODY IS PROTECTED, FOR THE CURES TO ALL ILLNESSES CAN BE FOUND IN NATURE.
Aspirin dates from even further back...
Hippocrates
IN WILLOWS IS A SUBSTANCE THAT EASES FEVER AND SOOTHES PAIN.
?
In 1829, Frenchman Henri Leroux isolated the active ingredient in willow bark: salicilin.
A few years later, the German Felix Hoffmann managed to isolate salicylic acid. Aspirin was born.
Bayer ASPIRIN tablets
BAYER
BAYER
This proved the Bayer company's greatest success, and marked the beginning of medical advertising.
An end to suffering
Aspirin is the most widely used medication in the world (more than 100,000 tons annually).
THEY SHOULD JUST PUT IT IN DRINKING WATER!

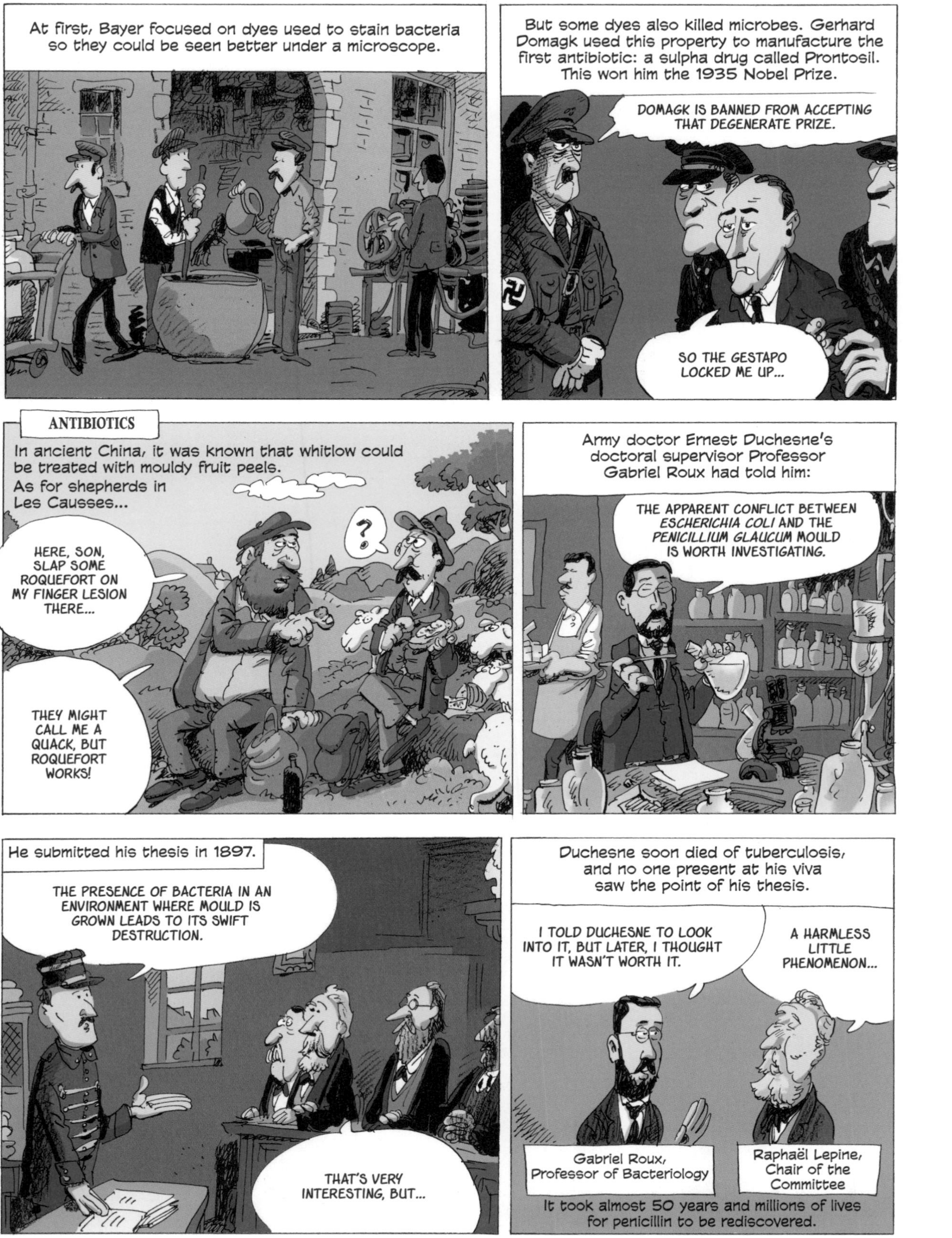
At first, Bayer focused on dyes used to stain bacteria so they could be seen better under a microscope.
But some dyes also killed microbes. Gerhard Domagk used this property to manufacture the first antibiotic: a sulpha drug called Prontosil. This won him the 1935 Nobel Prize.
DOMAGK IS BANNED FROM ACCEPTING THAT DEGENERATE PRIZE.
SO THE GESTAPO LOCKED ME UP...
ANTIBIOTICS
In ancient China, it was known that whitlow could be treated with mouldy fruit peels.
As for shepherds in Les Causses...
HERE, SON, SLAP SOME ROQUEFORT ON MY FINGER LESION THERE...
?
THEY MIGHT CALL ME A QUACK, BUT ROQUEFORT WORKS!
Army doctor Ernest Duchesne's doctoral supervisor Professor Gabriel Roux had told him:
THE APPARENT CONFLICT BETWEEN *ESCHERICHIA COLI* AND THE *PENICILLIUM GLAUCUM* MOULD IS WORTH INVESTIGATING.
He submitted his thesis in 1897.
THE PRESENCE OF BACTERIA IN AN ENVIRONMENT WHERE MOULD IS GROWN LEADS TO ITS SWIFT DESTRUCTION.
THAT'S VERY INTERESTING, BUT...
Duchesne soon died of tuberculosis, and no one present at his viva saw the point of his thesis.
I TOLD DUCHESNE TO LOOK INTO IT, BUT LATER, I THOUGHT IT WASN'T WORTH IT.
A HARMLESS LITTLE PHENOMENON...
Gabriel Roux, Professor of Bacteriology
Raphaël Lepine, Chair of the Committee
It took almost 50 years and millions of lives for penicillin to be rediscovered.

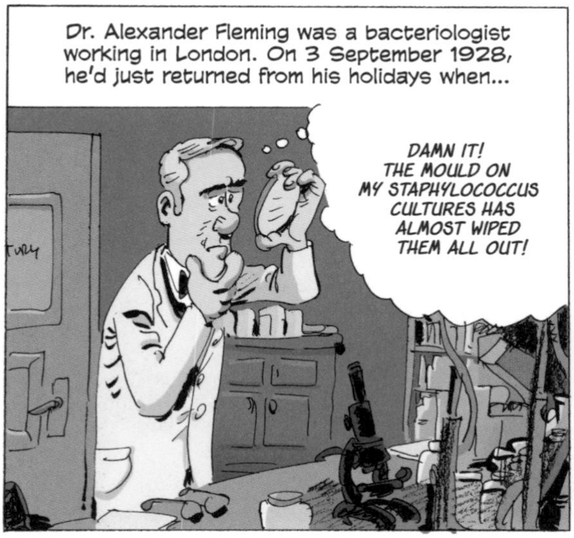
Dr. Alexander Fleming was a bacteriologist working in London. On 3 September 1928, he'd just returned from his holidays when...
DAMN IT! THE MOULD ON MY STAPHYLOCOCCUS CULTURES HAS ALMOST WIPED THEM ALL OUT!

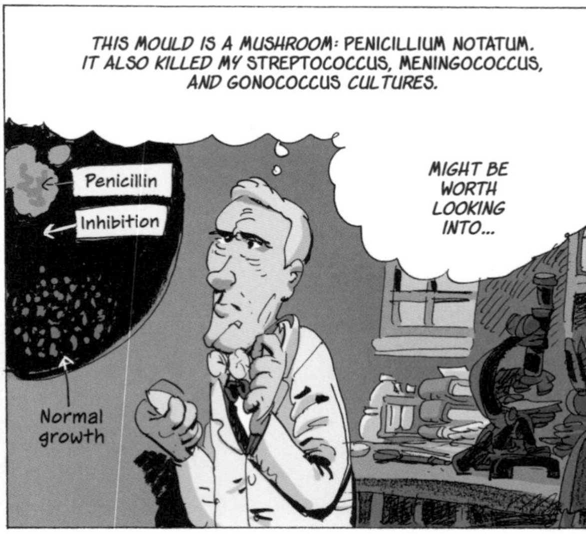
THIS MOULD IS A MUSHROOM: PENICILLIUM NOTATUM. IT ALSO KILLED MY STREPTOCOCCUS, MENINGOCOCCUS, AND GONOCOCCUS CULTURES.
Penicillin
Inhibition
Normal growth
MIGHT BE WORTH LOOKING INTO...

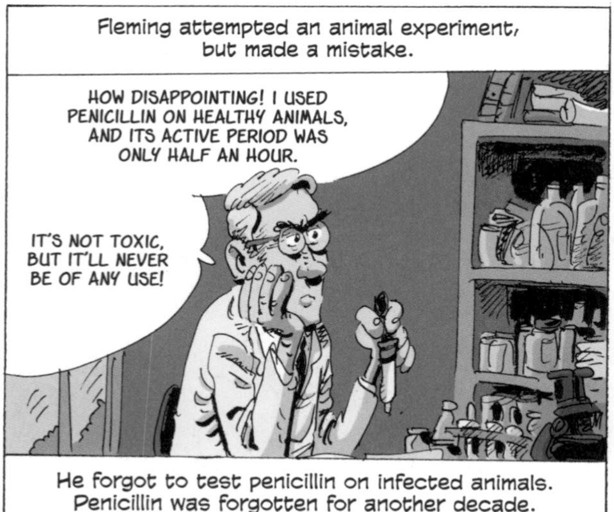
Fleming attempted an animal experiment, but made a mistake.
HOW DISAPPOINTING! I USED PENICILLIN ON HEALTHY ANIMALS, AND ITS ACTIVE PERIOD WAS ONLY HALF AN HOUR.
IT'S NOT TOXIC, BUT IT'LL NEVER BE OF ANY USE!
He forgot to test penicillin on infected animals. Penicillin was forgotten for another decade.

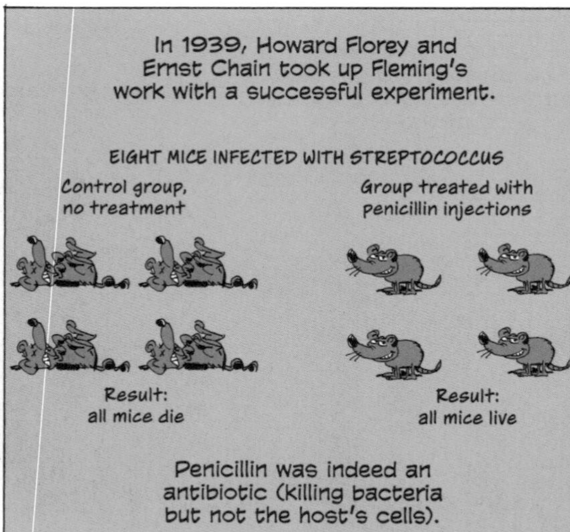
In 1939, Howard Florey and Ernst Chain took up Fleming's work with a successful experiment.
EIGHT MICE INFECTED WITH STREPTOCOCCUS
Control group, no treatment
Group treated with penicillin injections
Result: all mice die
Result: all mice live
Penicillin was indeed an antibiotic (killing bacteria but not the host's cells).

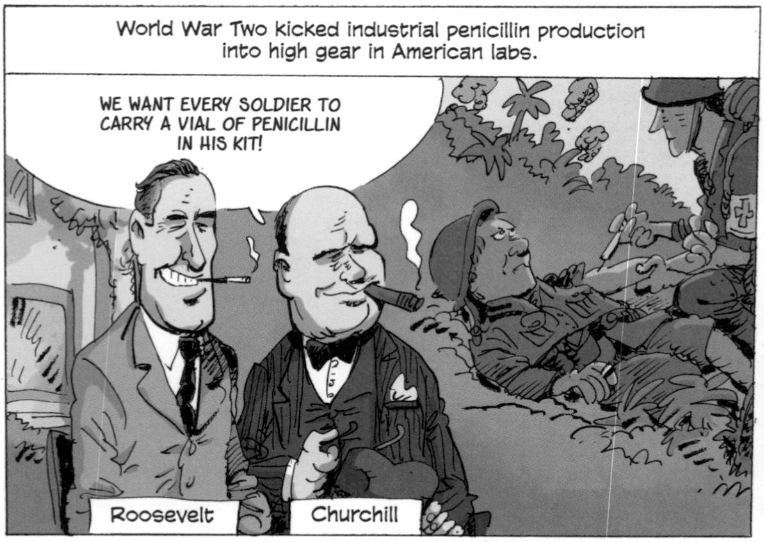
World War Two kicked industrial penicillin production into high gear in American labs.
WE WANT EVERY SOLDIER TO CARRY A VIAL OF PENICILLIN IN HIS KIT!
Roosevelt
Churchill

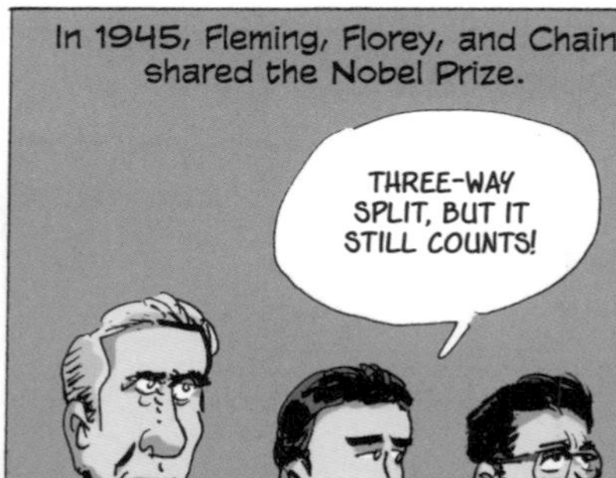
In 1945, Fleming, Florey, and Chain shared the Nobel Prize.
THREE-WAY SPLIT, BUT IT STILL COUNTS!

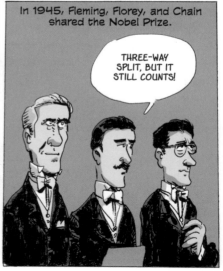

But penicillin proved inactive on Koch's bacillus.

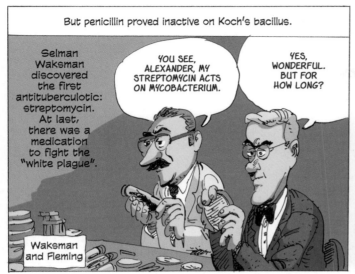

Selman Waksman discovered the first antituberculotic: streptomycin. At last, there was a medication to fight the "white plague".

YOU SEE, ALEXANDER, MY STREPTOMYCIN ACTS ON *MYCOBACTERIUM*.

YES, WONDERFUL. BUT FOR HOW LONG?

Waksman and Fleming

Fleming had observed the appearance of bacteria resistant to penicillin. Thus bacteria's talent for adaptation was discovered.

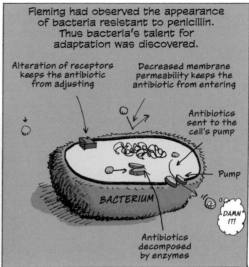

Alteration of receptors keeps the antibiotic from adjusting

Decreased membrane permeability keeps the antibiotic from entering

Antibiotics sent to the cell's pump

Pump

BACTERIUM

DAMN IT!

Antibiotics decomposed by enzymes

New antibiotics had to be constantly developed, and their prescription regulated to avoid resistance.

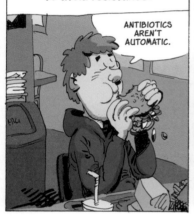

ANTIBIOTICS AREN'T AUTOMATIC.

HORMONES: ADRENALINE

From the start, humans have been able to react to stress thanks to a hormone secreted by the adrenal glands: adrenaline.

GRRR

RUN FOR YOUR LIFE!

Adrenaline speeds up the heart, increases the strength of its contractions, mobilizes stored energy, dilates the bronchia for easier breathing, and increases blood pressure to enhance physical effort.

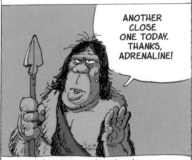

ANOTHER CLOSE ONE TODAY. THANKS, ADRENALINE!

Its secretion is thus "consumed" by the physical effort stress demands.

But in modern life, stress is everywhere...

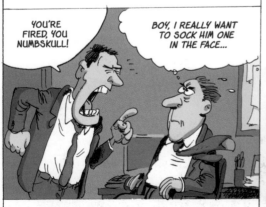

YOU'RE FIRED, YOU NUMBSKULL!

BOY, I REALLY WANT TO SOCK HIM ONE IN THE FACE...

And adrenaline secretions cannot always be used up by physical activity.

Which no doubt explains why stress is a risk factor in cardiovascular illnesses.

And why one of the best preventative measures is exercise.

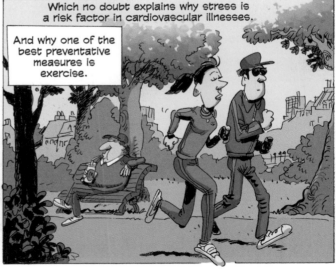

Adrenaline is first secreted by the adrenal glands...

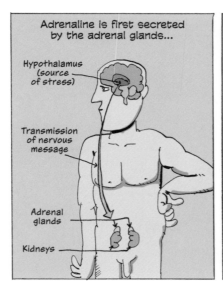

Hypothalamus (source of stress)

Transmission of nervous message

Adrenal glands

Kidneys

...and then attaches to specific receptors (alpha and beta) on numerous cells. Takamine Jōkichi discovered it in 1900 from adrenal samples.

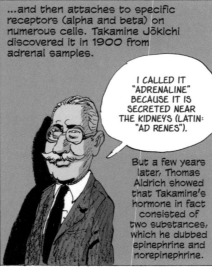

I CALLED IT "ADRENALINE" BECAUSE IT IS SECRETED NEAR THE KIDNEYS (LATIN: "AD RENES").

But a few years later, Thomas Aldrich showed that Takamine's hormone in fact consisted of two substances, which he dubbed epinephrine and norepinephrine.

Adrenaline remains the drug for shock and cardiorespiratory arrest.

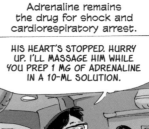

HIS HEART'S STOPPED. HURRY UP. I'LL MASSAGE HIM WHILE YOU PREP 1 MG OF ADRENALINE IN A 10-ML SOLUTION.

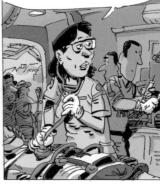

But to counter its negative effects on the cardiovascular system, beta blockers were developed in 1960.

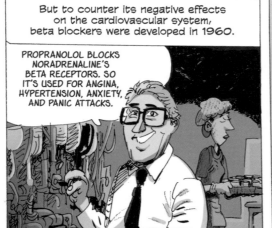

PROPRANOLOL BLOCKS NORADRENALINE'S BETA RECEPTORS. SO IT'S USED FOR ANGINA, HYPERTENSION, ANXIETY, AND PANIC ATTACKS.

Scotsman James Black, Nobel Prize, 1988

HORMONES: CORTISONE

In 1941, American intelligence found out the Germans had extracted, from the bovine adrenal cortex, a hormone that let pilots fly at high altitude without oxygen.

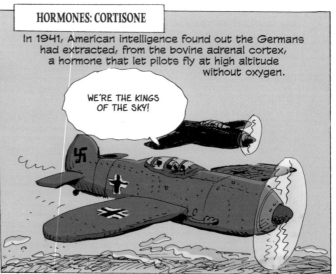

WE'RE THE KINGS OF THE SKY!

The army assigned Edward Kendall and the Merck company to isolate what they called "cortisone".

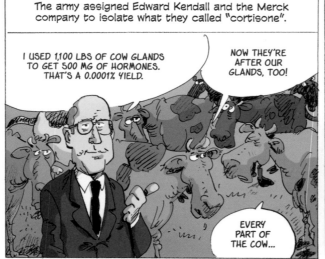

I USED 1,100 LBS OF COW GLANDS TO GET 500 MG OF HORMONES. THAT'S A 0.0001% YIELD.

NOW THEY'RE AFTER OUR GLANDS, TOO!

EVERY PART OF THE COW...

Merck managed to produce cortisone in sufficient quantities to attempt a clinical trial. Philip Hench, a Mayo Clinic rheumatologist, used the compound to treat a patient with rheumatoid polyarthritis.

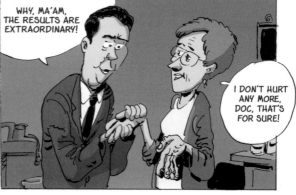

WHY, MA'AM, THE RESULTS ARE EXTRAORDINARY!

I DON'T HURT ANY MORE, DOC, THAT'S FOR SURE!

Cortisone was a genuine therapeutic revolution. It is a natural hormone that acts on specific receptors in many cells, and thus has many uses.
Cortex, source of cortisone
Medulla, source of adrenaline
It fights inflammation and allergies, and decreases immune response (against infection and rejection).
Adrenal gland (right)
Adrenal gland (left)
Kidney (right)
Kidney (left)
But it was soon clear that corticoids had many side effects.
AND I'VE GOT 'EM ALL!
Acne
Buffalo neck
Moon face
Bruising
Skin atrophy
Stomach ulcer
Stretch marks
Amenorrhoea
OR ALMOST!
And also weight gain, high blood pressure, diabetes, and mental disturbances.
Muscle wasting
Skin ulcers
HORMONES: INSULIN
The laboratory of Oskar Minkowski, Strasbourg, 1889...
SAY, BOSS!
IT'S WEIRD, BUT I TOOK OUT THIS DOG'S PANCREAS, AND NOW HE'S ALWAYS HUNGRY. PLUS, HIS URINE ATTRACTS FLIES!
YOU SURE, JOSEF?
Minkowski and Mering had just demonstrated the role of the pancreas in diabetes.
In 1921, Frederick Banting showed that cells from the islets of Langerhans in the pancreas produced a hormone that lowered blood sugar: insulin.
YOU SEE, CHARLES, WE'LL OBTAIN THE PUREST POSSIBLE PANCREAS SAMPLE FROM THIS DOG AND INJECT IT INTO A COMATOSE DIABETIC.
The first test, in Toronto on 11 January 1922, saved the life of a boy of 14.
BE BRAVE, LEONARD. SINCE YOU'RE VERY SKINNY, THIS COULD HURT.
These days, insulin is synthesized through the miracle of genetics.
Cell
Nucleus
D.N.A.
Injection
Extraction and purification of insulin
Isolation of insulin gene
G.M.O.
Introduction of gene into bacteria cells
Multiplication of bacteria to obtain a large number of genes

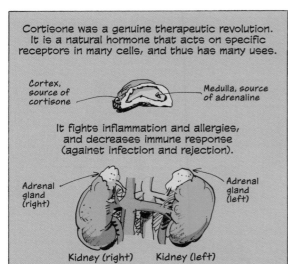

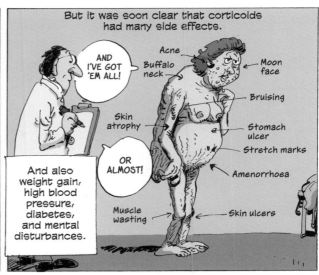

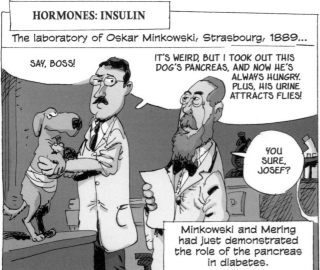

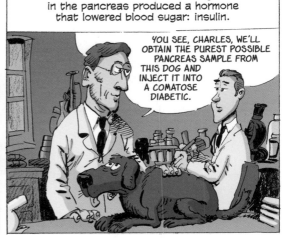

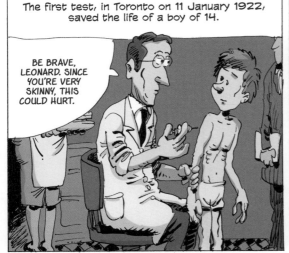

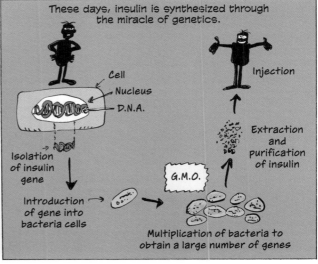

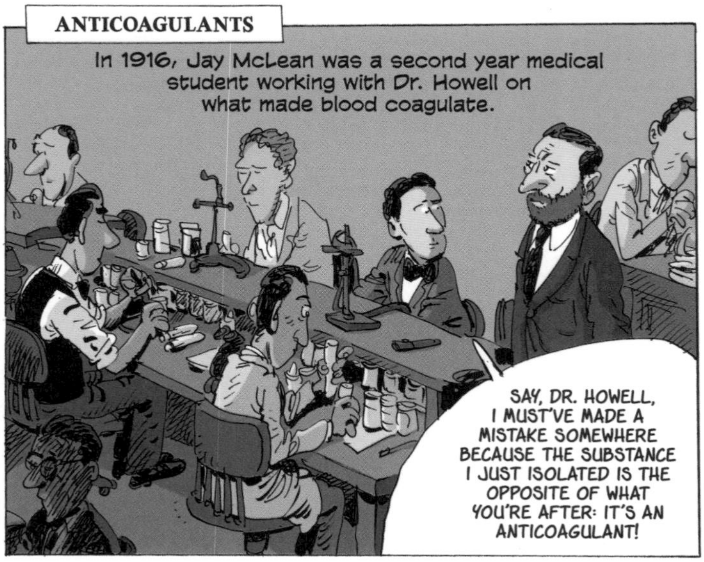
ANTICOAGULANTS
In 1916, Jay McLean was a second year medical student working with Dr. Howell on what made blood coagulate.
SAY, DR. HOWELL, I MUST'VE MADE A MISTAKE SOMEWHERE BECAUSE THE SUBSTANCE I JUST ISOLATED IS THE OPPOSITE OF WHAT YOU'RE AFTER: IT'S AN ANTICOAGULANT!

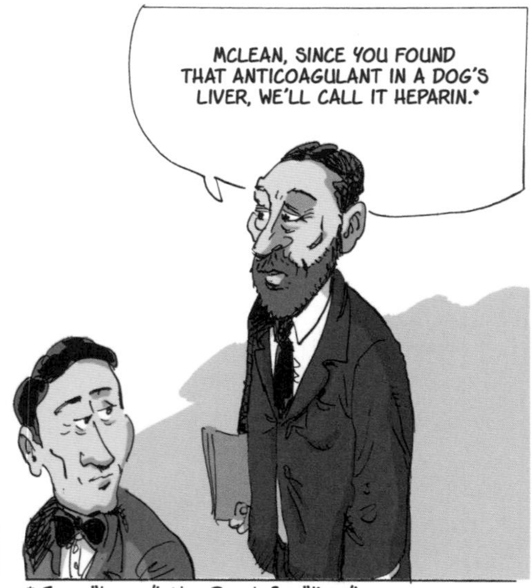
MCLEAN, SINCE YOU FOUND THAT ANTICOAGULANT IN A DOG'S LIVER, WE'LL CALL IT HEPARIN.*

* From "hepar", the Greek for "liver".

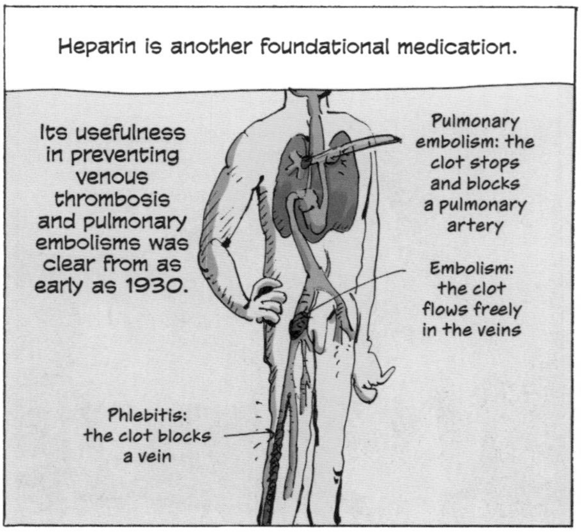
Heparin is another foundational medication.
Its usefulness in preventing venous thrombosis and pulmonary embolisms was clear from as early as 1930.
Pulmonary embolism: the clot stops and blocks a pulmonary artery
Embolism: the clot flows freely in the veins
Phlebitis: the clot blocks a vein

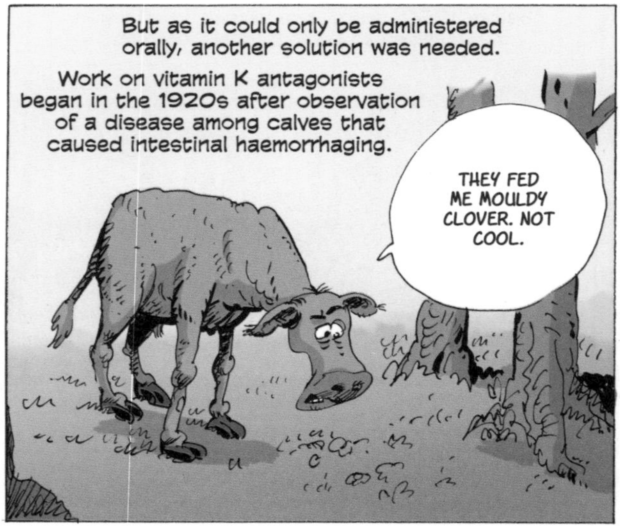
But as it could only be administered orally, another solution was needed.
Work on vitamin K antagonists began in the 1920s after observation of a disease among calves that caused intestinal haemorrhaging.
THEY FED ME MOULDY CLOVER. NOT COOL.

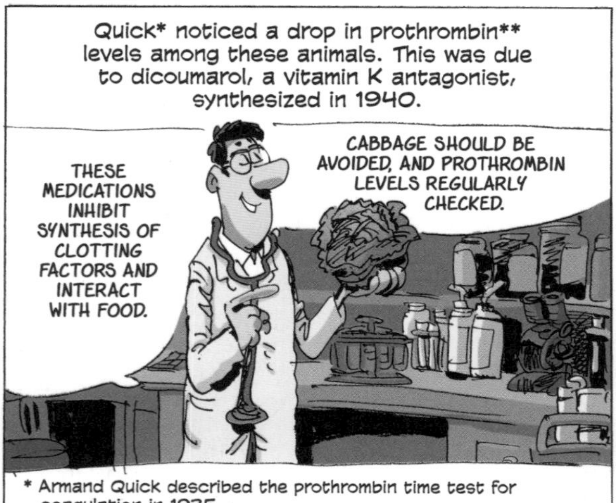
Quick* noticed a drop in prothrombin** levels among these animals. This was due to dicoumarol, a vitamin K antagonist, synthesized in 1940.
THESE MEDICATIONS INHIBIT SYNTHESIS OF CLOTTING FACTORS AND INTERACT WITH FOOD.
CABBAGE SHOULD BE AVOIDED, AND PROTHROMBIN LEVELS REGULARLY CHECKED.
* Armand Quick described the prothrombin time test for coagulation in 1935.
** The factor needed for coagulation.

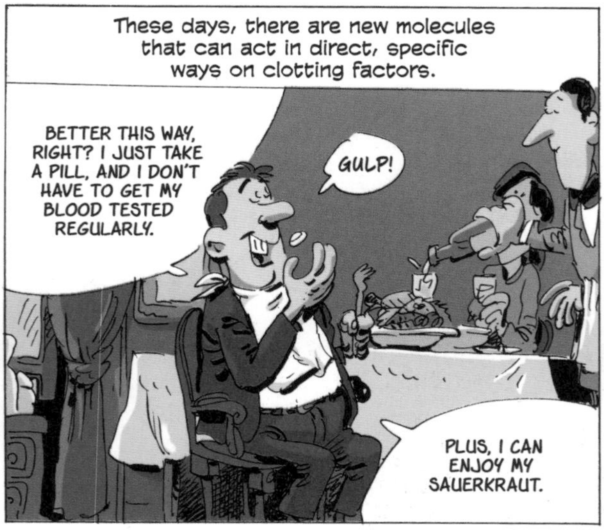
These days, there are new molecules that can act in direct, specific ways on clotting factors.
BETTER THIS WAY, RIGHT? I JUST TAKE A PILL, AND I DON'T HAVE TO GET MY BLOOD TESTED REGULARLY.
GULP!
PLUS, I CAN ENJOY MY SAUERKRAUT.

TREATMENT OF STOMACH ULCERS

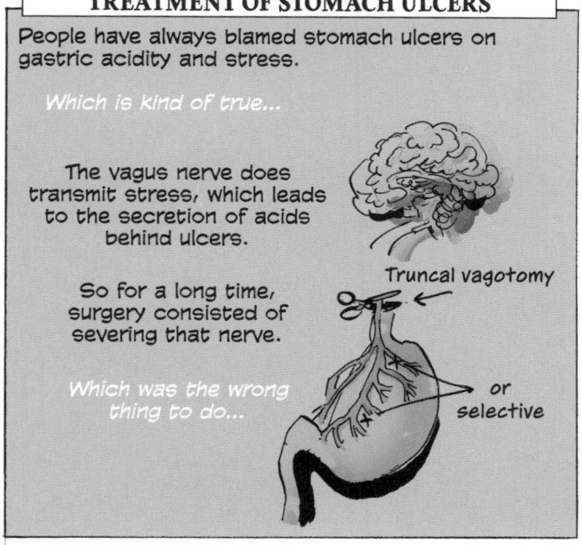
People have always blamed stomach ulcers on gastric acidity and stress.
Which is kind of true...
The vagus nerve does transmit stress, which leads to the secretion of acids behind ulcers.
So for a long time, surgery consisted of severing that nerve.
Truncal vagotomy
Which was the wrong thing to do...
or selective

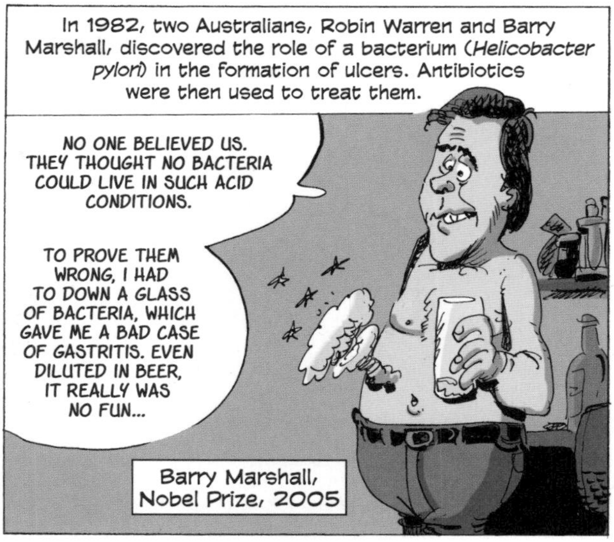
In 1982, two Australians, Robin Warren and Barry Marshall, discovered the role of a bacterium (Helicobacter pylori) in the formation of ulcers. Antibiotics were then used to treat them.
NO ONE BELIEVED US. THEY THOUGHT NO BACTERIA COULD LIVE IN SUCH ACID CONDITIONS.
TO PROVE THEM WRONG, I HAD TO DOWN A GLASS OF BACTERIA, WHICH GAVE ME A BAD CASE OF GASTRITIS. EVEN DILUTED IN BEER, IT REALLY WAS NO FUN...
Barry Marshall, Nobel Prize, 2005

PSYCHOTROPICS

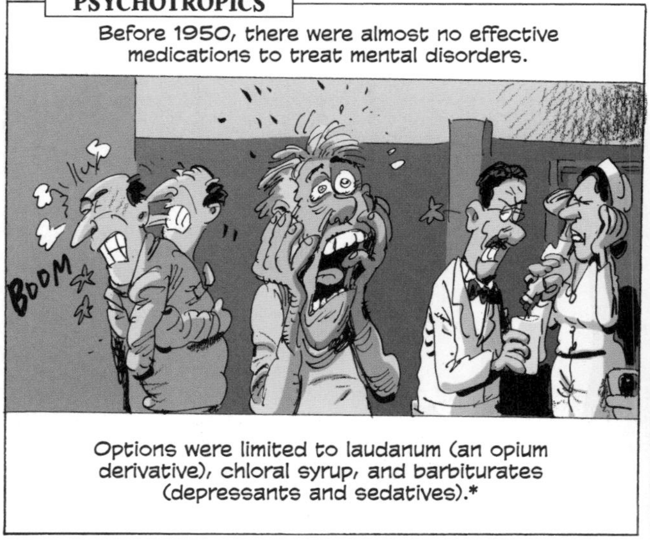
Before 1950, there were almost no effective medications to treat mental disorders.
BOOM
Options were limited to laudanum (an opium derivative), chloral syrup, and barbiturates (depressants and sedatives).*

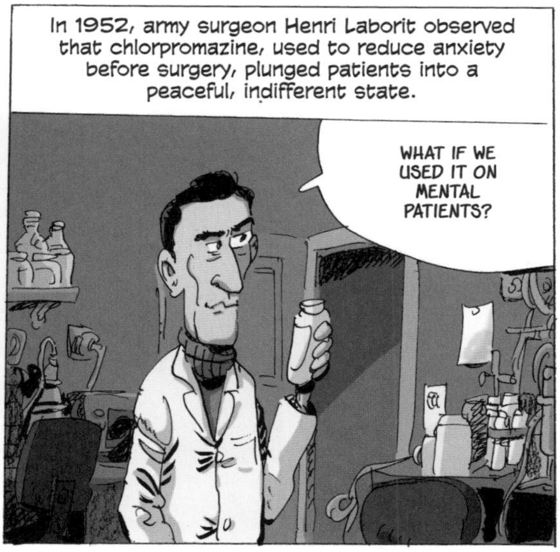
In 1952, army surgeon Henri Laborit observed that chlorpromazine, used to reduce anxiety before surgery, plunged patients into a peaceful, indifferent state.
WHAT IF WE USED IT ON MENTAL PATIENTS?

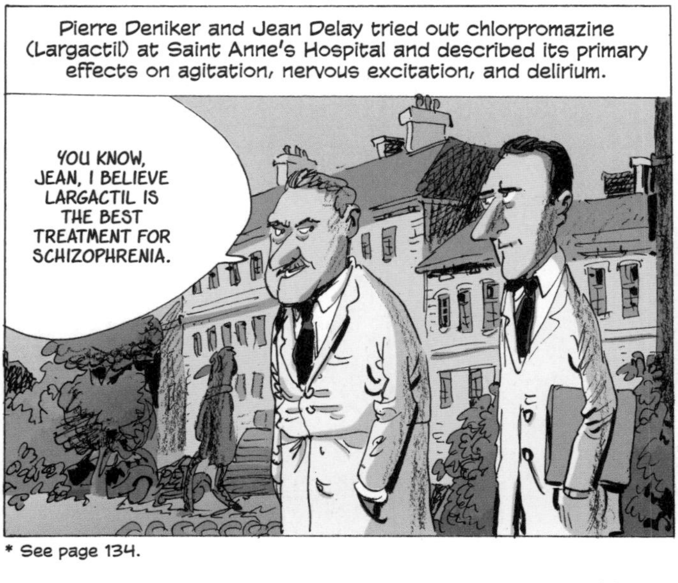
Pierre Deniker and Jean Delay tried out chlorpromazine (Largactil) at Saint Anne's Hospital and described its primary effects on agitation, nervous excitation, and delirium.
YOU KNOW, JEAN, I BELIEVE LARGACTIL IS THE BEST TREATMENT FOR SCHIZOPHRENIA.

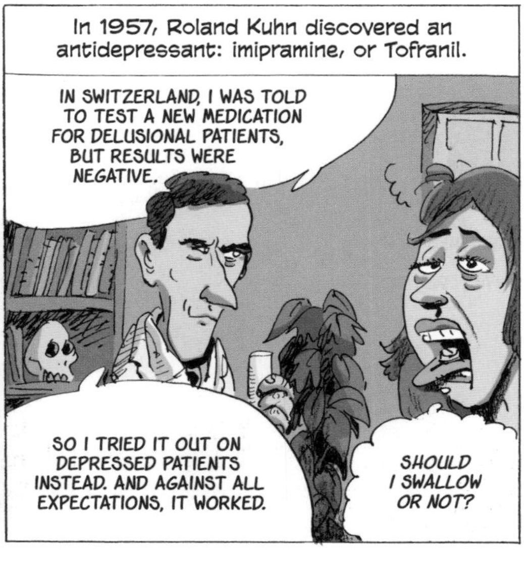
In 1957, Roland Kuhn discovered an antidepressant: imipramine, or Tofranil.
IN SWITZERLAND, I WAS TOLD TO TEST A NEW MEDICATION FOR DELUSIONAL PATIENTS, BUT RESULTS WERE NEGATIVE.
SO I TRIED IT OUT ON DEPRESSED PATIENTS INSTEAD. AND AGAINST ALL EXPECTATIONS, IT WORKED.
SHOULD I SWALLOW OR NOT?

* See page 134.

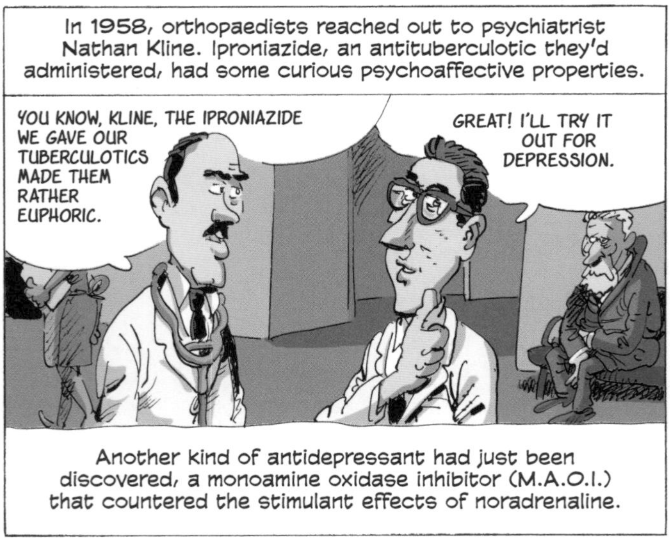
In 1958, orthopaedists reached out to psychiatrist Nathan Kline. Iproniazide, an antituberculotic they'd administered, had some curious psychoaffective properties.
YOU KNOW, KLINE, THE IPRONIAZIDE WE GAVE OUR TUBERCULOTICS MADE THEM RATHER EUPHORIC.
GREAT! I'LL TRY IT OUT FOR DEPRESSION.
Another kind of antidepressant had just been discovered, a monoamine oxidase inhibitor (M.A.O.I.) that countered the stimulant effects of noradrenaline.

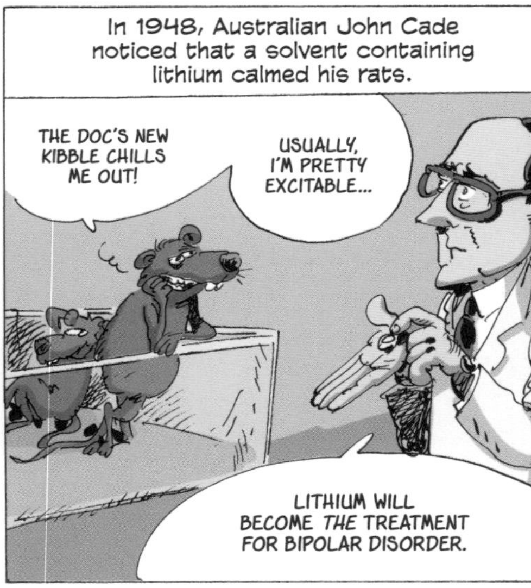
In 1948, Australian John Cade noticed that a solvent containing lithium calmed his rats.
THE DOC'S NEW KIBBLE CHILLS ME OUT!
USUALLY, I'M PRETTY EXCITABLE...
LITHIUM WILL BECOME *THE* TREATMENT FOR BIPOLAR DISORDER.

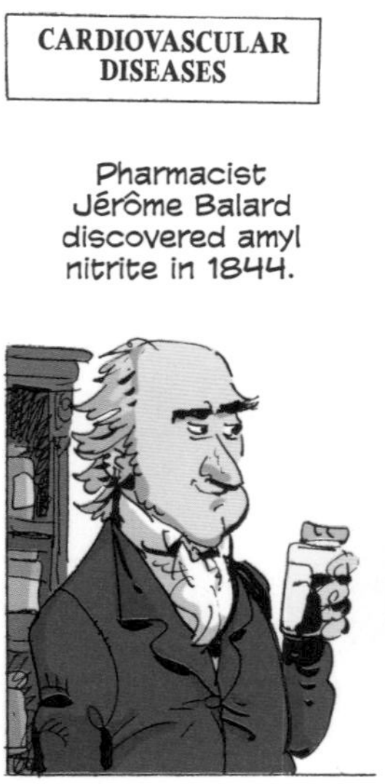
CARDIOVASCULAR DISEASES
Pharmacist Jérôme Balard discovered amyl nitrite in 1844.

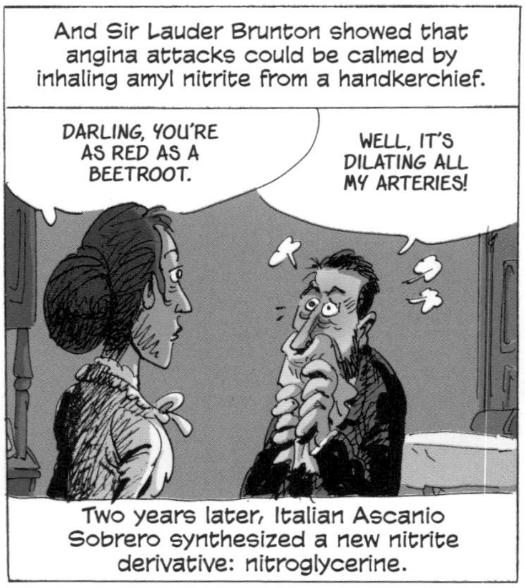
And Sir Lauder Brunton showed that angina attacks could be calmed by inhaling amyl nitrite from a handkerchief.
DARLING, YOU'RE AS RED AS A BEETROOT.
WELL, IT'S DILATING ALL MY ARTERIES!
Two years later, Italian Ascanio Sobrero synthesized a new nitrite derivative: nitroglycerine.

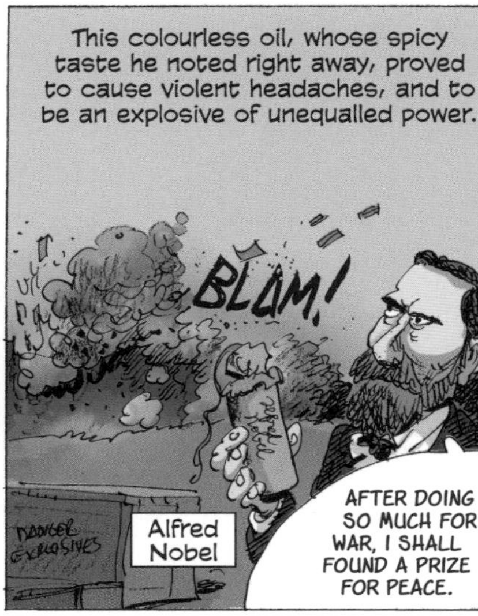
This colourless oil, whose spicy taste he noted right away, proved to cause violent headaches, and to be an explosive of unequalled power.
BLAM!
Alfred Nobel
AFTER DOING SO MUCH FOR WAR, I SHALL FOUND A PRIZE FOR PEACE.

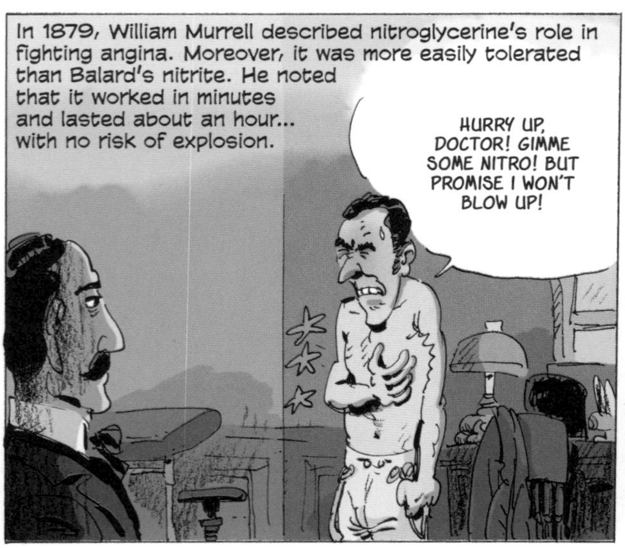
In 1879, William Murrell described nitroglycerine's role in fighting angina. Moreover, it was more easily tolerated than Balard's nitrite. He noted that it worked in minutes and lasted about an hour... with no risk of explosion.
HURRY UP, DOCTOR! GIMME SOME NITRO! BUT PROMISE I WON'T BLOW UP!

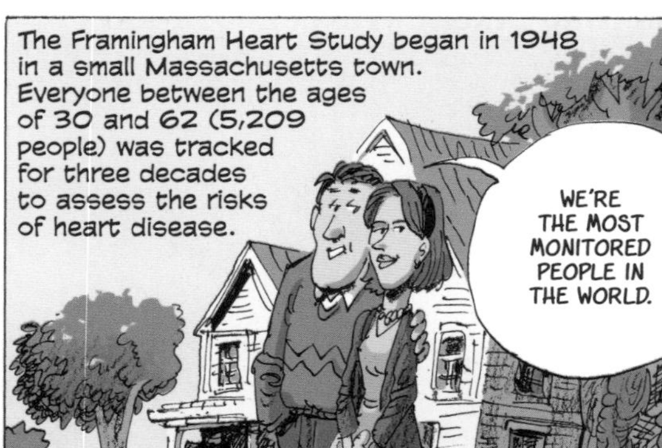
The Framingham Heart Study began in 1948 in a small Massachusetts town. Everyone between the ages of 30 and 62 (5,209 people) was tracked for three decades to assess the risks of heart disease.
WE'RE THE MOST MONITORED PEOPLE IN THE WORLD.

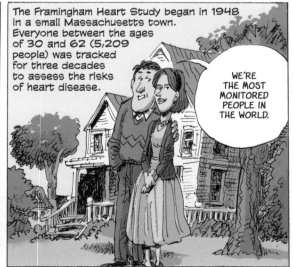

A certain number of risk factors showed statistically — isolated and, above all, associated.

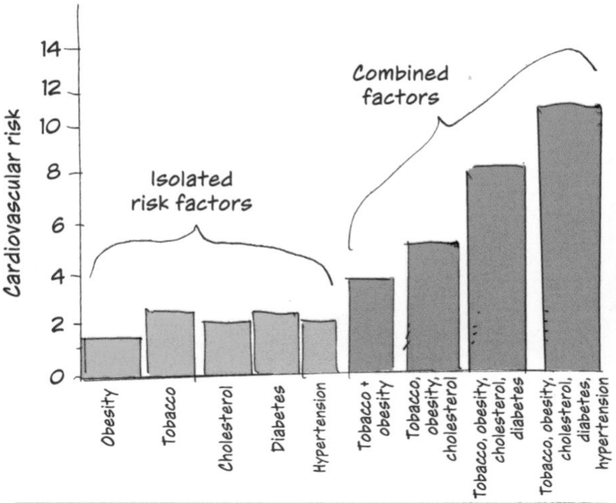
Cardiovascular risk
0
2
4
6
8
10
12
14
Isolated risk factors
Combined factors
Obesity
Tobacco
Cholesterol
Diabetes
Hypertension
Tobacco + obesity
Tobacco, obesity, cholesterol
Tobacco, obesity, cholesterol, diabetes
Tobacco, obesity, cholesterol, diabetes, hypertension

In the 1980s, Mediterranean diets were promoted as reducing the risk of heart disease.

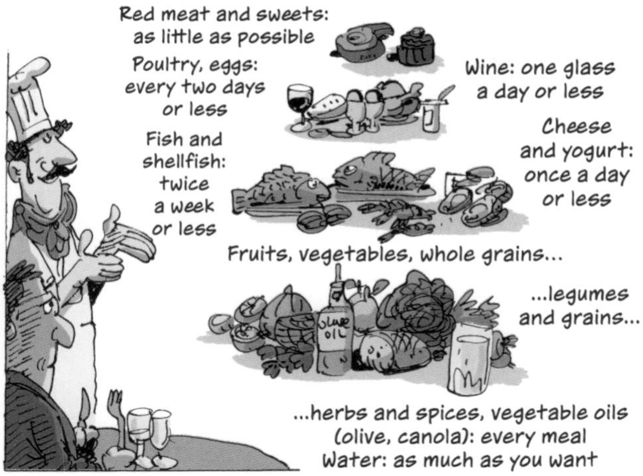
Red meat and sweets: as little as possible
Poultry, eggs: every two days or less
Wine: one glass a day or less
Fish and shellfish: twice a week or less
Cheese and yogurt: once a day or less
Fruits, vegetables, whole grains...
...legumes and grains...
...herbs and spices, vegetable oils (olive, canola): every meal
Water: as much as you want

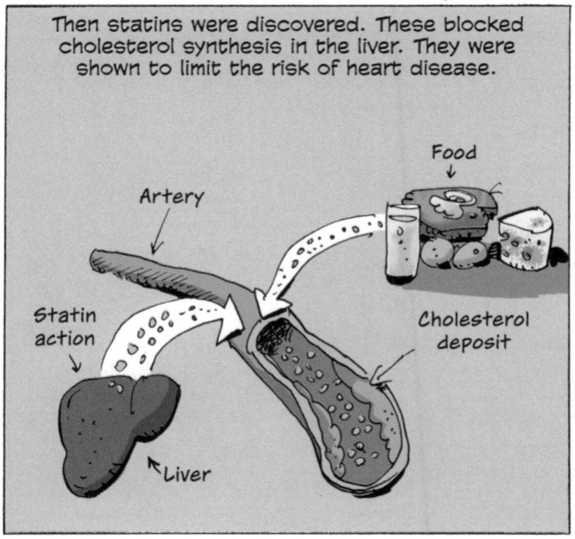
Then statins were discovered. These blocked cholesterol synthesis in the liver. They were shown to limit the risk of heart disease.
Food
Artery
Statin action
Cholesterol deposit
Liver

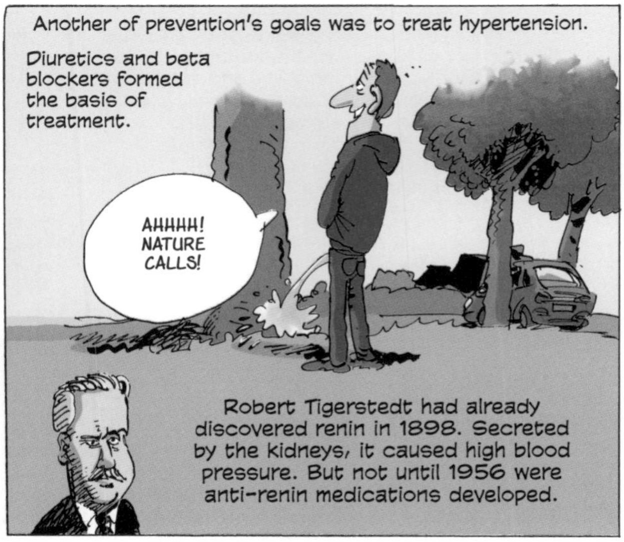
Another of prevention's goals was to treat hypertension.
Diuretics and beta blockers formed the basis of treatment.
AHHHH! NATURE CALLS!
Robert Tigerstedt had already discovered renin in 1898. Secreted by the kidneys, it caused high blood pressure. But not until 1956 were anti-renin medications developed.

FIGHTING CANCER WITH CHEMOTHERAPY

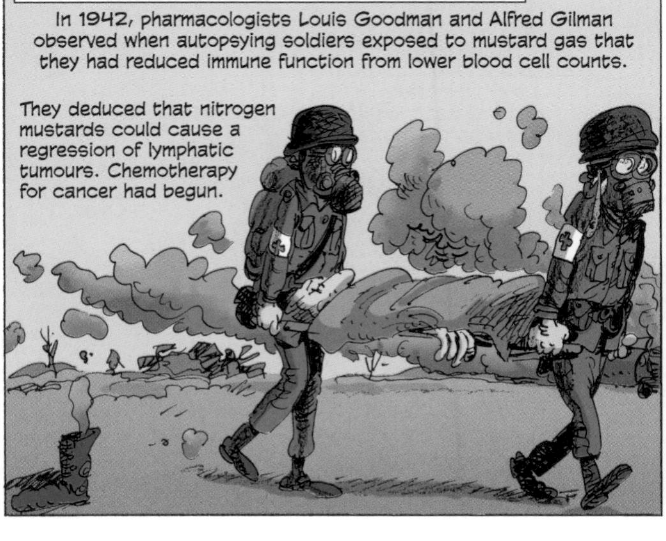
In 1942, pharmacologists Louis Goodman and Alfred Gilman observed when autopsying soldiers exposed to mustard gas that they had reduced immune function from lower blood cell counts.
They deduced that nitrogen mustards could cause a regression of lymphatic tumours. Chemotherapy for cancer had begun.

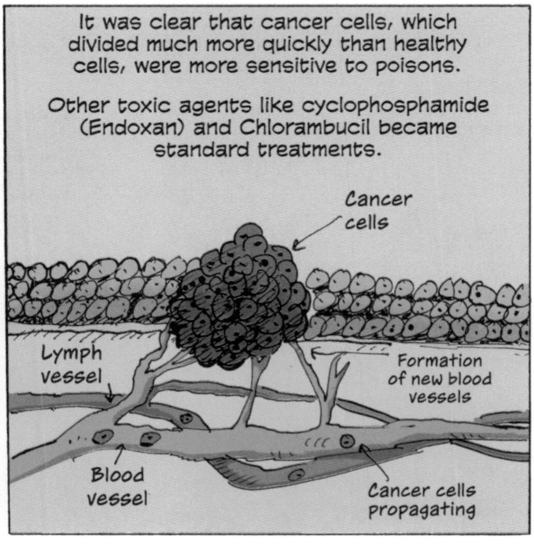
It was clear that cancer cells, which divided much more quickly than healthy cells, were more sensitive to poisons.
Other toxic agents like cyclophosphamide (Endoxan) and Chlorambucil became standard treatments.
Cancer cells
Lymph vessel
Formation of new blood vessels
Blood vessel
Cancer cells propagating

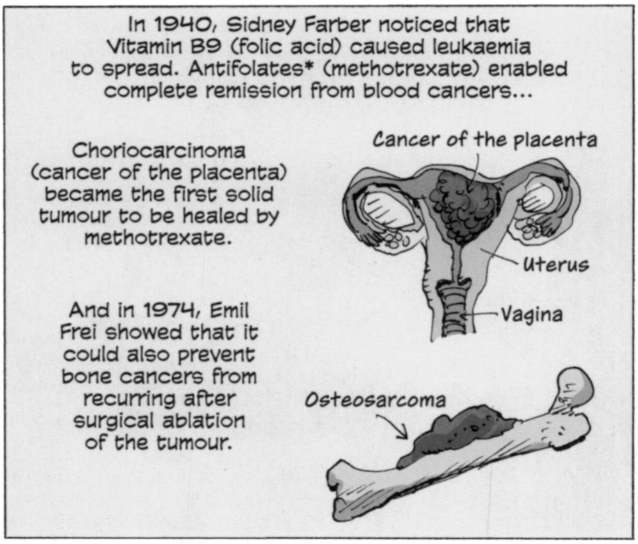
In 1940, Sidney Farber noticed that Vitamin B9 (folic acid) caused leukaemia to spread. Antifolates* (methotrexate) enabled complete remission from blood cancers...
Choriocarcinoma (cancer of the placenta) became the first solid tumour to be healed by methotrexate.
Cancer of the placenta
Uterus
Vagina
And in 1974, Emil Frei showed that it could also prevent bone cancers from recurring after surgical ablation of the tumour.
Osteosarcoma

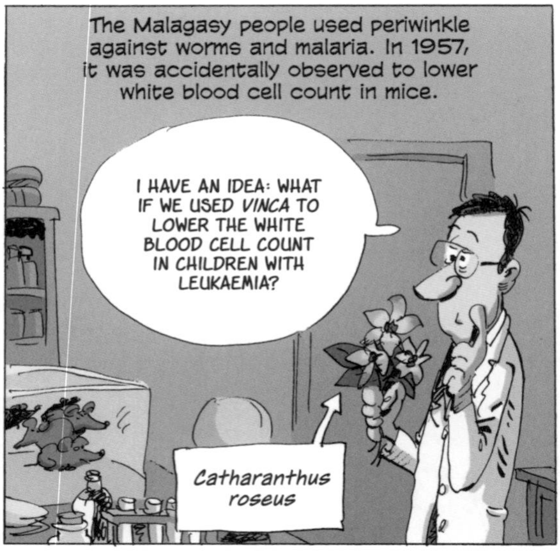
The Malagasy people used periwinkle against worms and malaria. In 1957, it was accidentally observed to lower white blood cell count in mice.
I HAVE AN IDEA: WHAT IF WE USED *VINCA* TO LOWER THE WHITE BLOOD CELL COUNT IN CHILDREN WITH LEUKAEMIA?
Catharanthus roseus

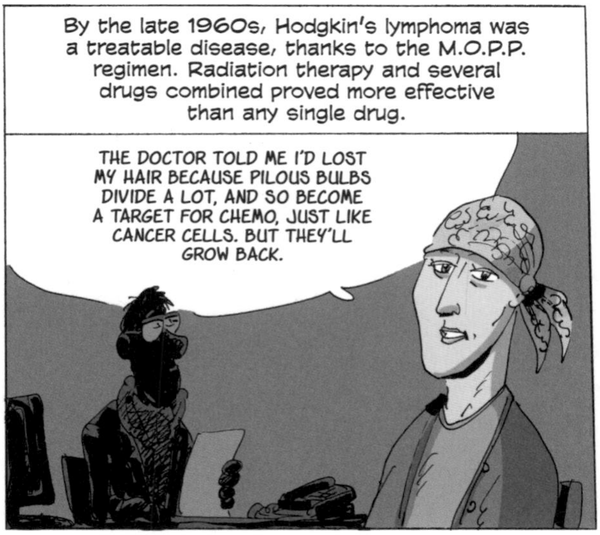
By the late 1960s, Hodgkin's lymphoma was a treatable disease, thanks to the M.O.P.P. regimen. Radiation therapy and several drugs combined proved more effective than any single drug.
THE DOCTOR TOLD ME I'D LOST MY HAIR BECAUSE PILOUS BULBS DIVIDE A LOT, AND SO BECOME A TARGET FOR CHEMO, JUST LIKE CANCER CELLS. BUT THEY'LL GROW BACK.

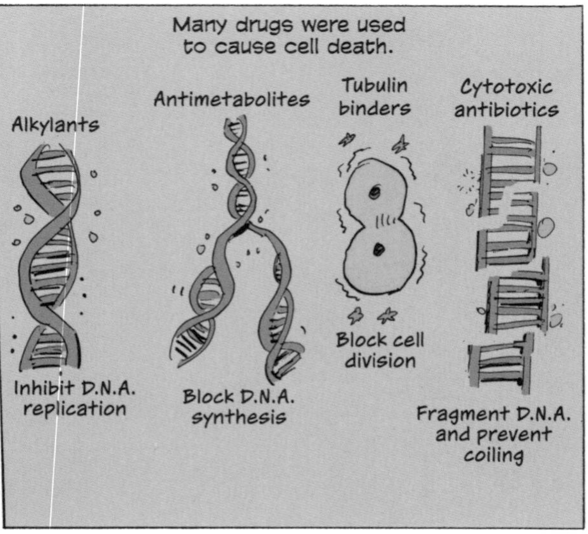
Many drugs were used to cause cell death.
Alkylants
Inhibit D.N.A. replication
Antimetabolites
Block D.N.A. synthesis
Tubulin binders
Block cell division
Cytotoxic antibiotics
Fragment D.N.A. and prevent coiling

In the early 1990s, the explosion in potential biological targets transformed cancer research, thanks to combinatorial chemical synthesis at major pharma companies.

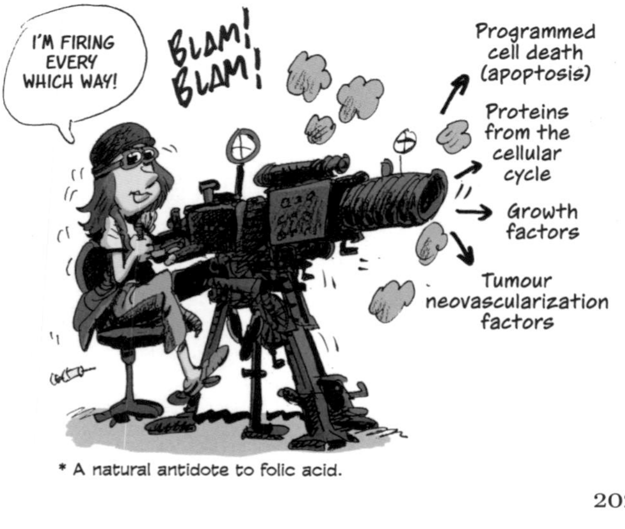
I'M FIRING EVERY WHICH WAY!
BLAM! BLAM!
Programmed cell death (apoptosis)
Proteins from the cellular cycle
Growth factors
Tumour neovascularization factors

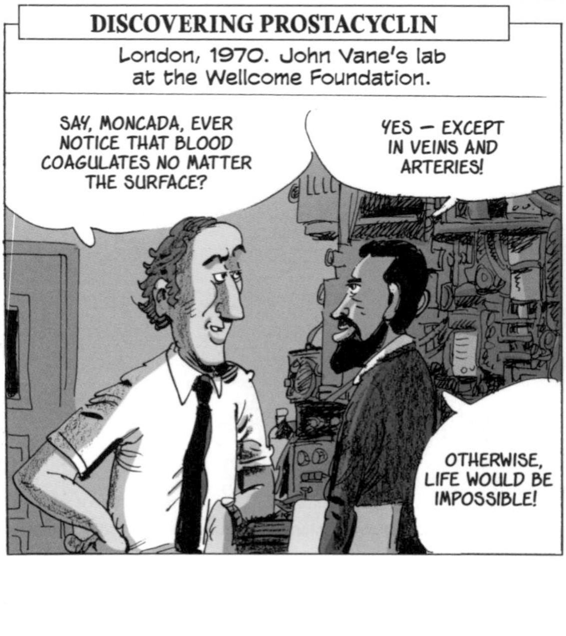
DISCOVERING PROSTACYCLIN
London, 1970. John Vane's lab at the Wellcome Foundation.
SAY, MONCADA, EVER NOTICE THAT BLOOD COAGULATES NO MATTER THE SURFACE?
YES — EXCEPT IN VEINS AND ARTERIES!
OTHERWISE, LIFE WOULD BE IMPOSSIBLE!

* A natural antidote to folic acid.

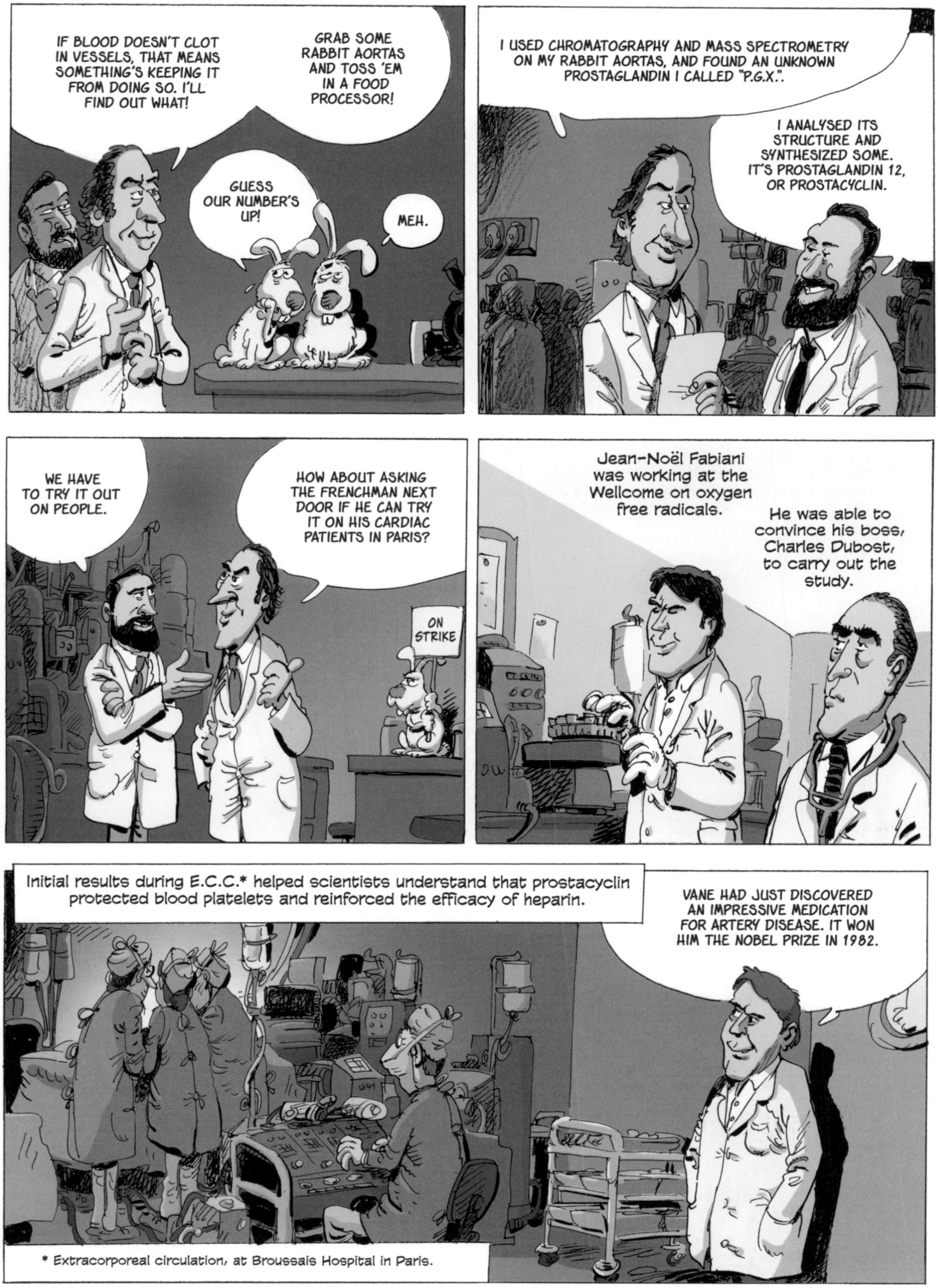
IF BLOOD DOESN'T CLOT IN VESSELS, THAT MEANS SOMETHING'S KEEPING IT FROM DOING SO. I'LL FIND OUT WHAT!
GRAB SOME RABBIT AORTAS AND TOSS 'EM IN A FOOD PROCESSOR!
GUESS OUR NUMBER'S UP!
MEH.
I USED CHROMATOGRAPHY AND MASS SPECTROMETRY ON MY RABBIT AORTAS, AND FOUND AN UNKNOWN PROSTAGLANDIN I CALLED "P.G.X.".
I ANALYSED ITS STRUCTURE AND SYNTHESIZED SOME. IT'S PROSTAGLANDIN 12, OR PROSTACYCLIN.
WE HAVE TO TRY IT OUT ON PEOPLE.
HOW ABOUT ASKING THE FRENCHMAN NEXT DOOR IF HE CAN TRY IT ON HIS CARDIAC PATIENTS IN PARIS?
ON STRIKE
Jean-Noël Fabiani was working at the Wellcome on oxygen free radicals.
He was able to convince his boss, Charles Dubost, to carry out the study.
Initial results during E.C.C.* helped scientists understand that prostacyclin protected blood platelets and reinforced the efficacy of heparin.
VANE HAD JUST DISCOVERED AN IMPRESSIVE MEDICATION FOR ARTERY DISEASE. IT WON HIM THE NOBEL PRIZE IN 1982.
* Extracorporeal circulation, at Broussais Hospital in Paris.

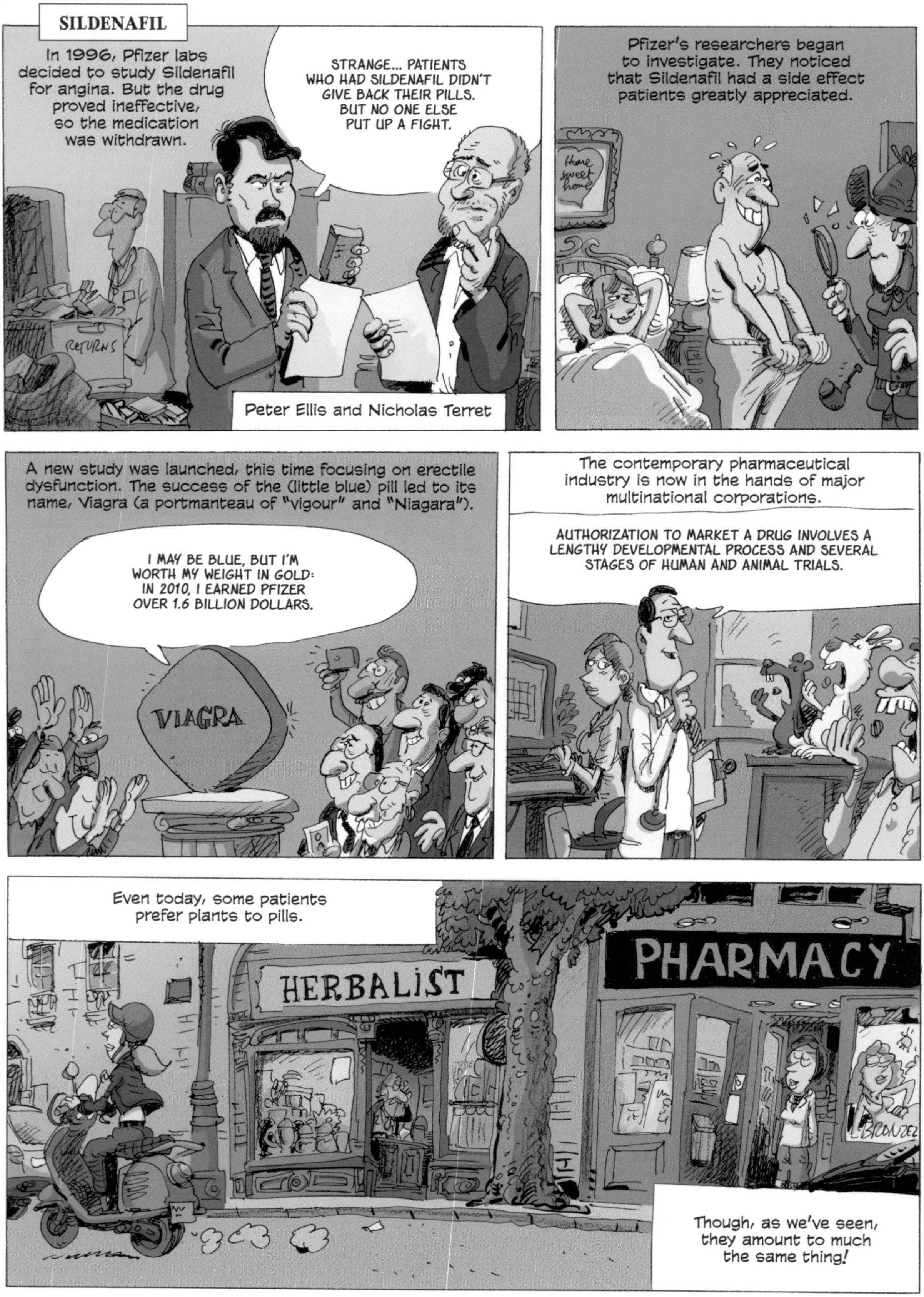
SILDENAFIL
In 1996, Pfizer labs decided to study Sildenafil for angina. But the drug proved ineffective, so the medication was withdrawn.
STRANGE... PATIENTS WHO HAD SILDENAFIL DIDN'T GIVE BACK THEIR PILLS. BUT NO ONE ELSE PUT UP A FIGHT.
RETURNS
Peter Ellis and Nicholas Terret
Pfizer's researchers began to investigate. They noticed that Sildenafil had a side effect patients greatly appreciated.
Home sweet home
A new study was launched, this time focusing on erectile dysfunction. The success of the (little blue) pill led to its name, Viagra (a portmanteau of "vigour" and "Niagara").
I MAY BE BLUE, BUT I'M WORTH MY WEIGHT IN GOLD: IN 2010, I EARNED PFIZER OVER 1.6 BILLION DOLLARS.
VIAGRA
The contemporary pharmaceutical industry is now in the hands of major multinational corporations.
AUTHORIZATION TO MARKET A DRUG INVOLVES A LENGTHY DEVELOPMENTAL PROCESS AND SEVERAL STAGES OF HUMAN AND ANIMAL TRIALS.
Even today, some patients prefer plants to pills.
HERBALIST
PHARMACY
Though, as we've seen, they amount to much the same thing!

CHAPTER 18

FORENSIC MEDICINE

Throughout history, physicians have found themselves involved in judicial matters, if only to perform autopsies.

But this involvement in criminal affairs was largely circumscribed by a conception of the brain's role. In the early 19th century, Franz Josef Gall espoused a theory according to which the brain was divided into zones that expressed tendencies and urges. Some people quickly adopted this hereditary conception of virtue and vice. Woe betide those whose skulls betrayed the bump of a murderer!

Alexandre Lacassagne's Lyons-based school of criminology, and his student Edmond Locard, led the way in devising the bases of scientific police work.

Surprisingly, Arthur Conan Doyle's fictional character Sherlock Holmes has long exerted a strange hold on a world that cares only about evidence and reality.

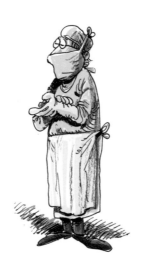

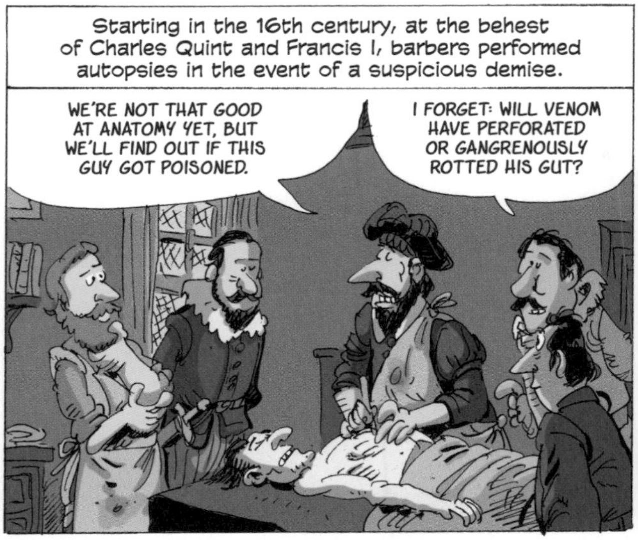
Starting in the 16th century, at the behest of Charles Quint and Francis I, barbers performed autopsies in the event of a suspicious demise.
WE'RE NOT THAT GOOD AT ANATOMY YET, BUT WE'LL FIND OUT IF THIS GUY GOT POISONED.
I FORGET: WILL VENOM HAVE PERFORATED OR GANGRENOUSLY ROTTED HIS GUT?

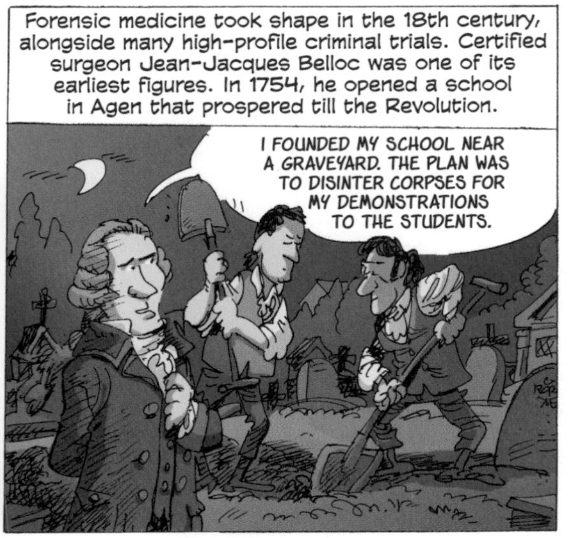
Forensic medicine took shape in the 18th century, alongside many high-profile criminal trials. Certified surgeon Jean-Jacques Belloc was one of its earliest figures. In 1754, he opened a school in Agen that prospered till the Revolution.
I FOUNDED MY SCHOOL NEAR A GRAVEYARD. THE PLAN WAS TO DISINTER CORPSES FOR MY DEMONSTRATIONS TO THE STUDENTS.

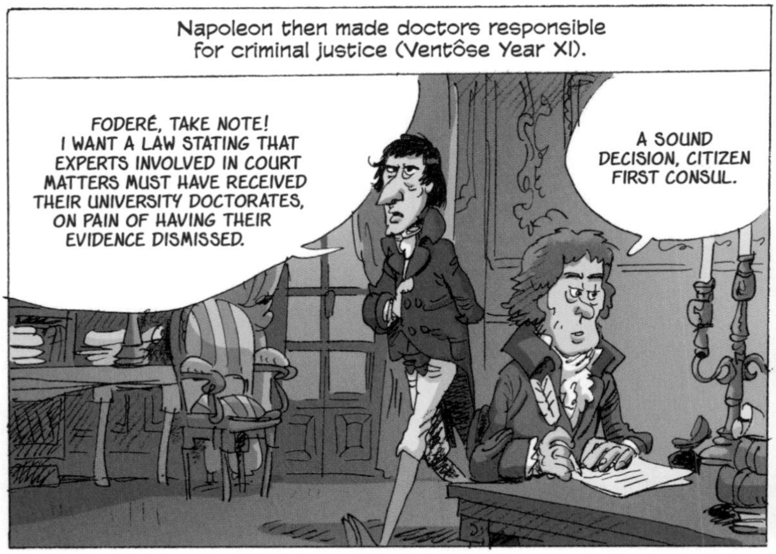
Napoleon then made doctors responsible for criminal justice (Ventôse Year XI).
FODERÉ, TAKE NOTE! I WANT A LAW STATING THAT EXPERTS INVOLVED IN COURT MATTERS MUST HAVE RECEIVED THEIR UNIVERSITY DOCTORATES, ON PAIN OF HAVING THEIR EVIDENCE DISMISSED.
A SOUND DECISION, CITIZEN FIRST CONSUL.

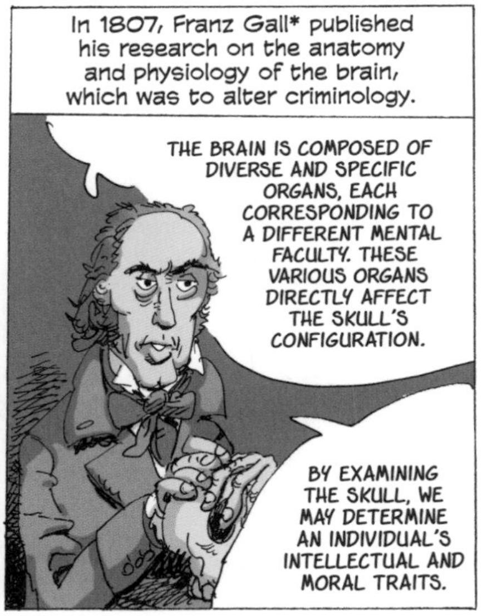
In 1807, Franz Gall* published his research on the anatomy and physiology of the brain, which was to alter criminology.
THE BRAIN IS COMPOSED OF DIVERSE AND SPECIFIC ORGANS, EACH CORRESPONDING TO A DIFFERENT MENTAL FACULTY. THESE VARIOUS ORGANS DIRECTLY AFFECT THE SKULL'S CONFIGURATION.
BY EXAMINING THE SKULL, WE MAY DETERMINE AN INDIVIDUAL'S INTELLECTUAL AND MORAL TRAITS.

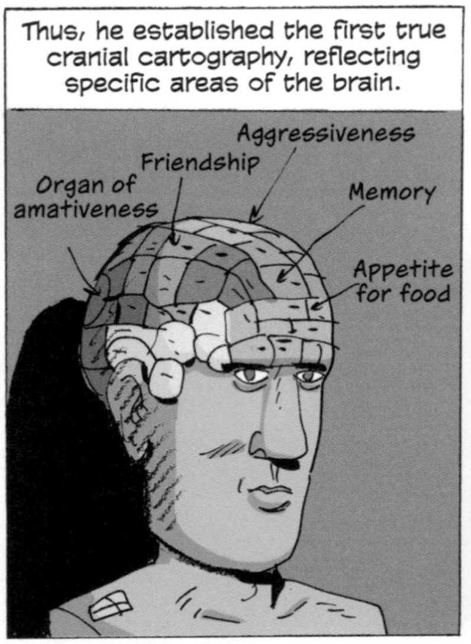
Thus, he established the first true cranial cartography, reflecting specific areas of the brain.
Aggressiveness
Friendship
Organ of amativeness
Memory
Appetite for food

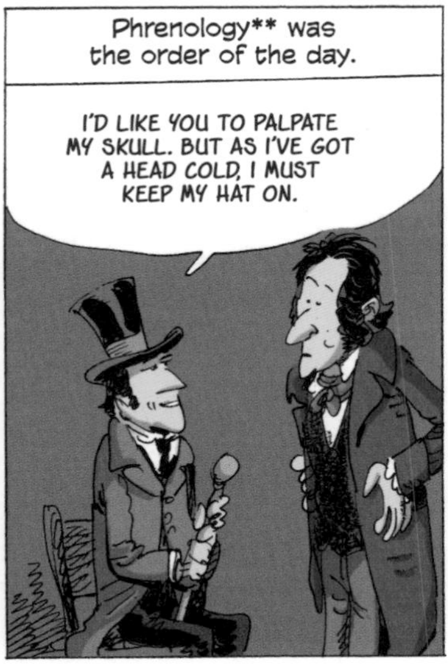
Phrenology** was the order of the day.
I'D LIKE YOU TO PALPATE MY SKULL. BUT AS I'VE GOT A HEAD COLD, I MUST KEEP MY HAT ON.

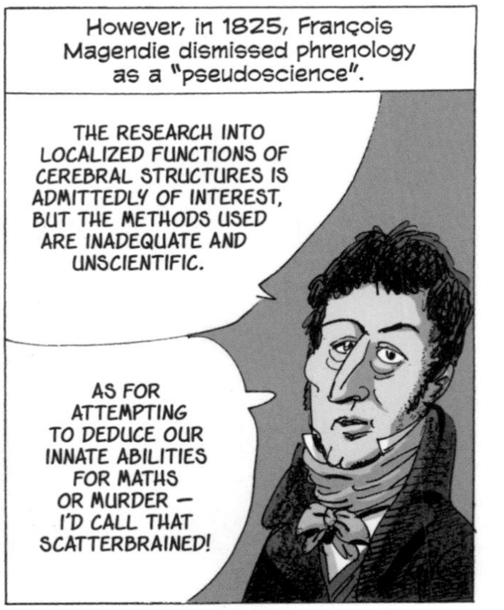
However, in 1825, François Magendie dismissed phrenology as a "pseudoscience".
THE RESEARCH INTO LOCALIZED FUNCTIONS OF CEREBRAL STRUCTURES IS ADMITTEDLY OF INTEREST, BUT THE METHODS USED ARE INADEQUATE AND UNSCIENTIFIC.
AS FOR ATTEMPTING TO DEDUCE OUR INNATE ABILITIES FOR MATHS OR MURDER — I'D CALL THAT SCATTERBRAINED!

* See pages 131 and 139.
** The study of the shape and size of the cranium as a supposed indication of character.

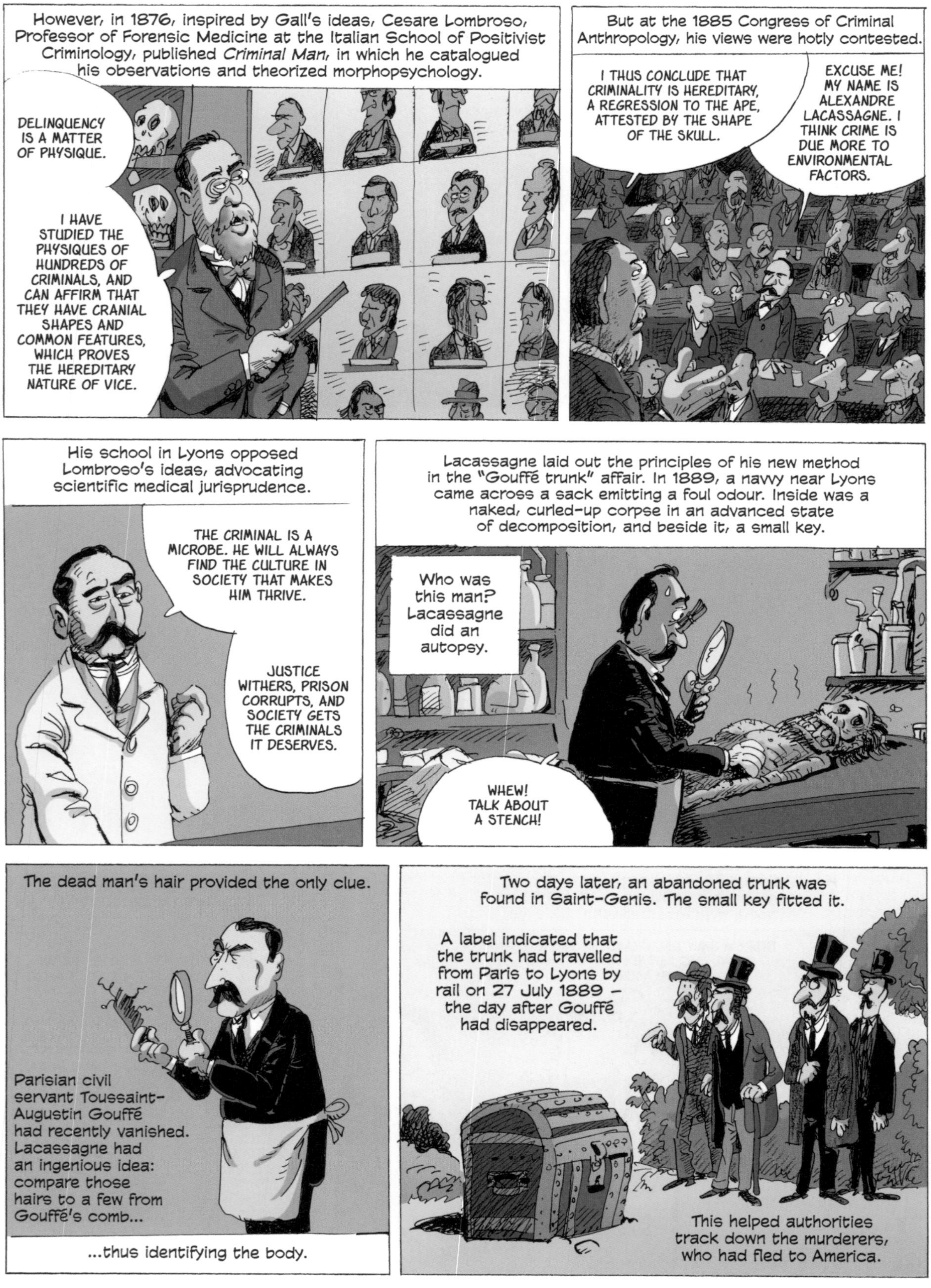
However, in 1876, inspired by Gall's ideas, Cesare Lombroso, Professor of Forensic Medicine at the Italian School of Positivist Criminology, published *Criminal Man*, in which he catalogued his observations and theorized morphopsychology.
DELINQUENCY IS A MATTER OF PHYSIQUE.
I HAVE STUDIED THE PHYSIQUES OF HUNDREDS OF CRIMINALS, AND CAN AFFIRM THAT THEY HAVE CRANIAL SHAPES AND COMMON FEATURES, WHICH PROVES THE HEREDITARY NATURE OF VICE.
But at the 1885 Congress of Criminal Anthropology, his views were hotly contested.
I THUS CONCLUDE THAT CRIMINALITY IS HEREDITARY, A REGRESSION TO THE APE, ATTESTED BY THE SHAPE OF THE SKULL.
EXCUSE ME! MY NAME IS ALEXANDRE LACASSAGNE. I THINK CRIME IS DUE MORE TO ENVIRONMENTAL FACTORS.
His school in Lyons opposed Lombroso's ideas, advocating scientific medical jurisprudence.
THE CRIMINAL IS A MICROBE. HE WILL ALWAYS FIND THE CULTURE IN SOCIETY THAT MAKES HIM THRIVE.
JUSTICE WITHERS, PRISON CORRUPTS, AND SOCIETY GETS THE CRIMINALS IT DESERVES.
Lacassagne laid out the principles of his new method in the "Gouffé trunk" affair. In 1889, a navvy near Lyons came across a sack emitting a foul odour. Inside was a naked, curled-up corpse in an advanced state of decomposition, and beside it, a small key.
Who was this man? Lacassagne did an autopsy.
WHEW! TALK ABOUT A STENCH!
The dead man's hair provided the only clue.
Parisian civil servant Toussaint-Augustin Gouffé had recently vanished. Lacassagne had an ingenious idea: compare those hairs to a few from Gouffé's comb...
...thus identifying the body.
Two days later, an abandoned trunk was found in Saint-Genis. The small key fitted it.
A label indicated that the trunk had travelled from Paris to Lyons by rail on 27 July 1889 – the day after Gouffé had disappeared.
This helped authorities track down the murderers, who had fled to America.

THE DISCOVERY OF TOXICOLOGY

In 1818, Mathieu Orfila, Professor of Forensic Medicine and Dean of the Faculty of Paris, published a major treatise on toxicology.

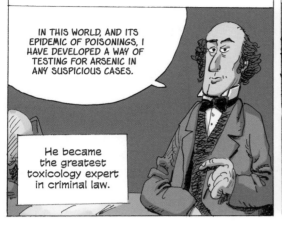

IN THIS WORLD, AND ITS EPIDEMIC OF POISONINGS, I HAVE DEVELOPED A WAY OF TESTING FOR ARSENIC IN ANY SUSPICIOUS CASES.

He became the greatest toxicology expert in criminal law.

He was called upon in the Lafarge case (1840). Marie Lafarge was accused of poisoning her husband with arsenic. But local experts had found no such traces in the body.

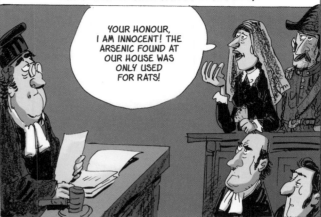

YOUR HONOUR, I AM INNOCENT! THE ARSENIC FOUND AT OUR HOUSE WAS ONLY USED FOR RATS!

Orfila used a test developed by chemist James Marsh, which he had modified.

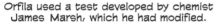

LAFARGE'S BODY INDISPUTABLY CONTAINS TRACES OF ARSENIC.

BUT THE PREVIOUS TESTS CAME UP NEGATIVE!

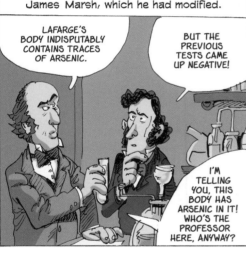

I'M TELLING YOU, THIS BODY HAS ARSENIC IN IT! WHO'S THE PROFESSOR HERE, ANYWAY?

Chemist François Raspail was called in too late as a defence witness.

ORFILA'S METHOD WOULD FIND ARSENIC ANYWHERE! IT'S NOT RELIABLE. ITS REAGENTS ARE VERY POOR.

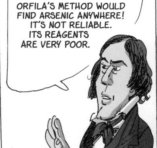

Marie Lafarge was sentenced to life imprisonment, no doubt erroneously. However, Orfila's attitude later discredited him.

To identify habitual criminals, Alphonse Bertillon proposed anthropometry in 1882.

STRICTLY FACE AND PROFILE. NOT VERY FLATTERING, BUT HIGHLY EFFECTIVE.

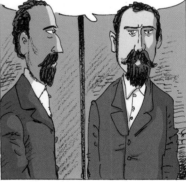

He developed "Bertillonage", a 14-point identification system, measuring waist, feet, hands, ears, arms, nose, distance between the eyes, etc.

THERE'S ONLY ONE CHANCE IN 286 MILLION THAT TWO INDIVIDUALS HAVE THE SAME MEASUREMENTS.

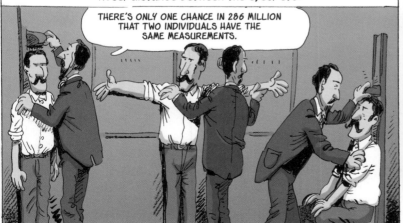

Meanwhile, Henry Faulds had discovered fingerprinting.

I PASSED MY OBSERVATIONS ON TO FRANCIS GALTON, WHO ESTIMATED THE CHANCE OF TWO PEOPLE SHARING FINGERPRINTS AS 1 IN 64 BILLION.

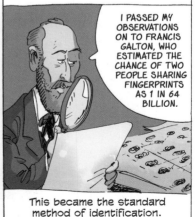

This became the standard method of identification.

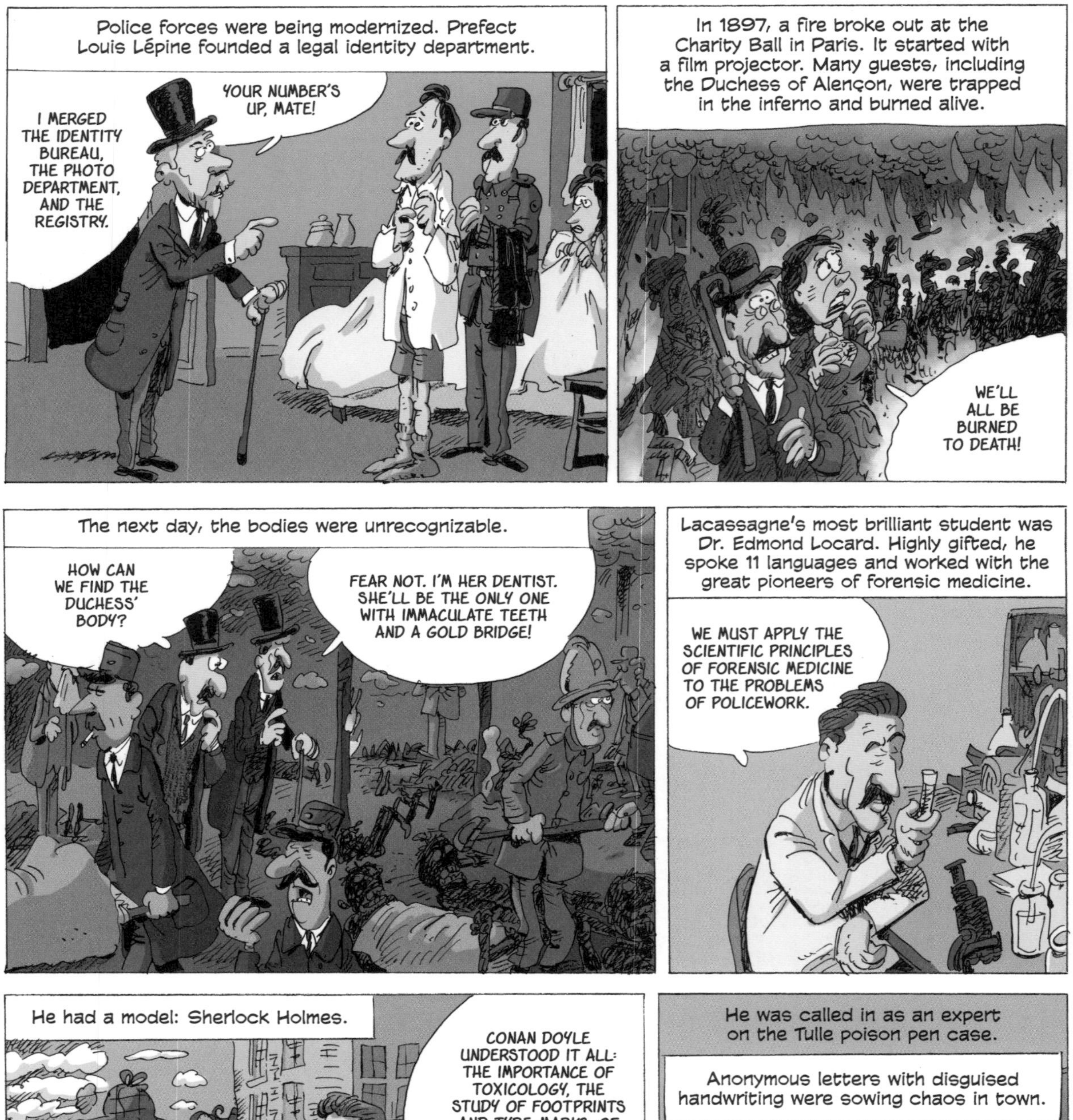
Police forces were being modernized. Prefect Louis Lépine founded a legal identity department.
I MERGED THE IDENTITY BUREAU, THE PHOTO DEPARTMENT, AND THE REGISTRY.
YOUR NUMBER'S UP, MATE!
In 1897, a fire broke out at the Charity Ball in Paris. It started with a film projector. Many guests, including the Duchess of Alençon, were trapped in the inferno and burned alive.
WE'LL ALL BE BURNED TO DEATH!
The next day, the bodies were unrecognizable.
HOW CAN WE FIND THE DUCHESS' BODY?
FEAR NOT. I'M HER DENTIST. SHE'LL BE THE ONLY ONE WITH IMMACULATE TEETH AND A GOLD BRIDGE!
Lacassagne's most brilliant student was Dr. Edmond Locard. Highly gifted, he spoke 11 languages and worked with the great pioneers of forensic medicine.
WE MUST APPLY THE SCIENTIFIC PRINCIPLES OF FORENSIC MEDICINE TO THE PROBLEMS OF POLICEWORK.
He had a model: Sherlock Holmes.
WINES
CONAN DOYLE UNDERSTOOD IT ALL: THE IMPORTANCE OF TOXICOLOGY, THE STUDY OF FOOTPRINTS AND TYRE-MARKS, OF DUST, BALLISTICS, AND HANDWRITING...
AND ABOVE ALL, FINGERPRINTS!
He was called in as an expert on the Tulle poison pen case.
Anonymous letters with disguised handwriting were sowing chaos in town.

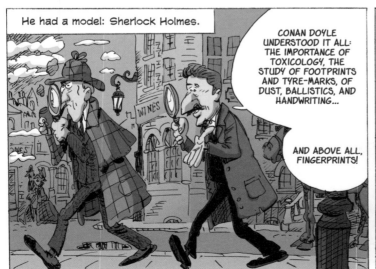

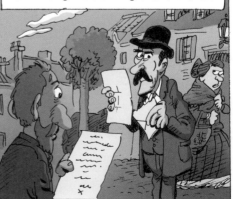

Locard organized a collective dictation session and caught out the perpetrator by forcing her to revert to her normal handwriting.

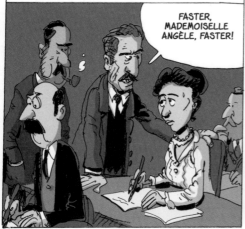

FASTER, MADEMOISELLE ANGÈLE, FASTER!

He took part in all the great cases of the time.

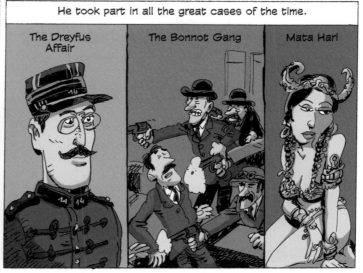

The Dreyfus Affair

The Bonnot Gang

Mata Hari

The discovery of D.N.A. naturally transformed police science. D.N.A. is an extremely stable and specific molecule. The Southern blot method allows for the identification of both bodies and sexual aggressors.

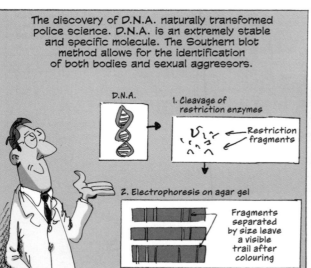

D.N.A.

1. Cleavage of restriction enzymes

Restriction fragments

2. Electrophoresis on agar gel

Fragments separated by size leave a visible trail after colouring

When the D.N.A. sample size is insufficient or altered, polymerase chain reaction (P.C.R.), or gene amplification, is used.

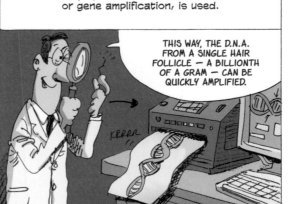

THIS WAY, THE D.N.A. FROM A SINGLE HAIR FOLLICLE — A BILLIONTH OF A GRAM — CAN BE QUICKLY AMPLIFIED.

KRRRR

Finally, forensic medicine can also help out with history.

Thanks to D.N.A., carbon-14, and scanning, we can perform diagnoses or even reconstruct ancient corpses.

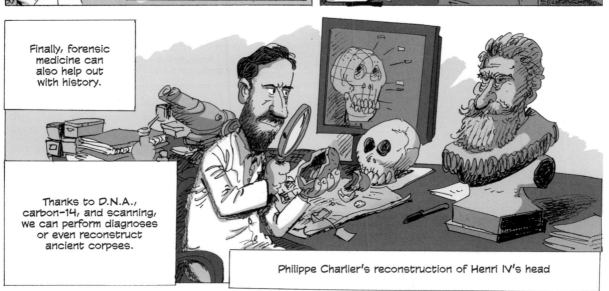

Philippe Charlier's reconstruction of Henri IV's head

CHAPTER 19

SOCIAL SECURITY AND HUMANITARIAN CARE

That diseases are often a great misfortune is something humankind knows all too well, having long suffered from them. That war and natural disaster can shatter lives has been common knowledge ever since humans learned how to use weapons.

But can we protect ourselves from such adversities in other ways, besides relying on our loved ones? To respond to this need and develop the notion of social welfare, societies had to grow up—for real. Principles of compassion, often religious in origin, had to transcend mere charity, and instead become an organized system of care. Corporations had to be made aware of the power they wielded, and their leaders had to understand that avoiding social conflict by looking after their workers was a better way of doing things. Nations had to adopt policies to protect mothers and children...

So it was that the major principles of social security and humanitarian aid arose at the same time. If one was the preserve of industry and the state, the other rushed into the breach opened by their lack, in order to spread a message of ideals and justice for all that transcended borders.

Long live Médecins sans Frontières!

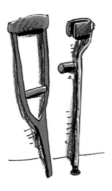

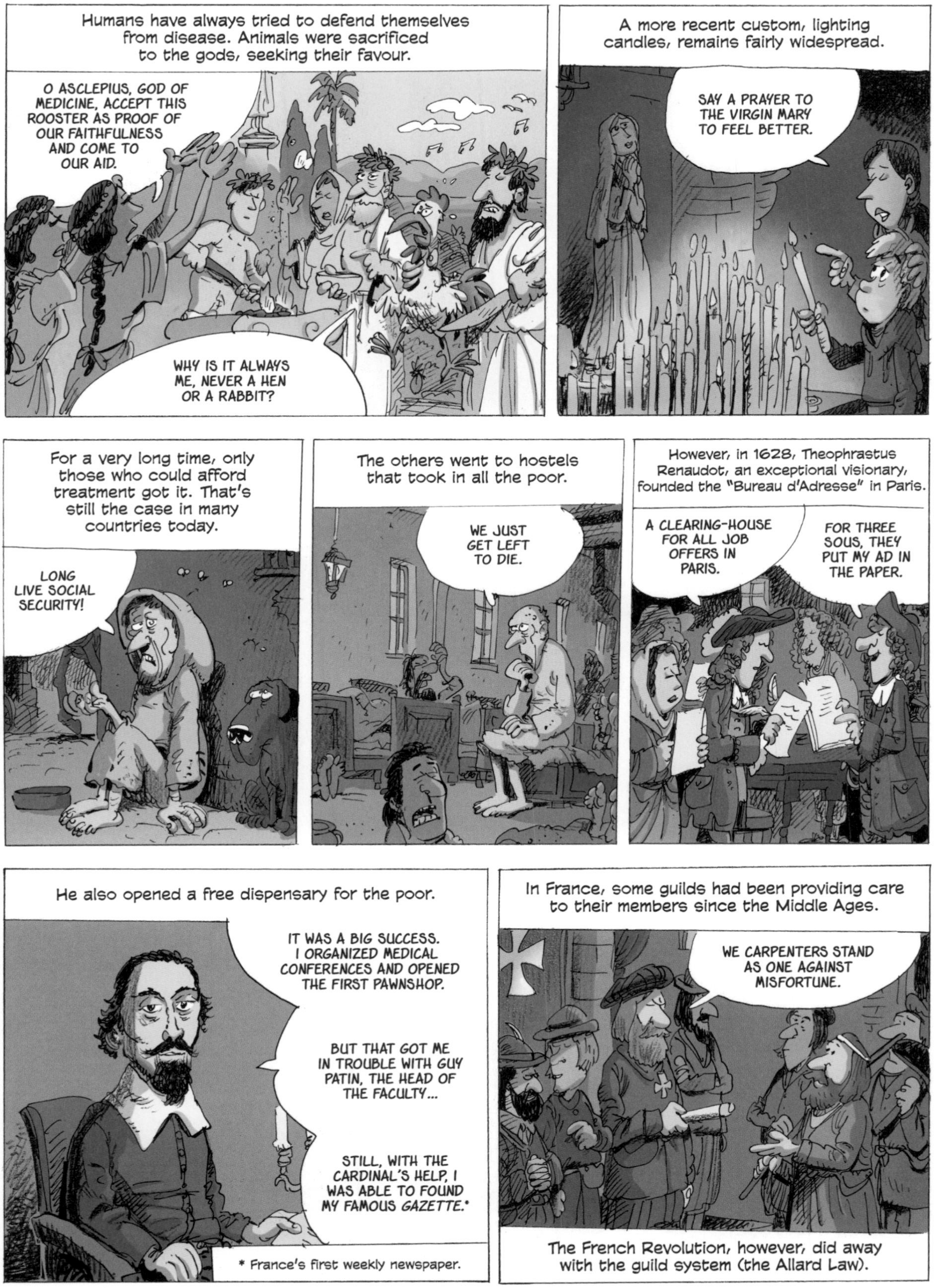
Humans have always tried to defend themselves from disease. Animals were sacrificed to the gods, seeking their favour.
O ASCLEPIUS, GOD OF MEDICINE, ACCEPT THIS ROOSTER AS PROOF OF OUR FAITHFULNESS AND COME TO OUR AID.
WHY IS IT ALWAYS ME, NEVER A HEN OR A RABBIT?
A more recent custom, lighting candles, remains fairly widespread.
SAY A PRAYER TO THE VIRGIN MARY TO FEEL BETTER.
For a very long time, only those who could afford treatment got it. That's still the case in many countries today.
LONG LIVE SOCIAL SECURITY!
The others went to hostels that took in all the poor.
WE JUST GET LEFT TO DIE.
However, in 1628, Theophrastus Renaudot, an exceptional visionary, founded the "Bureau d'Adresse" in Paris.
A CLEARING-HOUSE FOR ALL JOB OFFERS IN PARIS.
FOR THREE SOUS, THEY PUT MY AD IN THE PAPER.
He also opened a free dispensary for the poor.
IT WAS A BIG SUCCESS. I ORGANIZED MEDICAL CONFERENCES AND OPENED THE FIRST PAWNSHOP.
BUT THAT GOT ME IN TROUBLE WITH GUY PATIN, THE HEAD OF THE FACULTY...
STILL, WITH THE CARDINAL'S HELP, I WAS ABLE TO FOUND MY FAMOUS *GAZETTE*.*
* France's first weekly newspaper.
In France, some guilds had been providing care to their members since the Middle Ages.
WE CARPENTERS STAND AS ONE AGAINST MISFORTUNE.
The French Revolution, however, did away with the guild system (the Allard Law).

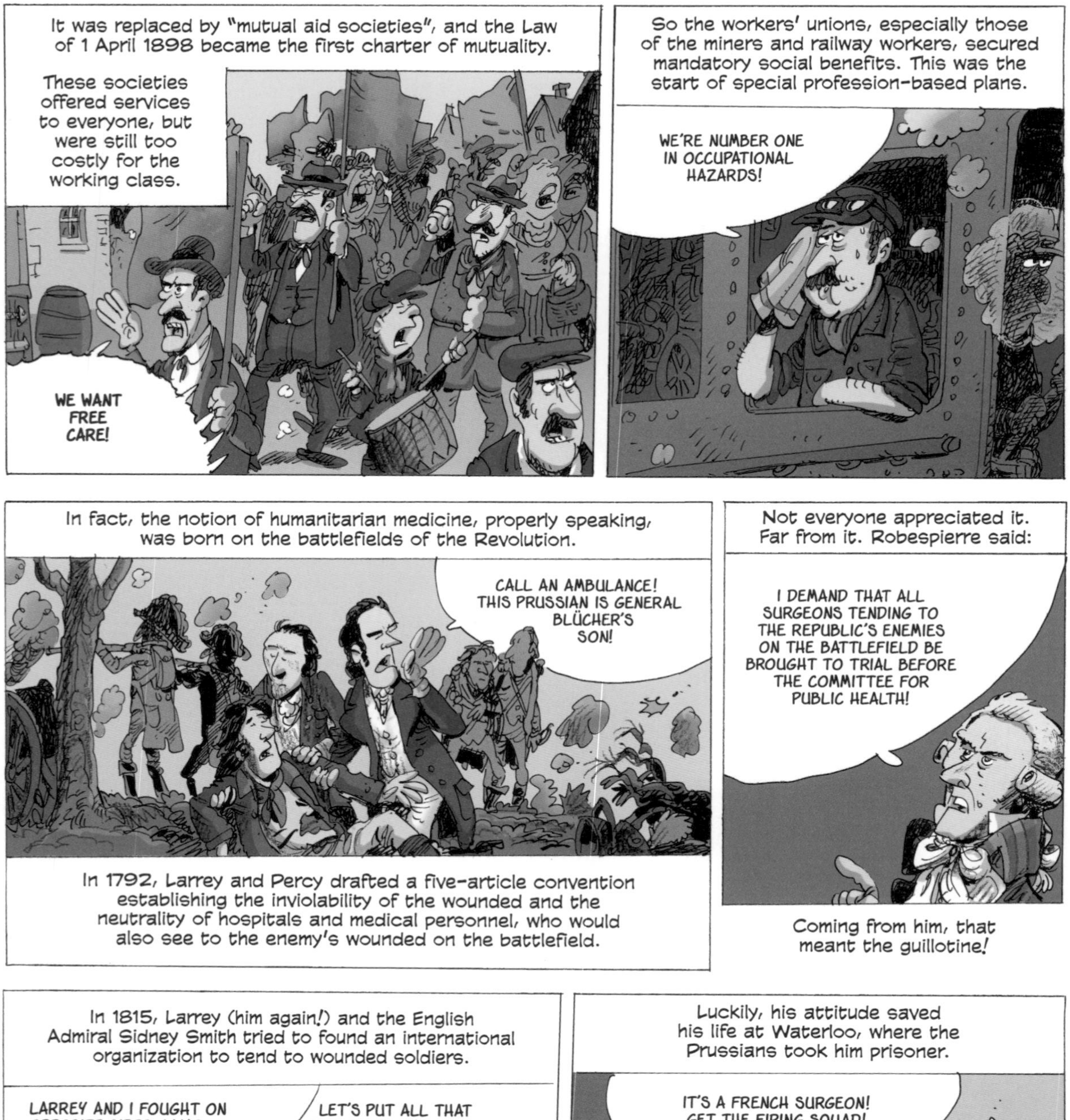
It was replaced by "mutual aid societies", and the Law of 1 April 1898 became the first charter of mutuality.
These societies offered services to everyone, but were still too costly for the working class.
WE WANT FREE CARE!
So the workers' unions, especially those of the miners and railway workers, secured mandatory social benefits. This was the start of special profession-based plans.
WE'RE NUMBER ONE IN OCCUPATIONAL HAZARDS!
In fact, the notion of humanitarian medicine, properly speaking, was born on the battlefields of the Revolution.
CALL AN AMBULANCE! THIS PRUSSIAN IS GENERAL BLÜCHER'S SON!
In 1792, Larrey and Percy drafted a five-article convention establishing the inviolability of the wounded and the neutrality of hospitals and medical personnel, who would also see to the enemy's wounded on the battlefield.
Not everyone appreciated it. Far from it. Robespierre said:
I DEMAND THAT ALL SURGEONS TENDING TO THE REPUBLIC'S ENEMIES ON THE BATTLEFIELD BE BROUGHT TO TRIAL BEFORE THE COMMITTEE FOR PUBLIC HEALTH!
Coming from him, that meant the guillotine!
In 1815, Larrey (him again!) and the English Admiral Sidney Smith tried to found an international organization to tend to wounded soldiers.
LARREY AND I FOUGHT ON OPPOSITE SIDES. I WAS AT SAINT-JEAN-D'ACRE AND ABUKIR.
LET'S PUT ALL THAT BEHIND US. IT'S TIME TO MAKE RULES FOR THOSE RENDERED "HORS DE COMBAT" BY THEIR WOUNDS.
Luckily, his attitude saved his life at Waterloo, where the Prussians took him prisoner.
IT'S A FRENCH SURGEON! GET THE FIRING SQUAD!

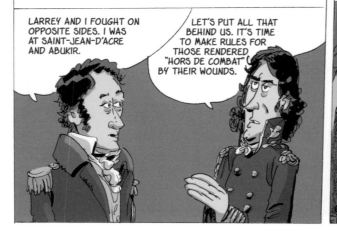

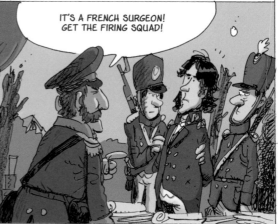

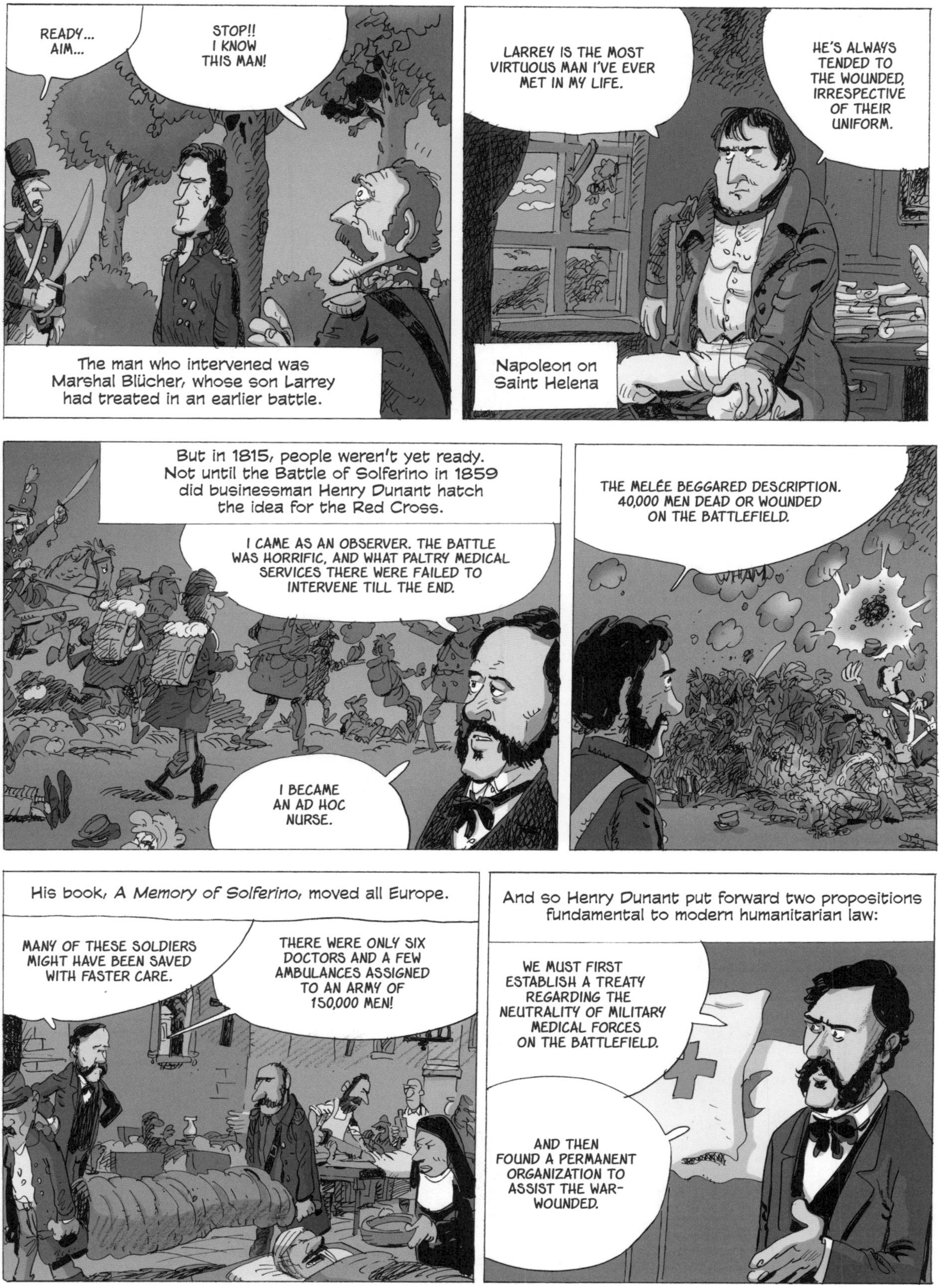
READY... AIM...
STOP!! I KNOW THIS MAN!
The man who intervened was Marshal Blücher, whose son Larrey had treated in an earlier battle.
LARREY IS THE MOST VIRTUOUS MAN I'VE EVER MET IN MY LIFE.
HE'S ALWAYS TENDED TO THE WOUNDED, IRRESPECTIVE OF THEIR UNIFORM.
Napoleon on Saint Helena
But in 1815, people weren't yet ready. Not until the Battle of Solferino in 1859 did businessman Henry Dunant hatch the idea for the Red Cross.
I CAME AS AN OBSERVER. THE BATTLE WAS HORRIFIC, AND WHAT PALTRY MEDICAL SERVICES THERE WERE FAILED TO INTERVENE TILL THE END.
I BECAME AN AD HOC NURSE.
THE MELÉE BEGGARED DESCRIPTION. 40,000 MEN DEAD OR WOUNDED ON THE BATTLEFIELD.
WHAM
His book, *A Memory of Solferino*, moved all Europe.
MANY OF THESE SOLDIERS MIGHT HAVE BEEN SAVED WITH FASTER CARE.
THERE WERE ONLY SIX DOCTORS AND A FEW AMBULANCES ASSIGNED TO AN ARMY OF 150,000 MEN!
And so Henry Dunant put forward two propositions fundamental to modern humanitarian law:
WE MUST FIRST ESTABLISH A TREATY REGARDING THE NEUTRALITY OF MILITARY MEDICAL FORCES ON THE BATTLEFIELD.
AND THEN FOUND A PERMANENT ORGANIZATION TO ASSIST THE WAR-WOUNDED.

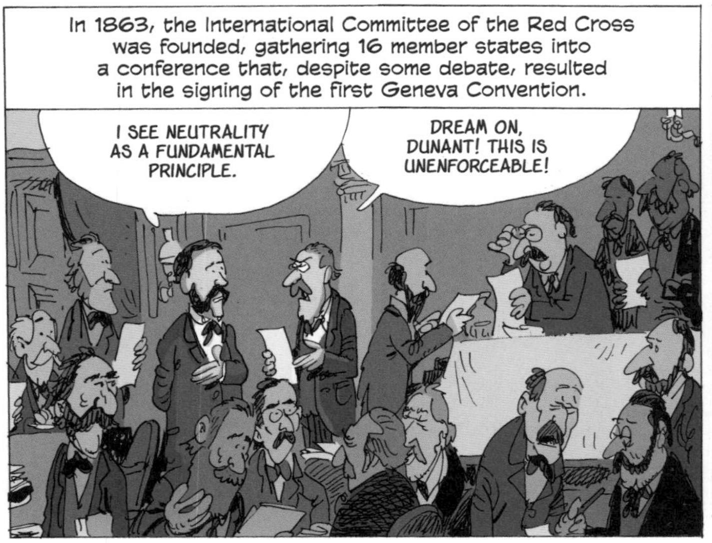
In 1863, the International Committee of the Red Cross was founded, gathering 16 member states into a conference that, despite some debate, resulted in the signing of the first Geneva Convention.
I SEE NEUTRALITY AS A FUNDAMENTAL PRINCIPLE.
DREAM ON, DUNANT! THIS IS UNENFORCEABLE!

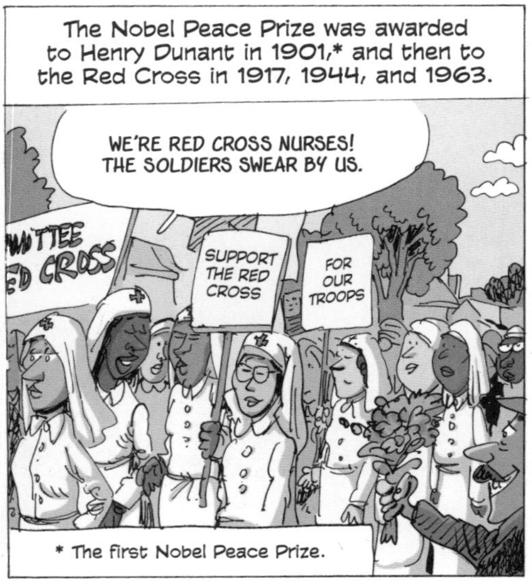
The Nobel Peace Prize was awarded to Henry Dunant in 1901,* and then to the Red Cross in 1917, 1944, and 1963.
WE'RE RED CROSS NURSES! THE SOLDIERS SWEAR BY US.
SUPPORT THE RED CROSS
FOR OUR TROOPS
* The first Nobel Peace Prize.

In addition to the Red Cross, some doctors saw it as their duty to bring aid to the world's underprivileged populations.

They took action in many different ways, such as colonial medicine and Dr. Schweitzer's legendary initiative.

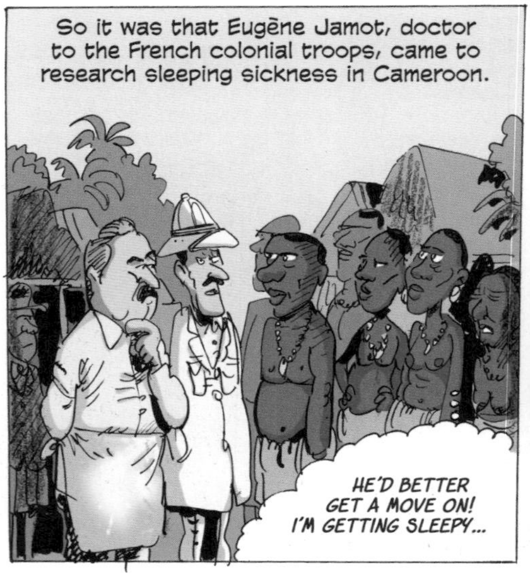
So it was that Eugène Jamot, doctor to the French colonial troops, came to research sleeping sickness in Cameroon.
HE'D BETTER GET A MOVE ON! I'M GETTING SLEEPY...

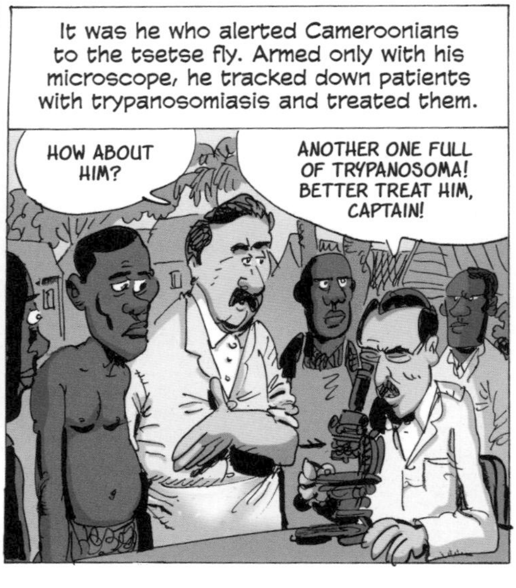
It was he who alerted Cameroonians to the tsetse fly. Armed only with his microscope, he tracked down patients with trypanosomiasis and treated them.
HOW ABOUT HIM?
ANOTHER ONE FULL OF TRYPANOSOMA! BETTER TREAT HIM, CAPTAIN!

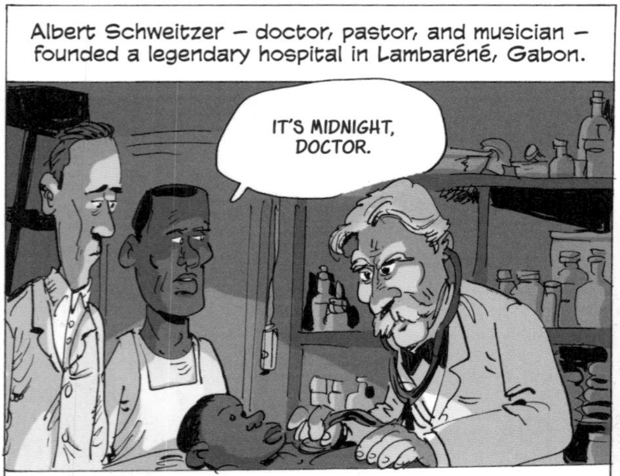
Albert Schweitzer – doctor, pastor, and musician – founded a legendary hospital in Lambaréné, Gabon.
IT'S MIDNIGHT, DOCTOR.
Extremely famous and popular, he won the Nobel Peace Prize in 1952.

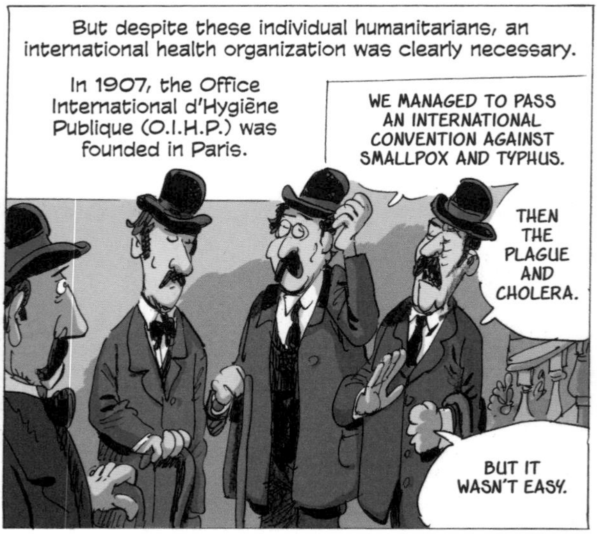
But despite these individual humanitarians, an international health organization was clearly necessary.
In 1907, the Office International d'Hygiène Publique (O.I.H.P.) was founded in Paris.
WE MANAGED TO PASS AN INTERNATIONAL CONVENTION AGAINST SMALLPOX AND TYPHUS.
THEN THE PLAGUE AND CHOLERA.
BUT IT WASN'T EASY.

1927 saw the founding of the U.N. Health Organization, headquartered in Geneva. In 1948, it was replaced by the World Health Organization (W.H.O.), a United Nations agency.

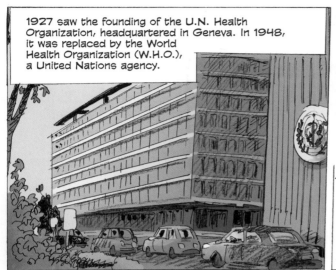

As for social benefits, Bismarck was the first to establish them in 1883 against illness, old age, and workplace accidents. The goal was to improve living conditions for the working class. These benefits depended on the workers' financial participation and were jointly overseen.

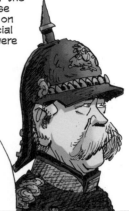

ABOVE ALL, I'M TRYING TO PULL THE RUG OUT FROM UNDER THE UNIONS AND THE SOCIALISTS.

Not until 1942 did economist William Beveridge propose a system of social benefits under the authority of the British government.

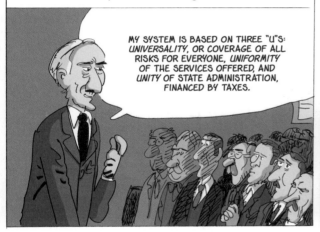

MY SYSTEM IS BASED ON THREE "U"S: *UNIVERSALITY*, OR COVERAGE OF ALL RISKS FOR EVERYONE, *UNIFORMITY* OF THE SERVICES OFFERED, AND *UNITY* OF STATE ADMINISTRATION, FINANCED BY TAXES.

In France, the laws of 19 October 1945 founded the social security system.

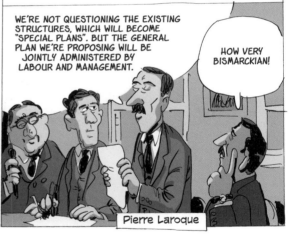

WE'RE NOT QUESTIONING THE EXISTING STRUCTURES, WHICH WILL BECOME "SPECIAL PLANS". BUT THE GENERAL PLAN WE'RE PROPOSING WILL BE JOINTLY ADMINISTERED BY LABOUR AND MANAGEMENT.

HOW VERY BISMARCKIAN!

Pierre Laroque

Over time, however, the limits of even the Red Cross became apparent. In 1967, the Nigerian Civil War led to a horrific famine...

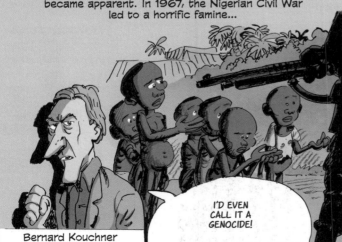

I'D EVEN CALL IT A GENOCIDE!

Bernard Kouchner

But the Red Cross refused to intervene in an internal conflict. Neutrality was paramount.

De Gaulle took a stance, calling for an unprecedented diplomatic act that forced the French Red Cross to take action.

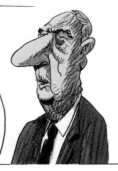

I WILL NOT HAVE IT SAID THAT FRANCE STOOD BY AND DID NOTHING WHEN TRAGEDY BEFELL THE GIANT OF AFRICA.

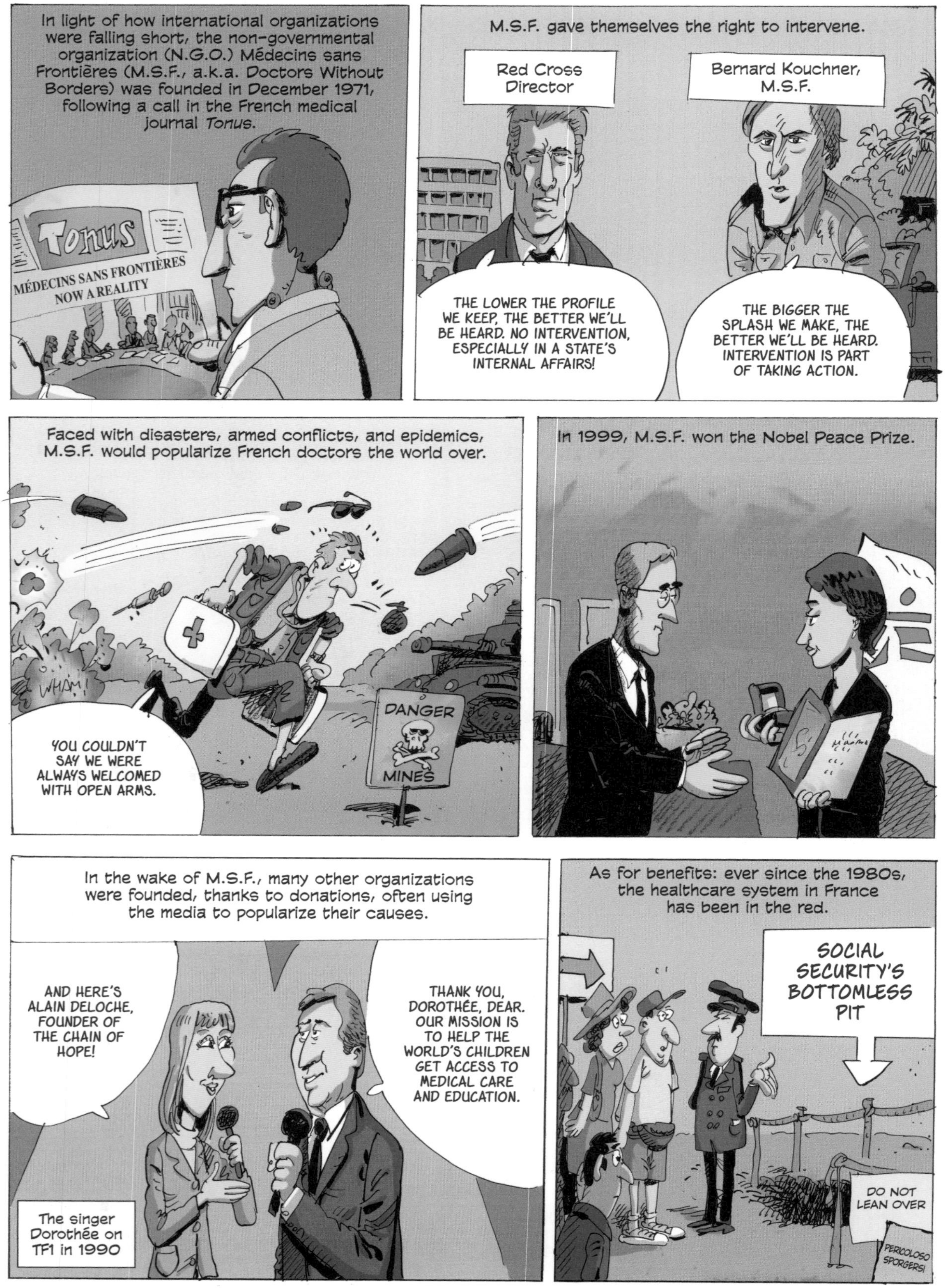
In light of how international organizations were falling short, the non-governmental organization (N.G.O.) Médecins sans Frontières (M.S.F., a.k.a. Doctors Without Borders) was founded in December 1971, following a call in the French medical journal *Tonus*.
Tonus
MÉDECINS SANS FRONTIÈRES NOW A REALITY
M.S.F. gave themselves the right to intervene.
Red Cross Director
Bernard Kouchner, M.S.F.
THE LOWER THE PROFILE WE KEEP, THE BETTER WE'LL BE HEARD. NO INTERVENTION, ESPECIALLY IN A STATE'S INTERNAL AFFAIRS!
THE BIGGER THE SPLASH WE MAKE, THE BETTER WE'LL BE HEARD. INTERVENTION IS PART OF TAKING ACTION.
Faced with disasters, armed conflicts, and epidemics, M.S.F. would popularize French doctors the world over.
WHAM!
DANGER MINES
YOU COULDN'T SAY WE WERE ALWAYS WELCOMED WITH OPEN ARMS.
In 1999, M.S.F. won the Nobel Peace Prize.
In the wake of M.S.F., many other organizations were founded, thanks to donations, often using the media to popularize their causes.
AND HERE'S ALAIN DELOCHE, FOUNDER OF THE CHAIN OF HOPE!
THANK YOU, DOROTHÉE, DEAR. OUR MISSION IS TO HELP THE WORLD'S CHILDREN GET ACCESS TO MEDICAL CARE AND EDUCATION.
The singer Dorothée on TF1 in 1990
As for benefits: ever since the 1980s, the healthcare system in France has been in the red.
SOCIAL SECURITY'S BOTTOMLESS PIT
DO NOT LEAN OVER
PERICOLOSO SPORGERSI

CHAPTER 20

A FEW MODERN PLAGUES

No sooner were the great epidemics of the Middle Ages contained than other plagues arose to claim the attention of doctors the world over.

Germs are great travellers. We know that much from cholera and the plague. When humans set out to discover the vast world in search of wealth and imperial conquest, by the same token they also encountered new diseases, previously unknown germs, and mysterious parasites.

We have already encountered Cortés with his syphilitic soldiers, and Eugène Jamot's battle against sleeping sickness. Now it is time to meet Alphonse Laveran, who discovered the protozoans that cause malaria, and Peter Piot, who grappled with the Ebola virus.

And finally, the scourge of 20th-century warfare provided many more medical challenges, from the *gueules cassées* ("shattered faces") of the World War One trenches to the pernicious after-effects of Hiroshima.

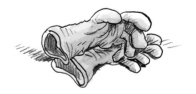

SCURVY

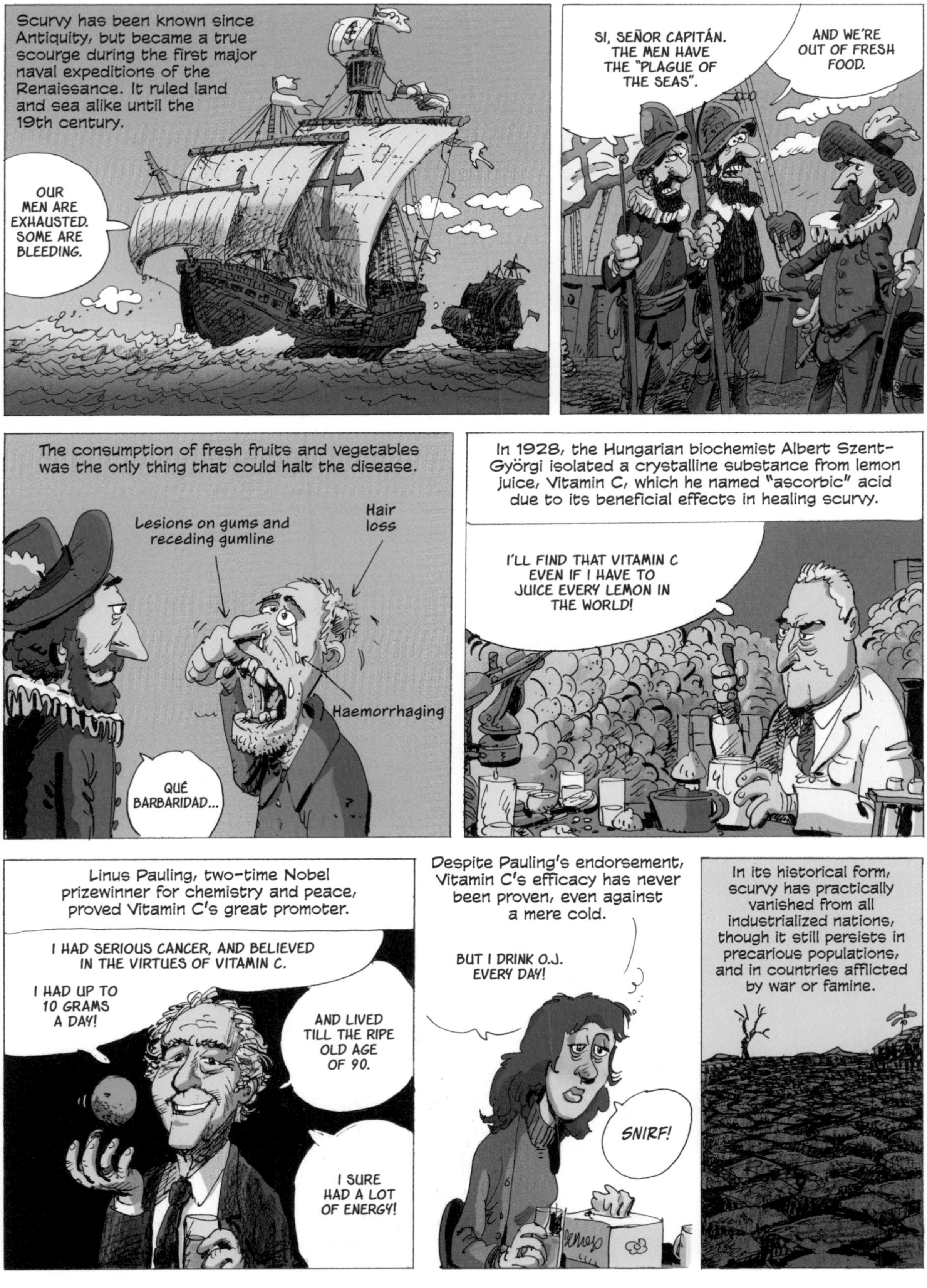

Scurvy has been known since Antiquity, but became a true scourge during the first major naval expeditions of the Renaissance. It ruled land and sea alike until the 19th century.
OUR MEN ARE EXHAUSTED. SOME ARE BLEEDING.
SI, SEÑOR CAPITÁN. THE MEN HAVE THE "PLAGUE OF THE SEAS".
AND WE'RE OUT OF FRESH FOOD.
The consumption of fresh fruits and vegetables was the only thing that could halt the disease.
Lesions on gums and receding gumline
Hair loss
Haemorrhaging
QUÉ BARBARIDAD...
In 1928, the Hungarian biochemist Albert Szent-Györgi isolated a crystalline substance from lemon juice, Vitamin C, which he named "ascorbic" acid due to its beneficial effects in healing scurvy.
I'LL FIND THAT VITAMIN C EVEN IF I HAVE TO JUICE EVERY LEMON IN THE WORLD!
Linus Pauling, two-time Nobel prizewinner for chemistry and peace, proved Vitamin C's great promoter.
I HAD SERIOUS CANCER, AND BELIEVED IN THE VIRTUES OF VITAMIN C.
I HAD UP TO 10 GRAMS A DAY!
AND LIVED TILL THE RIPE OLD AGE OF 90.
I SURE HAD A LOT OF ENERGY!
Despite Pauling's endorsement, Vitamin C's efficacy has never been proven, even against a mere cold.
BUT I DRINK O.J. EVERY DAY!
SNIRF!
In its historical form, scurvy has practically vanished from all industrialized nations, though it still persists in precarious populations, and in countries afflicted by war or famine.

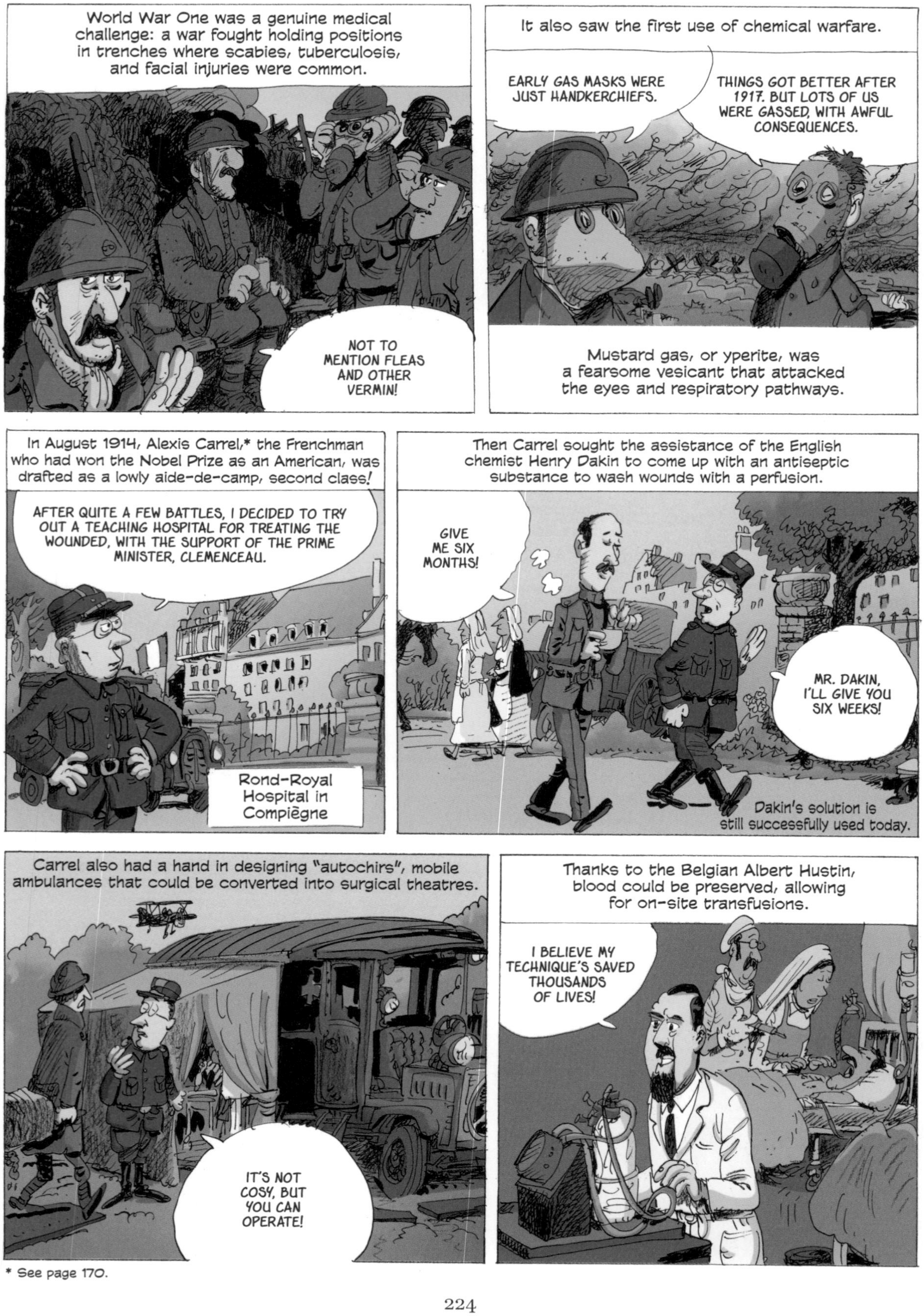
World War One was a genuine medical challenge: a war fought holding positions in trenches where scabies, tuberculosis, and facial injuries were common.
NOT TO MENTION FLEAS AND OTHER VERMIN!
It also saw the first use of chemical warfare.
EARLY GAS MASKS WERE JUST HANDKERCHIEFS.
THINGS GOT BETTER AFTER 1917. BUT LOTS OF US WERE GASSED, WITH AWFUL CONSEQUENCES.
Mustard gas, or yperite, was a fearsome vesicant that attacked the eyes and respiratory pathways.
In August 1914, Alexis Carrel,* the Frenchman who had won the Nobel Prize as an American, was drafted as a lowly aide-de-camp, second class!
AFTER QUITE A FEW BATTLES, I DECIDED TO TRY OUT A TEACHING HOSPITAL FOR TREATING THE WOUNDED, WITH THE SUPPORT OF THE PRIME MINISTER, CLEMENCEAU.
Rond-Royal Hospital in Compiègne
Then Carrel sought the assistance of the English chemist Henry Dakin to come up with an antiseptic substance to wash wounds with a perfusion.
GIVE ME SIX MONTHS!
MR. DAKIN, I'LL GIVE YOU SIX WEEKS!
Dakin's solution is still successfully used today.
Carrel also had a hand in designing "autochirs", mobile ambulances that could be converted into surgical theatres.
IT'S NOT COSY, BUT YOU CAN OPERATE!
Thanks to the Belgian Albert Hustin, blood could be preserved, allowing for on-site transfusions.
I BELIEVE MY TECHNIQUE'S SAVED THOUSANDS OF LIVES!

* See page 170.

The need to repair "shattered faces" led to the birth of plastic, cosmetic, and maxillofacial surgeries.

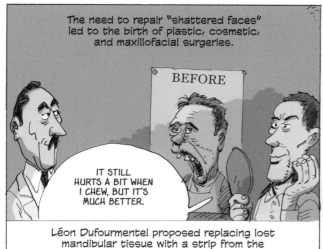

BEFORE

IT STILL HURTS A BIT WHEN I CHEW, BUT IT'S MUCH BETTER.

Léon Dufourmentel proposed replacing lost mandibular tissue with a strip from the scalp and bone grafts.

The war had already taken 1.4 million lives in combat, not counting the Spanish flu.* The H1N1 virus from China mutated in America, growing especially serious and contagious. American soldiers, arriving in France, passed it to their allies.

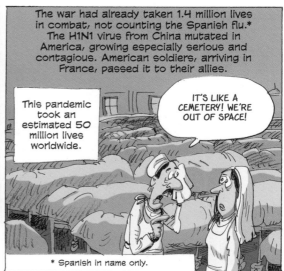

This pandemic took an estimated 50 million lives worldwide.

IT'S LIKE A CEMETERY! WE'RE OUT OF SPACE!

* Spanish in name only.

Ever since the work of Koch's students Pfeiffer and Kitasato, a bacterium was thought to be the cause of the flu. But in 1931, Richard Shope realized...

ODD. THESE PIGS HAVE A DISEASE NOT UNLIKE HUMAN FLU.

AND IT'S CAUSED BY A VIRUS.

I NOTE THAT A SERUM FROM FLU PATIENTS PROTECTS SWINE AGAINST THEIR OWN FLU.

SO HUMAN FLU MUST ALSO BE CAUSED BY A VIRUS.

In 1926, Christopher Andrews and William Smith managed to infect a ferret with human flu. One day, while sneezing, the ferret passed it to another researcher. So the sickness could be passed from humans to animals and vice versa!

THAT FERRET'S STILL WHEEZING!

IT'S YOUR FAULT. IF YOU HADN'T INFECTED ME IN THE FIRST PLACE...

SNIFF

The virus could be cultivated in chicken embryos, then observed with an electron microscope.

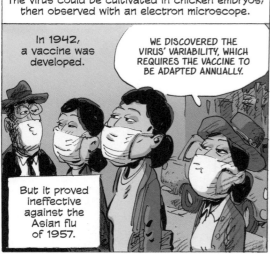

In 1942, a vaccine was developed.

WE DISCOVERED THE VIRUS' VARIABILITY, WHICH REQUIRES THE VACCINE TO BE ADAPTED ANNUALLY.

But it proved ineffective against the Asian flu of 1957.

In reality, wildfowl were reservoirs of the virus, which could recombine and mutate easily, and was the cause of so many different epidemics.

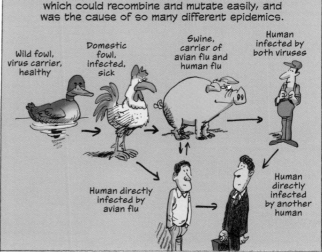

Wild fowl, virus carrier, healthy

Domestic fowl, infected, sick

Swine, carrier of avian flu and human flu

Human infected by both viruses

Human directly infected by avian flu

Human directly infected by another human

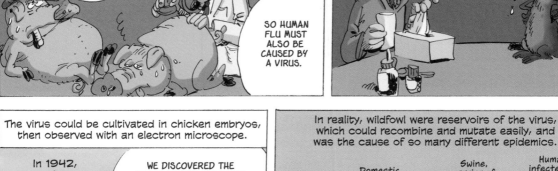

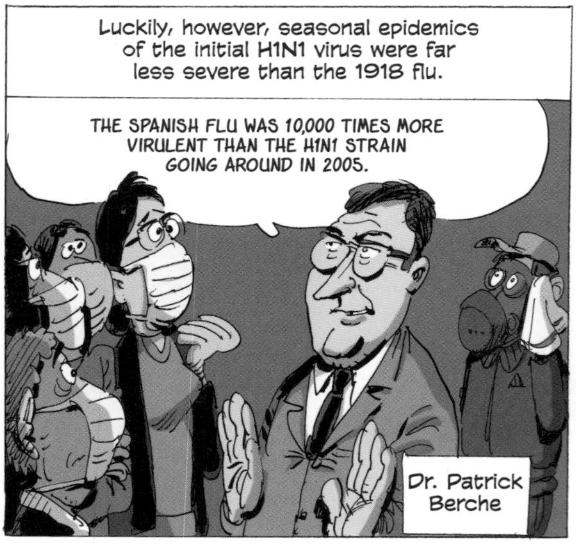
Luckily, however, seasonal epidemics of the initial H1N1 virus were far less severe than the 1918 flu.
THE SPANISH FLU WAS 10,000 TIMES MORE VIRULENT THAN THE H1N1 STRAIN GOING AROUND IN 2005.
Dr. Patrick Berche

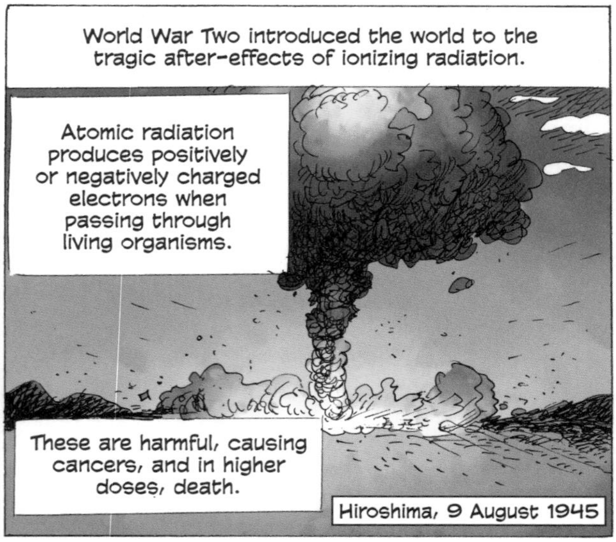
World War Two introduced the world to the tragic after-effects of ionizing radiation.
Atomic radiation produces positively or negatively charged electrons when passing through living organisms.
These are harmful, causing cancers, and in higher doses, death.
Hiroshima, 9 August 1945

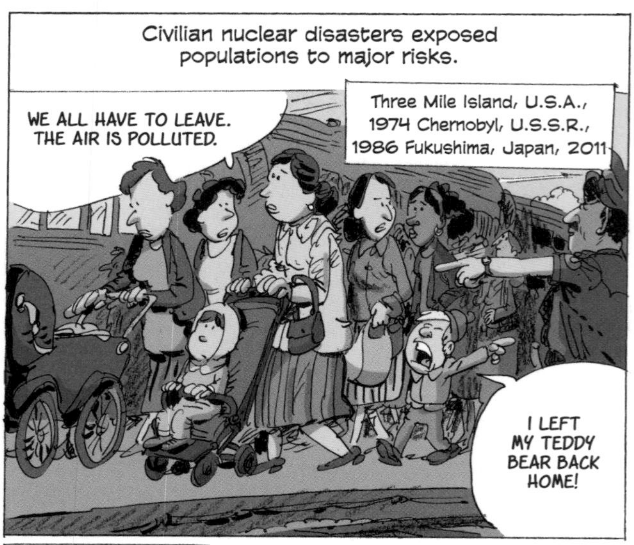
Civilian nuclear disasters exposed populations to major risks.
WE ALL HAVE TO LEAVE. THE AIR IS POLLUTED.
Three Mile Island, U.S.A., 1974 Chernobyl, U.S.S.R., 1986 Fukushima, Japan, 2011
I LEFT MY TEDDY BEAR BACK HOME!

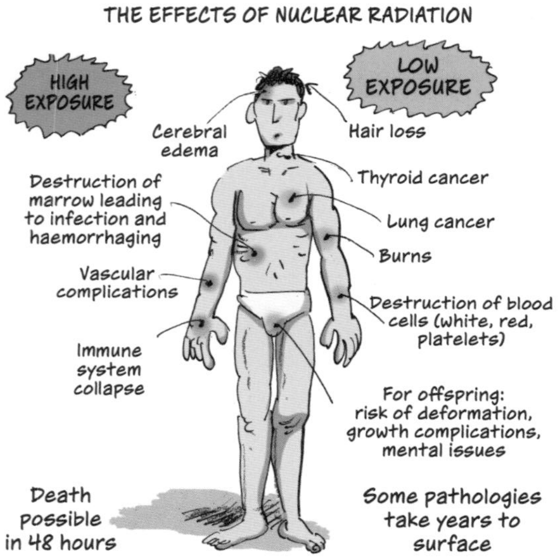
THE EFFECTS OF NUCLEAR RADIATION
HIGH EXPOSURE
LOW EXPOSURE
Cerebral edema
Hair loss
Destruction of marrow leading to infection and haemorrhaging
Thyroid cancer
Lung cancer
Burns
Vascular complications
Destruction of blood cells (white, red, platelets)
Immune system collapse
For offspring: risk of deformation, growth complications, mental issues
Death possible in 48 hours
Some pathologies take years to surface

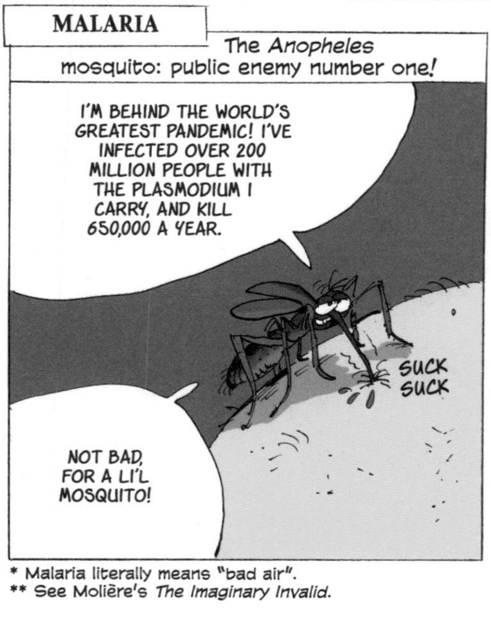
MALARIA
The *Anopheles* mosquito: public enemy number one!
I'M BEHIND THE WORLD'S GREATEST PANDEMIC! I'VE INFECTED OVER 200 MILLION PEOPLE WITH THE PLASMODIUM I CARRY, AND KILL 650,000 A YEAR.
SUCK SUCK
NOT BAD, FOR A LI'L MOSQUITO!

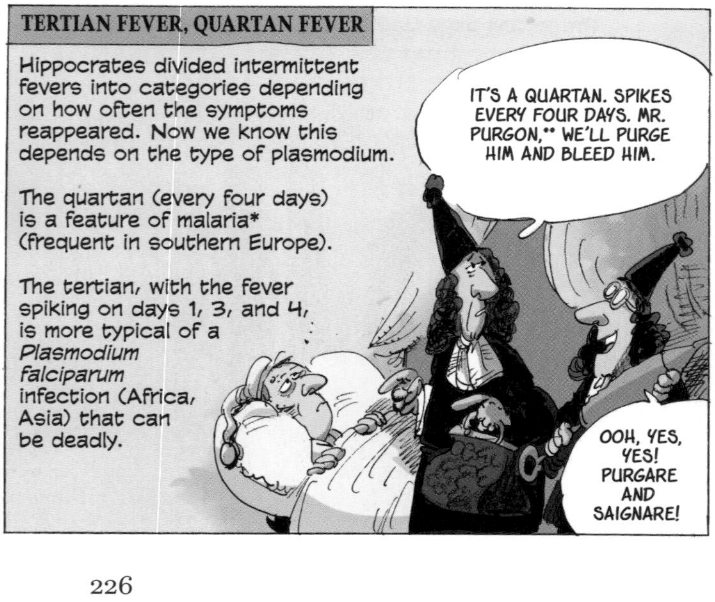
TERTIAN FEVER, QUARTAN FEVER
Hippocrates divided intermittent fevers into categories depending on how often the symptoms reappeared. Now we know this depends on the type of plasmodium.
The quartan (every four days) is a feature of malaria* (frequent in southern Europe).
The tertian, with the fever spiking on days 1, 3, and 4, is more typical of a *Plasmodium falciparum* infection (Africa, Asia) that can be deadly.
IT'S A QUARTAN. SPIKES EVERY FOUR DAYS. MR. PURGON,** WE'LL PURGE HIM AND BLEED HIM.
OOH, YES, YES! PURGARE AND SAIGNARE!

* Malaria literally means "bad air".
** See Molière's *The Imaginary Invalid*.

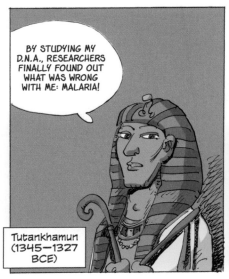

BY STUDYING MY D.N.A., RESEARCHERS FINALLY FOUND OUT WHAT WAS WRONG WITH ME: MALARIA!

Tutankhamun (1345—1327 BCE)

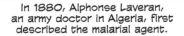

In 1880, Alphonse Laveran, an army doctor in Algeria, first described the malarial agent.

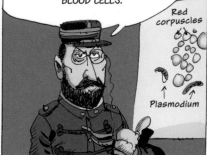

IN THE BLOOD OF A MALARIAL PATIENT, I DISCOVERED SPINDLY ELEMENTS MOVING ABOUT WITH GREAT SPEED, PUSHING ASIDE NEIGHBOURING RED BLOOD CELLS.

Red corpuscles

Plasmodium

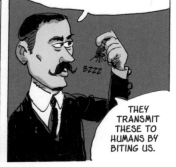

Ronald Ross, an English army doctor in India, proved that *Anopheles* had a role in the disease.

I DISSECTED HUNDREDS OF MOSQUITOES, AND PLASMODIA WERE FOUND IN THEIR SALIVARY GLANDS.

BZZZ

THEY TRANSMIT THESE TO HUMANS BY BITING US.

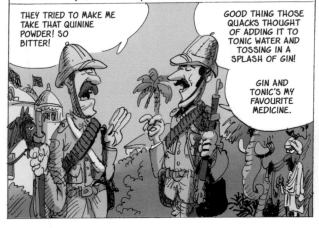

Quinine, synthesized by Pelletier and Canvetou, and known for reducing fever, also directly attacked the parasite. Exposed soldiers had only to receive preventative treatment.

THEY TRIED TO MAKE ME TAKE THAT QUININE POWDER! SO BITTER!

GOOD THING THOSE QUACKS THOUGHT OF ADDING IT TO TONIC WATER AND TOSSING IN A SPLASH OF GIN!

GIN AND TONIC'S MY FAVOURITE MEDICINE.

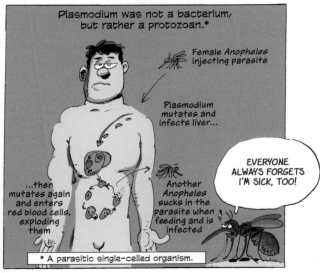

Plasmodium was not a bacterium, but rather a protozoan.*

Female *Anopheles* injecting parasite

Plasmodium mutates and infects liver...

...then mutates again and enters red blood cells, exploding them

Another *Anopheles* sucks in the parasite when feeding and is infected

EVERYONE ALWAYS FORGETS I'M SICK, TOO!

* A parasitic single-celled organism.

Prevention depended on eradicating *Anopheles*.

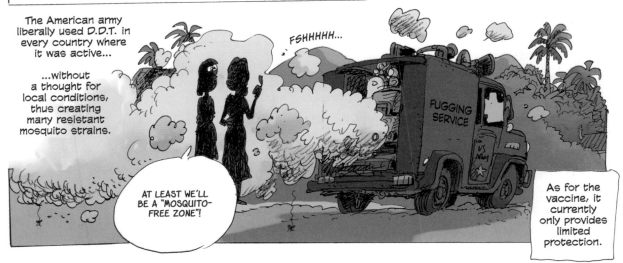

The American army liberally used D.D.T. in every country where it was active...

...without a thought for local conditions, thus creating many resistant mosquito strains.

FSHHHHH...

FUGGING SERVICE

AT LEAST WE'LL BE A "MOSQUITO-FREE ZONE"!

As for the vaccine, it currently only provides limited protection.

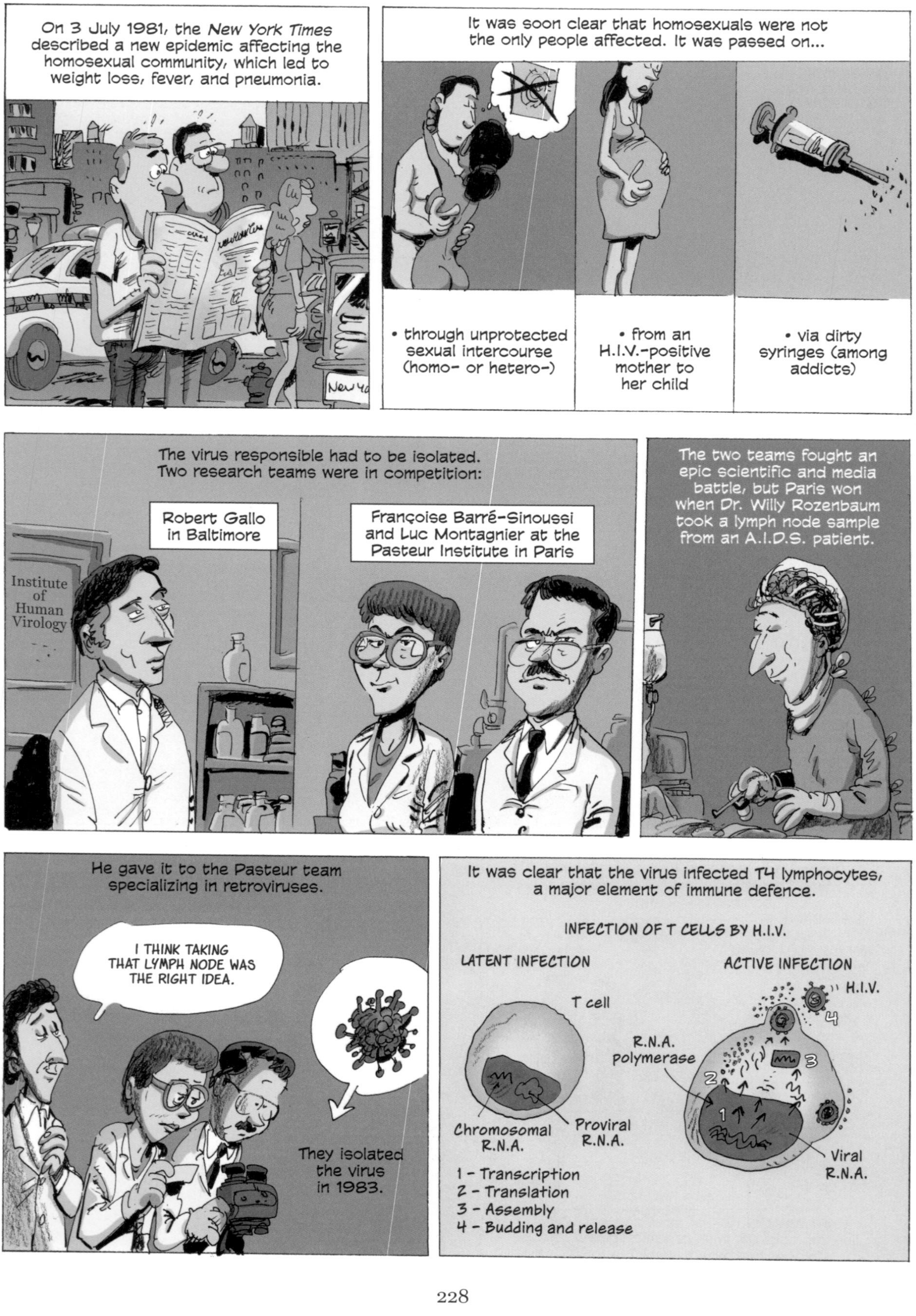
On 3 July 1981, the New York Times described a new epidemic affecting the homosexual community, which led to weight loss, fever, and pneumonia.
It was soon clear that homosexuals were not the only people affected. It was passed on...
• through unprotected sexual intercourse (homo- or hetero-)
• from an H.I.V.-positive mother to her child
• via dirty syringes (among addicts)
The virus responsible had to be isolated. Two research teams were in competition:
Robert Gallo in Baltimore
Institute of Human Virology
Françoise Barré-Sinoussi and Luc Montagnier at the Pasteur Institute in Paris
The two teams fought an epic scientific and media battle, but Paris won when Dr. Willy Rozenbaum took a lymph node sample from an A.I.D.S. patient.
He gave it to the Pasteur team specializing in retroviruses.
I THINK TAKING THAT LYMPH NODE WAS THE RIGHT IDEA.
They isolated the virus in 1983.
It was clear that the virus infected T4 lymphocytes, a major element of immune defence.
INFECTION OF T CELLS BY H.I.V.
LATENT INFECTION
T cell
Chromosomal R.N.A.
Proviral R.N.A.
ACTIVE INFECTION
H.I.V.
R.N.A. polymerase
Viral R.N.A.
1 - Transcription
2 - Translation
3 - Assembly
4 - Budding and release

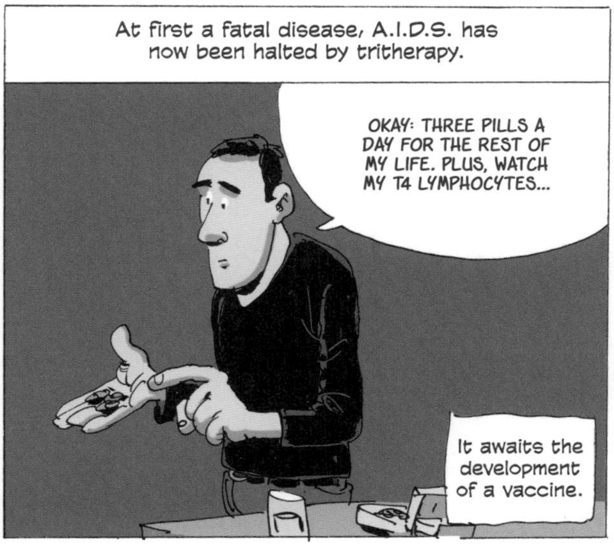
At first a fatal disease, A.I.D.S. has now been halted by tritherapy.
OKAY: THREE PILLS A DAY FOR THE REST OF MY LIFE. PLUS, WATCH MY T4 LYMPHOCYTES...
It awaits the development of a vaccine.

THE EBOLA VIRUS

This virus causes haemorrhagic fevers that often prove deadly.

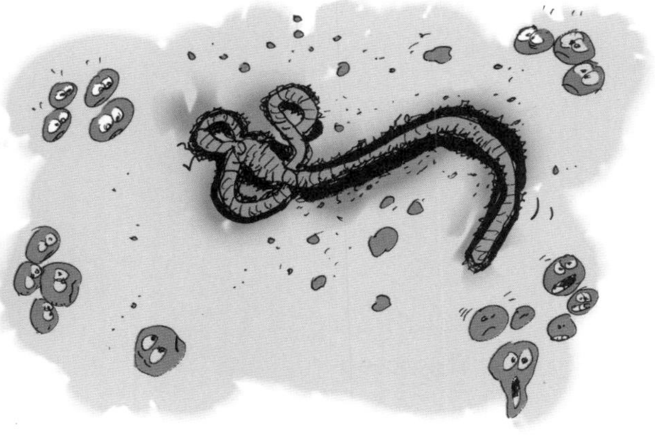

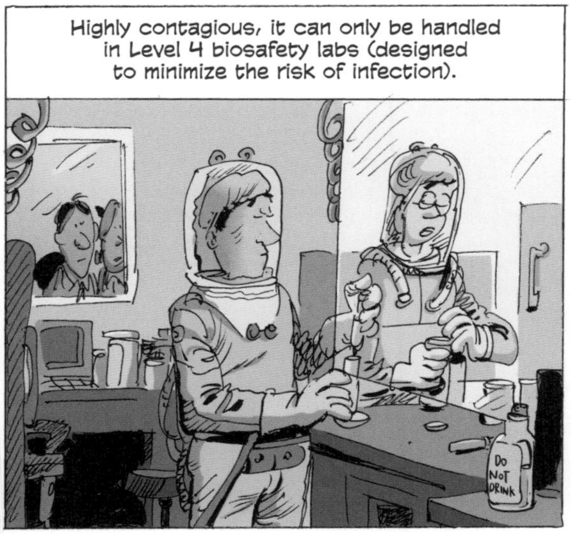
Highly contagious, it can only be handled in Level 4 biosafety labs (designed to minimize the risk of infection).
DO NOT DRINK

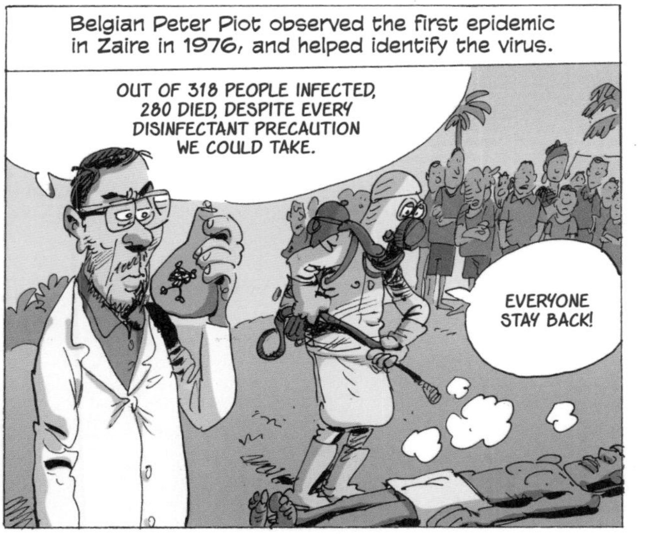
Belgian Peter Piot observed the first epidemic in Zaire in 1976, and helped identify the virus.
OUT OF 318 PEOPLE INFECTED, 280 DIED, DESPITE EVERY DISINFECTANT PRECAUTION WE COULD TAKE.
EVERYONE STAY BACK!

The 2014 epidemic was the worst on record, and posed a risk of spreading by air travel. Airlines even refused to land in Conakry.

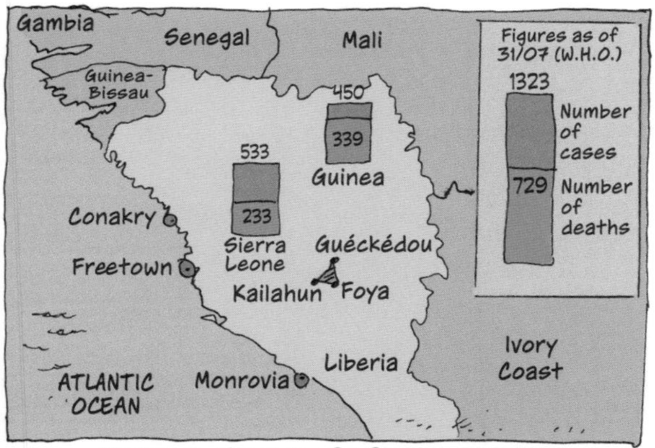
Gambia
Senegal
Mali
Guinea-Bissau
Figures as of 31/07 (W.H.O.)
1323
Number of cases
729
Number of deaths
450
339
Guinea
533
233
Sierra Leone
Conakry
Freetown
Guéckédou
Kailahun
Foya
Liberia
Ivory Coast
ATLANTIC OCEAN
Monrovia

However, the risk of infection outside of contact with organic liquids (blood, diarrhoea, vomit) is low.

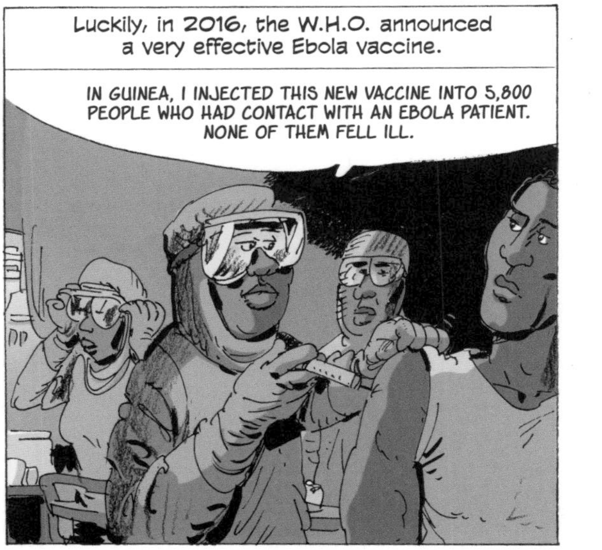
Luckily, in 2016, the W.H.O. announced a very effective Ebola vaccine.
IN GUINEA, I INJECTED THIS NEW VACCINE INTO 5,800 PEOPLE WHO HAD CONTACT WITH AN EBOLA PATIENT. NONE OF THEM FELL ILL.

CHAPTER 21

ADVANCES IN RESEARCH

And research marches on.

There are still so many things yet to discover. No sooner do doctors solve one problem than they are confronted with others that lead them to contemplate still further mysteries. No sooner is a vaccine devised, an antibiotic concocted, or a surgery proposed than new difficulties arise. The vaccine is suspected of causing disease, bacteria find a way to fight off the antibiotic, and the operation reveals its limitations.

What a mad, desperate, and exciting headlong dash medicine is—and one whose pace has only picked up over the last hundred years, swallowing up vast amounts of money as it goes, but for a cause that no one could argue against, since it concerns the welfare of the human race...

And yet the mysteries of medicine are those of life itself. Tackling them means constantly running up against fundamental questions. Science has no intrinsic morality; it merely expresses facts as they are. And these do not always correspond with the ethics of our societies. Should we pursue cloning for therapeutic purposes? Should we manipulate genes to heal hereditary illnesses? Should we strive officiously to keep hopeless cases alive, claiming constant medical advances in our defence?

There are profound changes in medicine to come, and the precedent of the past helps us imagine future progress. What will become of medicine as we have known it through the ages in the era of telehealth, nanotechnology, robotics, and artificial intelligence?

An inspiring story is waiting to be told...

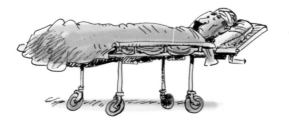

CARDIOPULMONARY BYPASS

Beginning in 1937, John and Mary Gibbon developed the first heart-lung machine, which enabled cardiac surgery by stopping the heart and lungs.

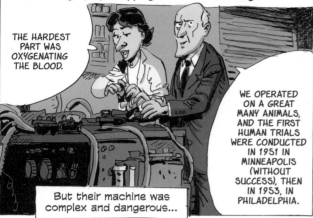

THE HARDEST PART WAS OXYGENATING THE BLOOD.

WE OPERATED ON A GREAT MANY ANIMALS, AND THE FIRST HUMAN TRIALS WERE CONDUCTED IN 1951 IN MINNEAPOLIS (WITHOUT SUCCESS), THEN IN 1953, IN PHILADELPHIA.

But their machine was complex and dangerous...

So that in 1953, Walton Lillehei was still operating on children's hearts by using cross-circulation with a parent.

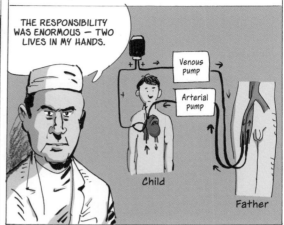

THE RESPONSIBILITY WAS ENORMOUS — TWO LIVES IN MY HANDS.

Venous pump

Arterial pump

Child

Father

Another method was to induce hypothermia via immersion in a bathtub of freezing water.

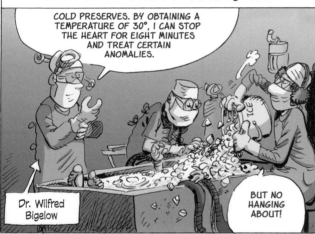

COLD PRESERVES. BY OBTAINING A TEMPERATURE OF 30°, I CAN STOP THE HEART FOR EIGHT MINUTES AND TREAT CERTAIN ANOMALIES.

Dr. Wilfred Bigelow

BUT NO HANGING ABOUT!

The heart-lung machine eventually proved superior, once it had been modified by Lillehei and Richard DeWall.

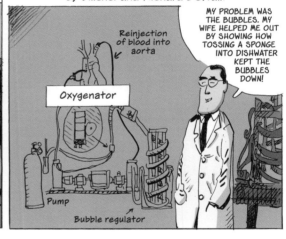

MY PROBLEM WAS THE BUBBLES. MY WIFE HELPED ME OUT BY SHOWING HOW TOSSING A SPONGE INTO DISHWATER KEPT THE BUBBLES DOWN!

Reinjection of blood into aorta

Oxygenator

Pump

Bubble regulator

And in 1956, cardiac surgery could at last begin in earnest...

By Lillehei and DeWall, then John Kirklin and Cooley in the U.S.

And by Charles Dubost and DeWall at Marie-Lannelongue in Europe.

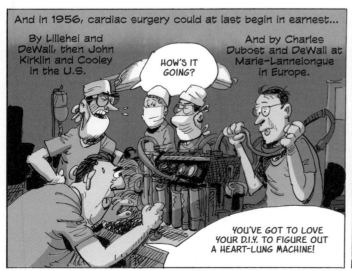

HOW'S IT GOING?

YOU'VE GOT TO LOVE YOUR D.I.Y. TO FIGURE OUT A HEART-LUNG MACHINE!

Kolff, the inventor of the artificial kidney, invented a membrane to ensure better oxygenation. It also allowed oxygenation over longer periods of time for patients with respiratory insufficiency.

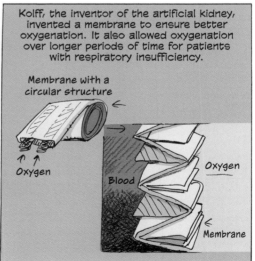

Membrane with a circular structure

Oxygen

Oxygen

Blood

Membrane

The only thing left was to protect the heart, which remained out of the loop. This was the first cardioplegia.
HANS-JÜRGEN BRETSCHNEIDER PROPOSED A COLD IONIC SOLUTION, BUCKBERG A WARM BLOOD-BASED ONE, AND OURS WAS BLOOD-BASED, COLD, AND RETROGRADE.
Anterograde injection into aorta
Retrograde injection in right auricle
BUT THE IMPORTANT PART? PARALYSING THE HEART!
J.-N. Fabiani, 1982
THE CORONARY ADVENTURE
It all began in 1959, when F. Mason Sones performed the first selective coronary angiography.
I WAS TRYING TO INJECT SOMETHING INTO THE AORTA, BUT MY HAND SLIPPED, AND THE CATHETER WENT INTO THE CORONARY ARTERY.
THAT WAS WHEN I NOTICED THE GREAT VIEW IT GAVE ME OF THE ARTERIES AND THEIR POTENTIAL CONSTRICTIONS.
Since 1967, heart surgeons have been performing bypasses on narrowed arteries to avoid the risk of heart attacks.
I PICKED A PATIENT'S LEG VEIN AND GRAFTED IT ONTO HIS HEART.
Obstructed coronary artery
Saphenous vein used to bypass diseased coronary artery
René Favaloro, Argentine surgeon working in Cleveland, U.S.A.
The operation was a worldwide success.
But in September 1977, in Zurich, Andreas Gruentzig conceived the idea of performing the first dilation of a narrowed artery by arterial balloon catheter.
IT WAS A HUGE LEAP FORWARD. UNFORTUNATELY, CONSTRICTIONS HAVE A TENDENCY TO RECUR.
Plaque
A
Balloon
Catheter
B
Inflated balloon
C
Remaining plaque
To prevent this restenosis, engineer Hans Wallsten invented the stent* in 1982.
IT'S JUST A LITTLE MESH THAT SAVES LIVES.
I COULD'VE CALLED IT THE WALLSTENT!
WE DARED TO PUT A STENT IN A CORONARY ARTERY. OF COURSE, THAT NECESSITATES ANTIPLATELET DRUGS FOR LIFE.
Hans Wallsten, Lausanne
Jacques Puel, Toulouse, 1986
But the story went on, for despite stents, restenosis was still common after angioplasty. An active stent, or drug-eluting stent, was put forward to chemically prevent renewed narrowing.
Active substance
THIS NEW GENERATION CAN CAUSE CLOTS AND NECESSITATES DUAL ANTIPLATELET THERAPY FOR AT LEAST SIX MONTHS.
BUT WE'RE PAVING THE WAY FOR THE FUTURE: RESORBABLE STENTS...

* Named after Charles T. Stent (1807—1885), an English dentist.

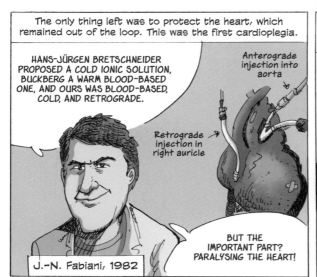

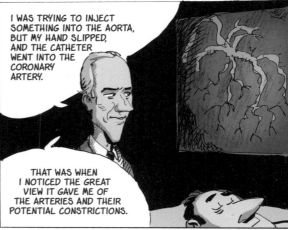

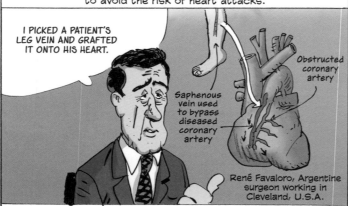

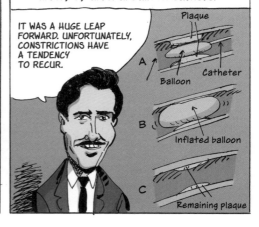

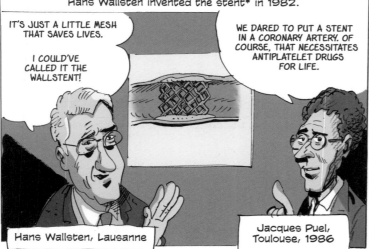

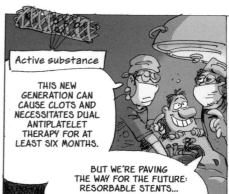

ENDOSCOPY
Claude Bernard's contemporary Antonin Desormeaux developed the first endoscope in 1852.
THE INNOVATION I BROUGHT TO THE TABLE WAS TO USE A GAS-POWERED LAMP TO MAKE THINGS MORE VISIBLE THAN EVER.
Lamp
Rigid tube
Lens
This invention was to revolutionize medicine.
Considerable progress permitted the exploration of the digestive tract, the genito-urinary system, and the major cavities.
THE 1930S SAW THE DEVELOPMENT OF SEMI-FLEXIBLE TUBES FOR STUDYING THE INSIDE OF THE STOMACH.
20 YEARS LATER, THE INTRODUCTION OF LIGHT-GUIDING FIBRE-OPTIC BUNDLES ALLOWED ENDOSCOPES TO BECOME COMPLETELY FLEXIBLE.
OKAY, DOC — SAVE THE HISTORY LESSON AND LET'S WRAP UP THE EXAM!
Miniature cameras and advances in video technology paved the way for endoscopic surgery, allowing actions to be seen in real time on a screen.
MY EYE IS THE CAMERA.
AND MY INSTRUMENTS ARE INSIDE THE PATIENT.
Videosurgery would lead to robotic surgery. Robotics, an evergreen military fantasy, began developing in earnest in 1995.
An assistant fixes instruments to the robot's arms
The surgeon operates remotely via a 3-D console
I COULD WORK FROM HOME...
IN FACT, THE ROBOT BETWEEN MY HANDS AND THE PATIENT IS A COMPUTER THAT AIDS AND RECONSTRUCTS MY ACTIONS.
I AM A SLAVE. I DO ONLY AS MY MASTER THE SURGEON COMMANDS.
AND I'M THE PATIENT. JUST FOUR LITTLE HOLES TO TAKE CARE OF MY ANEURYSM!
TELEMEDICINE, NANOTECH, AND ARTIFICIAL INTELLIGENCE
Telemedicine allows patients to be examined remotely, obviating travel.
At the exam centre, a technician performs an ultrasound.
At the expert centre, the cardiologist reviews the exam and makes a diagnosis.

1999: the first robotically assisted aneurysm operation

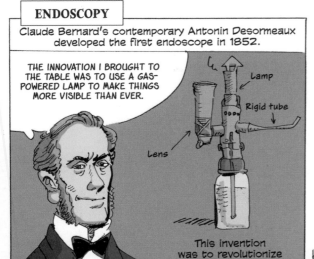

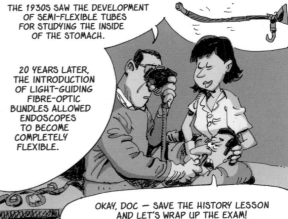

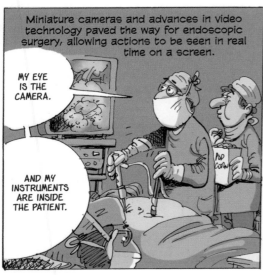

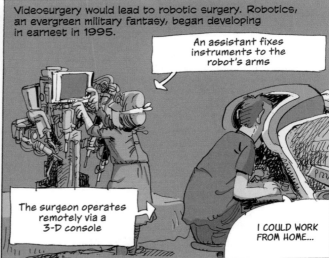

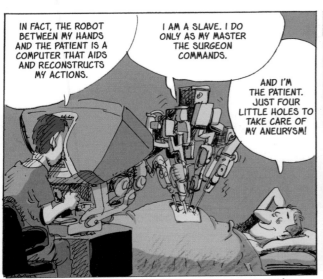

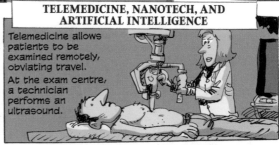

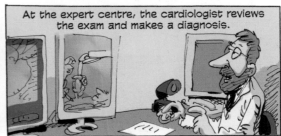

Implantable chips have revolutionized the surveillance of chronic cardiac patients or those undergoing chemotherapy.

1. The implant can detect many substances in the body

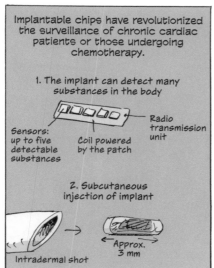

Sensors: up to five detectable substances

Coil powered by the patch

Radio transmission unit

2. Subcutaneous injection of implant

Intradermal shot

Approx. 3 mm

3. The patch gathers data from the sensors

Implant   Patch

4. Transmission of data by Bluetooth via phone network

5. Data reaches doctor's computer

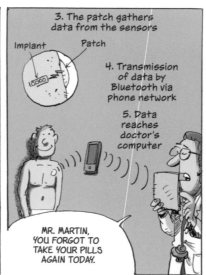

MR. MARTIN, YOU FORGOT TO TAKE YOUR PILLS AGAIN TODAY.

Artificial intelligence's areas of expertise will multiply.

I CAN INTERPRET THESE SCANS AS EFFICIENTLY AS THE 10 FINEST EXPERTS IN THE WORLD.

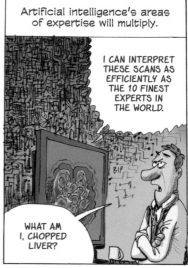

BIP

WHAT AM I, CHOPPED LIVER?

Nanobiotechnologies are concerned with distances on an atomic scale.

Nanoparticles will:
— improve resolution of images obtained during scans;
— serve to identify the nature of a microorganism or spot a genetic anomaly;
— specifically address medication to target tissue.

Nanoparticles in contact with red blood cells

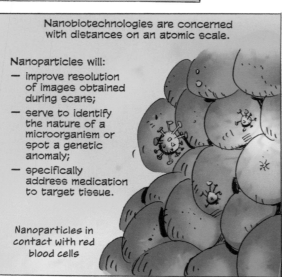

Example: nanoparticles and cancer

Nanoshells

Cancer cells

Nanoshells

Cancer cells

Healthy cells

Infrared rays

Healthy cells

Dead cancer cells

Healthy cells

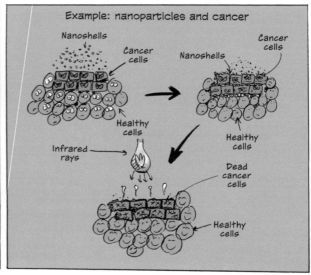

In this highly technological future, industry will play a fundamental role.

SIR, I'VE JUST DISCOVERED A NEW SUBSTANCE TO TREAT A DOZEN CHILDREN SUFFERING FROM—

YOU MUST BE JOKING! YOU KNOW HOW MUCH DEVELOPMENT AND CLINICAL TRIALS COST FOR A NEW DRUG? I NEED PROFITABLE MARKETS!

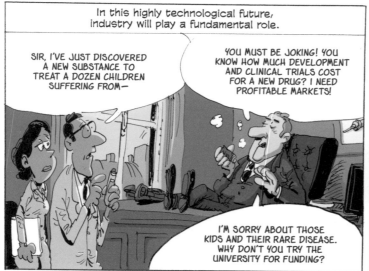

I'M SORRY ABOUT THOSE KIDS AND THEIR RARE DISEASE. WHY DON'T YOU TRY THE UNIVERSITY FOR FUNDING?

And the General Practitioner, who remains at the centre of all these changes, will always be irreplaceable.

WELL, MR. MARTIN, HOW DID THOSE EXAMS I ORDERED GO?

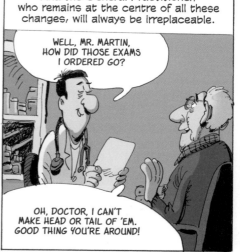

OH, DOCTOR, I CAN'T MAKE HEAD OR TAIL OF 'EM. GOOD THING YOU'RE AROUND!

Jean-Noël Fabiani
Philippe Bercovici

SELECT BIBLIOGRAPHY

Ameisen, Jean-Claude, with Berche, Patrick, Brohard, Yvan, and Kahn, Axel,
Une histoire de la médecine, ou le Souffle d'Hippocrate (La Martinière, 2011)

Ariès, Philippe, *L'Enfant et la vie familiale sous l'Ancien Régime* (Le Seuil, 2014)

Bariéty, Maurice, and Coury, Charles, *Histoire de la médecine* (Fayard, 1963)

Becchi, Egle, and Dominique, Julia, *Histoire de l'enfance en Occident* (Le Seuil, 1998)

Binet, Léon, *Médecins, biologistes et chirurgiens* (SEGEP, 1954)

Bonn, Gérard, *Du clystère au stéthoscope* (Glyphe, 2015)

Canguilhem, Georges, *Le Normal et le Pathologique* (PUF, 1966)

Chastel, Claude, *Une petite histoire de la médecine* (Ellipses, 2004)

Chastel, Claude, and Cénac, Arnaud, *Histoire de la médecine, introduction à l'épistémologie* (Ellipses, 1998)

Chevalier, Patrick, with Rullière, Roger, and Heymans, Georges, *Abrégé d'histoire de la médecine* (Masson, 1981)

Coninck, Philippe de, *Le Roman de la chirurgie* (Fayard, 1959)

Coppens, Yves, *L'Histoire de l'homme* (Odile Jacob, 1990)

Dachez, Roger, *Histoire de la médecine: de l'Antiquité à nos jours* (Tallandier, 2012)

Duhamel, Pierre, *Histoire des médecins français* (Plon, 1993)

Fabiani, Jean-Noël, *30 histoires insolites qui ont fait la médecine* (Plon, 2017)

Foucault, Michel, *Naissance de la clinique* (PUF, 1972)

Gilbert-Dreyfus, *Origines et devenir de la médecine* (Calmann-Lévy, 1968)

Gorny, Philippe, *L'Aventure de la médecine* (J.-C. Lattès, 1991)

Grmek, Mirko D., *Histoire de la pensée médicale en Occident*, 3 vols (Le Seuil, 2014)

Halioua, Bruno, *Abrégé d'histoire de la médecine* (Masson, 2009)

Hecketsweiler, Philippe, *Histoire de la médecine, des malades, des médecins, des soins et de l'éthique biomédicale* (Ellipses, 2010)

Landry, Yves, *Petite histoire des médicaments : de l'Antiquité à nos jours* (Dunod, 2011)

Lichtenthaler, Charles, *Histoire de la médecine* (Fayard, 1978)

Lyons, Albert, and Petrucelli, Joseph, *Histoire illustrée de la médecine* (Presses de la Renaissance, 1979)

Mondor, Henri, *Anatomistes et chirurgiens* (Fragrance, 1949)

Parker, Steve, *Médecine: Histoire illustrée de l'Antiquité à nos jours* (Larousse, 2017)

Perez, Stanis, *Histoire des médecins* (Tempus, 2018)

Pickover, Clifford A., *Le Beau Livre de la médecine. Des sorciers guérisseurs à la microchirurgie* (Dunod, 2013)

Schlogel, Gilbert, *Les princes du sang* (Fayard, 1994)

Sournia, Jean-Charles, *Histoire de la médecine* (La Découverte, 2004)

Tubiana, Maurice, *Histoire de la pensée médicale* (Flammarion, 1999)

Vigarello, Georges, *Histoire des pratiques de santé* (Le Seuil, 1993)

Thank you to Laurent Muller and my publisher Arènes
for deciding to take a risk on this comic.
Thank you to Philippe Bercovici for bringing his talent and humour to it.

Jean-Noël Fabiani